RELATIONAL PROCESSES AND DSM-V

Neuroscience, Assessment, Prevention, and Intervention

RELATIONAL PROCESSES AND DSM-V

Neuroscience, Assessment, Prevention, and Intervention

Edited by

Steven R. H. Beach, Ph.D.
Marianne Z. Wamboldt, M.D.
Nadine J. Kaslow, Ph.D.
Richard E. Heyman, Ph.D.
Michael B. First, M.D.
Lynn G. Underwood, Ph.D.
David Reiss, M.D.

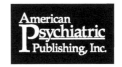

Washington, DC
London, England

Copyright © 2006 American Psychiatric Publishing, Inc.
ALL RIGHTS RESERVED

Manufactured in the United States of America on acid-free paper
14   13   5   4
First Edition

Typeset in Adobe's Frutiger and AGaramond.

American Psychiatric Publishing, Inc.
1000 Wilson Boulevard
Arlington, VA 22209-3901
www.appi.org

Library of Congress Cataloging-in-Publication Data
Relational processes and DSM-V : neuroscience, assessment, prevention, and
    treatment / edited by Steven R. H. Beach . . . [et al.].—1st ed.
        p. ; cm.
    Includes bibliographical references and index.
    ISBN 1-58562-238-9 (pbk. : alk. paper)
    1. Psychology, Pathological. 2. Mental illness—Diagnosis. 3. Interpersonal
relations. I. Beach, Steven R. H. II. Diagnostic and statistical manual of mental
disorders.
    [DNLM: 1. Mental Disorders—diagnosis. 2. Interpersonal Relations.
3. Mental Disorders—therapy. WM 141 R382 2006]
    RC454.R45 2006
    616.89—dc22
                                                          2006016136

British Library Cataloguing in Publication Data
A CIP record is available from the British Library.

CONTENTS

I

Biological Underpinnings

II
Assessment

III
Prevention and Treatment

IV
Summary and Implications for Future Research

CONTRIBUTORS

Steven R. H. Beach, Ph.D.
Director, Institute for Behavioral Research, University of Georgia, Athens, Georgia

Theodore P. Beauchaine, Ph.D.
Associate Professor of Psychology, University of Washington, Seattle, Washington

Lorna Smith Benjamin, Ph.D.
Professor of Psychology, IRT Clinic, University Neuropsychiatric Institute, Salt Lake City, Utah

Guillermo Bernal, Ph.D.
Director, University Center for Psychological Services and Research (CUSEP), and Professor, Department of Psychology, University of Puerto Rico, Rio Piedras Campus, San Juan, Puerto Rico

George W. Brown, Ph.D.
Professor Emeritus, Department of Social Psychiatry, Institute of Psychiatry, Kings College London, St. Thomas' Hospital Campus, London, United Kingdom

Lisa M. Christian, M.A.
Doctoral Candidate, Department of Psychology, Department of Molecular Virology, Immunology, and Medical Genetics, Ohio State University College of Medicine, Columbus, Ohio

Kenneth L. Critchfield, Ph.D.
IRT Clinic, University Neuropsychiatric Institute, Salt Lake City, Utah

Eduardo Cumba-Avilés, Ph.D.
Assistant Research Scientist, University Center for Psychological Services and Research (CUSEP), University of Puerto Rico, Rio Piedras, San Juan, Puerto Rico

Jennifer E. Graham, Ph.D.
Postdoctoral Fellow, Department of Molecular Virology, Immunology, and Medical Genetics, Institute for Behavioral Medicine Research, Ohio State University College of Medicine, Columbus, Ohio

Richard E. Heyman, Ph.D.
Research Professor, Department of Psychology, State University of New York, Stony Brook, New York

Jill M. Hooley, D.Phil.
Professor of Psychology, Department of Psychology, Harvard University, Cambridge, Massachusetts

Nadine J. Kaslow, Ph.D.
Professor and Chief Psychologist, Emory School of Medicine, Department of Psychiatry and Behavioral Sciences, Grady Health System, Atlanta, Georgia

Janice K. Kiecolt-Glaser, Ph.D.
S. Robert Davis Chair of Medicine, Professor and Director, Division of Health Psychology, Department of Psychiatry, Ohio State University College of Medicine, Columbus, Ohio

Miranda M. Lim, Ph.D.
Postdoctoral Research Fellow, Department of Psychiatry and Behavioral Sciences, Center for Behavioral Neuroscience, Yerkes National Research Center, Emory University School of Medicine, Atlanta, Georgia

William R. McFarlane, M.D.
Director, Center for Psychiatric Research, University of Vermont at Maine Medical Center, Portland, Maine

David J. Miklowitz, Ph.D.
Professor of Psychology and Psychiatry, Department of Psychology, University of Colorado at Boulder, Boulder, Colorado

Paul M. Plotsky, Ph.D.
GlaxoSmithKline Professor and Director, Stress Neurobiology Laboratory, Department of Psychiatry and Behavioral Sciences, Emory University School of Medicine, Atlanta, Georgia

David Reiss, M.D.
Vivian Gill Distinguished Professor of Research, George Washington University Medical Center, Center for Family Research, Department of Psychiatry and Behavioral Sciences, Washington, DC

Emily Sáez-Santiago, Ph.D.
Assistant Research Scientist, University Center for Psychological Services and Research (CUSEP), University of Puerto Rico, Rio Piedras Campus, San Juan, Puerto Rico

Irwin N. Sandler, Ph.D.
Regents' Professor, Prevention Research Center, Psychology North, Arizona State University, Tempe, Arizona

Clorinda Schenck, Ph.D.
Research Assistant, Prevention Research Center, Psychology North, Arizona State University, Tempe, Arizona

Amy M. Smith Slep, Ph.D.
Research Associate Professor, Family Translational Research Group, Department of Psychology, State University of New York at Stony Brook, Stony Brook, New York

Nelson K. B. Totah, B.S.
Research Specialist, Stress Neurobiology Laboratory, Department of Psychiatry and Behavioral Sciences, Emory University School of Medicine, Atlanta, Georgia

Lynn G. Underwood Ph.D.
Professor of Biomedical Humanities and Director of the Center for Literature, Medicine and the Health Care Professions, Hiram College, Hiram, Ohio

Marianne Z. Wamboldt, M.D.
Vice Chair for Child Psychiatry, University of Colorado at Denver and Health Sciences Center, and Chair, Psychiatry and Behavioral Science, The Children's Hospital of Denver, Denver, Colorado

Mark A. Whisman, Ph.D.
Associate Professor of Psychology, University of Colorado at Boulder, Department of Psychology, Boulder, Colorado

Emily B. Winslow, Ph.D.
Faculty Research Associate, Prevention Research Center, Psychology North, Arizona State University, Tempe, Arizona

Sharlene A. Wolchik, Ph.D.
Professor, Prevention Research Center, Psychology North, Arizona State University, Tempe, Arizona

Larry J. Young, Ph.D.
Associate Professor, Department of Psychiatry and Behavioral Sciences, Center for Behavioral Neuroscience, Yerkes National Research Center, Emory University School of Medicine, Atlanta, Georgia

PREFACE

Work on the next edition of the *Diagnostic and Statistical Manual of Mental Disorders* (DSM-V) is not expected to begin until late 2006, with eventual publication anticipated for 2011. The American Psychiatric Association, which oversees the development of the DSM, initiated a DSM-V research planning process with the goal of enriching the empirical database in preparation for the eventual start of the DSM-V revision process. In the first phase of the planning process, the American Psychiatric Association (APA), in partnership with the National Institute of Mental Health, the National Institute on Alcohol Abuse and Alcoholism, and the National Institute on Drug Abuse commissioned a series of white papers with the goal of developing a research agenda to improve the scientific basis for future revisions of DSM and the *International Classification of Diseases* (ICD). Research planning workgroups were appointed to consider the following five topic areas:

- Basic nomenclature issues (e.g., definition of mental disorder)
- Advances in developmental science, mental disorders and disability
- Basic and clinical neuroscience and genetics research
- Culture and psychiatric diagnosis
- Gaps in DSM-IV

The six papers were published together in 2002 as a monograph entitled *A Research Agenda for DSM-V* (Kupfer et al. 2002) and is available from American Psychiatric Publishing, Inc.

The white paper developed by the Gaps in DSM-IV group considered the problems with the DSM-IV categorical method for diagnosing personality disorders and the limited provision for the diagnosis of relational disorders to be "two of the most important gaps in the current DSM-IV" (First et al. 2002, p. 123). The inadequacy of the classification of relational disorders was recognized by the DSM-IV Task Force (Frances et al. 1997) and led to the commissioning of literature reviews on the utility and definitional features of a number of relational disorders, including relational problems associated with high expressed emotion (Goldstein et al. 1997), parent inadequate discipline (Chamberlain et al. 1997), marital and family communication difficulties (Clarkin and Miklowitz 1997), partner relational problems with physical abuse (O'Leary and Jacobson 1997), sibling relational problems (Kahn and Monks 1997), physical abuse and neglect of children (Knutson and Schartz 1997), and incest (Kaplan and Pelcovitz 1997). Ultimately, the DSM-IV Task Force determined that the available empirical database was insufficiently developed to justify including relational disorders in the DSM-IV.

As work started on planning a research agenda for DSM-V, it was decided that this topic should be revisited and that a research agenda for stimulating further research in this area needed to be included in the chapter on "Gaps in DSM-IV" (which was ultimately renamed "Personality Disorders and Relational Disorders: A Research Agenda for Addressing Crucial Gaps in DSM" in the published monograph). Specific recommendations in the proposed research agenda included developing assessment modules; determining the clinical utility of relational disorders; determining the role of relational disorders in the etiology and maintenance of individual mental disorders; and considering aspects of relational disorders that might be modulated by individual mental disorders.

The second phase of the DSM-V research planning process consists of 11 research planning conferences (plus a methods conference) that are scheduled to be convened during the period 2004 to 2007 under the title "The Future of Psychiatric Diagnosis: Refining the Research Agenda." These conferences are being organized with the assistance and support of the World Health Organization and are cofunded by the NIMH, NIAAA, and NIDA. Unlike the white papers in the first phase, which focused on general cross-cutting issues, these conferences for the most part will focus on specific diagnostic topics. Conference topics were selected after consultation with U.S. and international experts. Finite resources, however, necessitated that the number of APA-NIH–sponsored conferences be limited to a total of 11, leaving out a number of potentially important topics, such as relational disorders.

For this reason, the APA has been encouraging researchers to conduct additional research planning conferences to cover additional topic areas and has offered to establish liaison connections to ensure that research coming from these conferences is integrated into the DSM-V process. The Fetzer Institute–sponsored conference on relational disorders that is the source of the contributions to the present monograph was modeled after the DSM-V research planning conferences and has achieved the same high level of quality in terms of both the plenary presentations and the discussions. We are hopeful that the chapters contained in this monograph will spur on the necessary research to allow for more empirically informed deliberations about the role of relational disorders in DSM-V.

Michael B. First, M.D.
Columbia University
New York State Psychiatric Institute
New York, New York

References

Chamberlain P, Reid JB, Ray J, et al: Parent inadequate discipline, in DSM-IV Sourcebook, Vol 3. Edited by Widiger TA, Frances AJ, Pincus HA, et al. Washington, DC, American Psychiatric Association, 1997, pp 569–630

Clarkin JF, Miklowitz DJ: Marital and family communication difficulties, in DSM-IV Sourcebook, Vol 3. Edited by Widiger TA, Frances AJ, Pincus HA, et al. Washington, DC, American Psychiatric Association, 1997, pp 631–672

First MB, Bell CC, Cuthbert B, et al: Personality disorders and relational disorders: a research agenda for addressing crucial gaps in DSM, in A Research Agenda for DSM-V. Edited by Kupfer DJ, First MB, Regier DA. Washington, DC, American Psychiatric Association, 2002, pp 123–199

Frances AJ, Clarkin JF, Ross R: Family/relational problems, in DSM-IV Sourcebook, Vol 3. Edited by Widiger TA, Frances AJ, Pincus HA, et al. Washington, DC, American Psychiatric Association, 1997, pp 521–530

Goldstein MJ, Strachan AM, Wynne LC: Relational problem related to a mental disorder or general medical condition, in DSM-IV Sourcebook, Vol 3. Edited by Widiger TA, Frances AJ, Pincus HA, et al. Washington, DC, American Psychiatric Association, 1997, pp 531–560

Kahn MD, Monks G: Sibling relational problems, in DSM-IV Sourcebook, Vol 3. Edited by Widiger TA, Frances AJ, Pincus HA, et al. Washington, DC, American Psychiatric Association, 1997, pp 693–712

Kaplan S, Pelcovitz D: Incest, in DSM-IV Sourcebook, Vol 3. Edited by Widiger TA, Frances AJ, Pincus HA, et al. Washington, DC, American Psychiatric Association, 1997, pp 805–860

Knutson JF, Schartz HA: Physical abuse and neglect of children, in DSM-IV Sourcebook, Vol 3. Edited by Widiger TA, Frances AJ, Pincus HA, et al. Washington, DC, American Psychiatric Association, 1997, pp 713–804

Kupfer DA, First MB, Regier DA (eds): A Research Agenda for DSM-V. Washington, DC, American Psychiatric Association, 2002

O'Leary KD, Jacobson NS: Partner relational problems with physical abuse, in DSM-IV Sourcebook, Vol 3. Edited by Widiger TA, Frances AJ, Pincus HA, et al. Washington, DC, American Psychiatric Association, 1997, pp 673–692

INTRODUCTION

Recent developments in psychiatry have been guided by dramatic growth in our knowledge about the biological underpinnings of disordered human behavior. By basing diagnosis of mental health problems on an increasingly solid foundation of biological science, the study of mental health has been able to follow the lead of other branches of medicine and rely increasingly on technical expertise and sophisticated research methodologies. This has led to rapid advances in both understanding and intervention. Unfortunately, this emphasis on the brain and biology has also resulted in a loss of focus on relationship-centered care.

Indeed, one potential casualty of an exclusive focus on biological psychiatry is the negation of the crucial role of interpersonal relationships in our conceptualization of both mental health and recovery from mental illness. In the context of diagnosis, a biologically based framework for behavioral problems has very nearly supplanted an interpersonally based understanding, contributing to a potential lack of balance between the different levels of analysis that have traditionally guided the biopsychosocial approach to psychiatric practice. This imbalance is reflected in the current version of the *Diagnostic and Statistical Manual of Mental Disorders* (DSM), and it is the purpose of the current volume to facilitate the process of addressing and correcting the imbalance.

As we approach the next reformulation of the diagnostic system that guides all mental health care in the United States and that informs diagnosis and intervention in many other countries in the world, there is a growing danger that psychiatric diagnosis will ignore the larger human context of mental illness. If so, the practice of psychiatry would forgo the substantial benefits that may arise from synthesizing technical advances in biology with a substantially enhanced appreciation of the relational and sociocultural framework within which psychiatric disorders occur. The DSM can either facilitate the increasing division between biological processes and relational (and larger environmental) processes or it can be revised to make it more likely that mental health care workers at all levels will harness the generative and healing properties of intimate relationships and make them a focus of clinical practice. Similarly, if the DSM can be revised in a manner that helps practitioners better assess relationships, and understand when relationship problems are associated with disease expressed either in the body or the mind, practitioners in all the various fields that are influenced by the DSM may be more willing to practice relationship-centered care, and practitioners in other medical specialties may be better able to see the relevance of psychiatry for their own disciplines.

Why Highlight Relationships?

Individuals who experience the diverse array of mental health problems often are confronted with a marked decline in traditional sources of support, coping, and interconnection with others. Recent research suggests that marital/couple relationships are less satisfying, family interactions are less regular and less supportive, and many people are less involved in their communities than was the case in previous decades. As a result, the relationship context of human suffering has become increasingly important and relevant to good diagnosis, treatment, and prevention. It would be ironic and disappointing if advances in psychiatric diagnosis came at the price of a decreased emphasis on the value of relationship context in mental health problems. A better outcome would be increased attention in DSM-V on ways to include information and guidance about relational processes and the role of relational interventions as a component of thorough assessment and comprehensive intervention recommendations.

Intimate relationships have been shown to be associated with many significant mental health outcomes. Close relationships—such as those in families—appear highly relevant for mental health outcomes, whether the focus is the basic psychopathology of mental disorders (Reiss and Wamboldt, Chapter 6), factors influencing maintenance and relapse of disorder (Brown, Chapter 7; Hooley et al., Chapter 11), sources of burden for family members (Whisman, Chapter 14), guiding family-based intervention (McFarlane, Chapter 5), interventions that deal with the consequences of family processes (Sandler et al., Chapter 12), or broader cultural issues (Bernal et al., Chapter 13). High-quality intimate relationships promote effective coping, resiliency in the face of stressors, better recovery from illness, and therefore better ability to contribute to the world at large. Conversely, poor quality intimate relationships are associated with poorer recovery from medical illnesses, less-efficient healing processes, and poorer outcomes for psychiatric illnesses (see Graham et al., Chapter 4; Hooley et al., Chapter 11; Whisman, Chapter 14). At the same time, problems in intimate relationships confer as much disability and suffering in their own right as do many psychiatric illnesses.

Intimate adult relationships (e.g., Brown, Chapter 7; Hooley et al., Chapter 11; Graham et al., Chapter 4) and caregiver-child relationships (Totah and Plotsky, Chapter 3) are particularly powerful in their effects on psychopathology. This suggests that sound measurement of problematic intimate partner and caregiver-child relationships may be particularly important in guiding future research and intervention. Indeed, the salience of family relationships and family events may arise because humans are "hard-wired" to respond to certain types of relationship events (Lim and

Young, Chapter 2), suggesting that these relationships may require special descriptive attention in a revised DSM.

Why Not Highlight Relationships?

For many it may seem so natural for mental health professionals to focus on promoting healthy relationships that it would not seem to require any special effort to foster a relational focus within the diagnostic manual that guides research and clinical practice. However, a number of objections already have been raised with regard to an increased focus on relational processes, and particularly to the idea of relational disorders. Accordingly, it will be essential to attend to these objections if an enhanced emphasis on relational processes in the DSM is to have any chance of success.

Objections focus primarily on four areas. First, some potential decision-makers believe that a biologically based diagnostic system will confer greater prestige and status within the medical health care system than would a system highlighting relational processes. One goal of the current book is to provide readers with the data to counter such arguments. By tying relational processes to basic research on psychopathology, we hope to overcome this objection and demonstrate that a better outcome than the triumph of biological psychiatry would be a true integration of two separate streams of research, linking the hard brain sciences with a sensitive and sophisticated understanding of the self-organizing and self-sustaining characteristics of relationships. The chapters in the current volume dealing with basic research go a long way toward achieving this integration.

Second, some decision-makers believe that a focus on relationship disorders and relational processes related to mental health will frighten third-party payers and preclude parity of reimbursement between mental health problems and physical health problems. The current volume offers information about the utility of attention to relational disorders and the potential for enhanced efficacy and effectiveness when interventions attend to relational context (e.g., McFarlane, Chapter 5; Hooley et al., Chapter 11; Sandler et al., Chapter 12). Likewise, by showing that relational processes are integral to understanding physical health (e.g., Graham et al., Chapter 4), as well as mental health, we provide information that can be used to counter these concerns. Finally, by highlighting the value of relational processes for treatment implementation and maintenance of gains (e.g., McFarlane, Chapter 5; Hooley et al., Chapter 11), the potential synergy of biological and relational perspectives should become clearer to decision-makers.

Third, some researchers believe that all genuine progress in behavioral diagnosis depends on the judicious application of neuroscience and genetics. The current volume helps to dispel this view by providing a forum for the presentation of new empirical findings on the study of relational processes. These findings include recent advances in the assessment of relational processes over time (Brown, Chapter 7), research showing that relationships play a role in regulating neurobiology (and genetic expression), and investigations demonstrating that relationships are critical for understanding the course and evolution of schizophrenia, conduct disorders, antisocial personality, eating disorders, and other disorders. These advances can help counteract the perspective that biology alone should provide the foundation of the diagnostic system.

Finally, some interest groups have a legitimate concern that an increased focus on relational processes would lead to labeling a variety of normative relationship difficulties as "disordered," and so would contribute to stigmatizing patients or their families rather than to helping them. This is particularly likely when relational categories are very poorly or vaguely defined as in the current DSM. Likewise, it is particularly likely when categories use evaluative terms rather than behavioral terms as diagnostic criteria. The current volume helps to address these issues by reviewing assessment practices and evidence that these processes are important for prediction of clinical outcomes. It is in no way the intention of the editors or authors to "blame" families for their loved one's difficulties. Quite the contrary. Rather, it is hoped that the increased focus on relationships will underscore the powerful role that family can play in ensuring the best possible outcome for a family member who is diagnosed with a psychiatric disorder.

How to Use This Volume

One aim of the current volume is to develop a shared commitment on the part of clinicians, researchers, psychopathologists, consumers, and advocates who have an interest in the revision of the DSM to take seriously the issue of relational processes as they relate to diagnoses within the DSM. A critical constituency in this process will be practicing clinicians who can speak to the salience of relational processes in their work and the value of a diagnostic manual that illuminates these processes and integrates them with other important treatment considerations. However, it is clear that influencing the development of the DSM-V will require a very broadly based alliance of researchers and practitioners across areas as diverse as neuroscience, applied assessment, intervention, prevention, and policy. The current volume is meant to speak to each of these groups and to indicate that their input is both welcomed and desired as the current project moves forward and grows. At the same time, the current volume is meant to be useful to clinicians and clinical researchers who are interested in the substantive issue of how to integrate greater sensitivity to relational processes in their own work. In addition, it is hoped that the information provided in this volume will further inform consumers and family members, and their thoughtful insights will be crucial in advancing our efforts to sensitively develop a more broad-based and contextually grounded conceptualization of psychosocial disability and its assessment and treatment. A more comprehensive perspective will ensure more appropriate diagnoses and better treatments, which in turn will be associated with greater recovery and quality of life for individuals whose challenges result in their receiving a DSM diagnosis. Toward this end, the book is divided into several sections.

The introductory chapter provides a definition of relational processes, describes their current treatment in the DSM, and explains why this treatment is inadequate. It then goes on to articulate several ways that the DSM could be improved as we move toward DSM-V. The next group of chapters provides a discussion of research linking relational processes to basic research in neuroscience, neurobiology, health outcomes, intervention research, prevention research, and genetics. These chapters collectively make the point that a true integration of research linking basic biological processes with a sensitive and sophisticated understanding of the self-organizing and self-sustaining characteristics of relationships is both possible and necessary. The conclusion that attention to relational processes is important, even for the correct specification of biological outcomes, will not be a surprise to most practicing clinicians. However, the sophistication of the empirical evidence that is already available on these topics may be surprising to many. We know far more about the genetics, neuroscience, and biology of relational processes than is commonly recognized. A greater appreciation of these results has the potential to allow for greater communication and synergy between biologically oriented colleagues and those who are more focused on family and relationship context.

For clinicians interested in sampling, but not exhausting the first group of chapters dealing with basic processes, Chapter 2, on the neurobiology of the social brain, may be an excellent choice. Alternatively, for those whose area of emphasis is physical health and illness, the chapter on marriage, health, and immune function (Chapter 4), provides an engaging look at the intimate interconnections of relational processes, depression, and health. We predict that many readers will return to this section in the future for the wealth of insights and background material. Each of the chapters in this section has much to offer. Chapter 3 provides a detailed description of the link between relational processes and the neurobiology of trauma. Chapter 5 examines the critical role of family processes in the development and management of psychosis. Chapter 6 offers an excellent overview of our emerging understanding of the role of genetics in relational processes, as well as the role of relational processes in the development of disorders that have a genetic component.

The chapters in Parts II and III will have greater initial appeal to many because the issues are more immediately compelling and more directly tied to the context of assessment or treatment. In Part II, Chapters 7, 9, and 11 raise a number of issues about best approaches to the assessment of relational processes with clear clinical significance such as a history of child abuse, ongoing partner abuse, and expressed emotion. These chapters will be of great interest to those attempting to refine their approach to assessment in these areas, and the authors provide a number of suggestions that may be applicable to many aspects of assessment of relational processes. Chapter 8 provides a simple introduction to the methodology of taxometrics, an approach that is likely to be important in future discussions of DSM categories. Those who want to know whether key relational disorders are categories that may be present or absent or whether they are dimensions that vary from a little to a lot will find this chapter quite informative. Chapter 10 overviews the links between relational processes and psychiatric outcomes and will be valuable for those people looking for a theoretical foundation for the discussion of links between relational processes and psychopathology.

In Part III, Chapter 12 describes an example of the relevance of relational processes to prevention of disorder, a topic of increasing interest. Chapter 13 discusses the role of culture in understanding psychopathology in general and relational processes in particular. This chapter will be of particular interest to those fascinated by the way that cultural context may modify decision making processes. Chapter 14 will be particularly relevant to those who wonder about the potential efficacy of relational interventions in the context of commonly diagnosed and treated disorders, such as depression.

The current volume is not exhaustive of the valuable work being conducted on the assessment of relational processes, but it is illustrative of the potential for assessment in this area to be reliable and valid and capable of guiding clinical intervention.

The concluding chapter, Chapter 15, presents implications for future research as well as an overview of the conclusions that can be drawn from the collection of chapters as a whole. This chapter is likely to be relevant to everyone who reads the book, whether their interest is primarily related to clinical work, research, policy, or the DSM-V revision. Persons working on DSM-V subcommittees may wish to start with Chapter 15 and sample backward through the book.

However you approach reading the current volume, we hope you will enjoy the book and that it will stimulate discussion of the myriad important issues related to the role of relational processes in psychopathology—issues that are quickly becoming critical as we head into the DSM revision process. It is time to begin greater discussion of the relevance of relational processes for psychiatric diagnosis, outcomes, treatment, and prevention. It is our hope that by including a wide range of individuals interested in relational processes, we will influence the dialogue in a way that leads to better guidance for assessment of relational processes in the DSM-V, as well as for the treatment of mental health problems unfolding in the context of relational processes.

Steven R. H. Beach, Ph.D.
Marianne Z. Wamboldt, M.D.
Nadine J. Kaslow, Ph.D.
Richard E. Heyman, Ph.D.
David Reiss, M.D.

ACKNOWLEDGMENTS

Any undertaking of the magnitude of the current volume involves contributions in addition to those of the editors of the volume and the authors of the chapters. There are also the less public contributions of those who initiate, coordinate, and maintain the effort over time. Despite these roles being less public, they are no less important, and we were especially fortunate to have a number of people who made special contributions to the process throughout the time this volume has been incubating.

We are especially grateful for the good humor and unflagging energy of Heidi Ihrig, who organized the Relational Process conference and represented the Fetzer Institute. Without her involvement, the current volume would certainly be very different, and much impoverished. She allowed the planning committee to focus on conceptual issues and made the practical details of hotel rooms, flight reservations, booklets, presentations, equipment, and coordination of schedules seem easy. Her presence was one of the several ways in which the Fetzer Institute helped to support the conference and sustain the process that eventually led to this volume.

We would also like to give special mention to Lynn Underwood, who played a pivotal role in launching the discussion of relational processes in mental health. She also helped to highlight the importance of relationships in the healing process. We are grateful for the help she provided at critical moments in the process, as well as her input on substantive issues.

Likewise, David Miklowitz played a crucial role in helping finish the volume by taking the lead role on summarizing the research recommendations of the conference participants. His ability to lay out the big picture, suggest broad future directions, and build consensus was invaluable, and we feel fortunate that we had his involvement.

Also calling for special mention are Bruce Cuthbert and Michael First, who, as members of the American Psychiatric Association's steering committee overseeing the planning for the DSM-V, were very helpful in providing advice and direction. In particular, they helped keep the Relational Process conference parallel to the 10 other conferences in the APA series and kept the planning focused on refining the research agenda for relational processes in mental health.

The core members of the planning committee are a diverse group, including both psychiatrists and psychologists, and have been working for the past 3 years under the leadership of David Reiss. As we have collaborated, we have developed special bonds of friendship and mutual respect. The result has been an auspicious beginning for an effort that will necessarily involve close collaboration across the usual disciplinary divides. As the current collection of papers demonstrates, there is a very broad range of material encompassed under the umbrella of relational processes in mental health.

We have been especially heartened by the good will and overwhelmingly positive response of the contributors to the current volume. Representing a true collaboration of psychiatrists, and psychologists, basic and applied researchers, clinical and prevention researchers, neuroscientists and behavioral geneticists, the current volume captures a cross-cutting dialogue that will engage all the stakeholders in the DSM revision process.

A particular source of gratification for us has been the strong resonance running from basic neuroscience through assessment and prevention and intervention. As became clear during the conference discussions, no area has greater potential to spark translational research or stimulate breakthroughs in prevention and intervention than does the study of relational processes in mental health. The available research is compelling, but we have barely begun to tap its potential.

We extend our deepest appreciation to all those who generously donated their time to attend the conference and participate in the detailed, probing, and engaging dialogues. All the participants played a pivotal role in the unfolding workgroup discussions that provided the basis for the recommendations chapter in the current volume. Their involvement also was central in refining the chapters and will continue to be critical as we move forward to the next phase of discussion on the revision of the DSM. We extend our special thanks to Drs. Theodore Beauchaine, Lorna Smith Benjamin, Ellen Berman, Guillermo Bernal, George Brown, E. Jane Costello, Judith Crowell, Mark Eddy, Robert Emde, Rise Goldstein, Christine Heim, Kristen Holm, Jill Hooley, Evan Imber-Black, Allan Josephson, Janice Kiecolt-Glaser, Kenneth Leonard, William McFarlane, David Miklowitz, Velma McBride, Jenae Neiderhiser, Lisa Onken, Emeline Otey, Daniel Pine, Paul Plotsky, Irwin Sandler, Erica Spotts, Mark Stanton, Frederick Wamboldt, Karen Wampler, Myrna Weissman, Beatrice Wood, and Larry Young.

CHAPTER 1

RELATIONAL PROCESSES AND MENTAL HEALTH

A Bench-to-Bedside Dialogue to Guide DSM-V

Steven R. H. Beach, Ph.D.
Marianne Z. Wamboldt, M.D.
Nadine J. Kaslow, Ph.D.
Richard E. Heyman, Ph.D.
David Reiss, M.D.

Relational processes are integral to the underlying biology of mental disorder. Thus, they must be given a prominent role in the ongoing revision of DSM. Marital and parenting relationships are particularly important, but a range of other relational processes are important as well for understanding the development and maintenance of a disorder and its appropriate management. In this chapter, we discuss four key issues and so set the stage for other chapters in the current volume. First, we highlight the need for continued integration of basic bench science with research on relational processes. Second, we review the way in which relational processes are currently described in DSM-IV (American Psychiatric Association 1994) and its text revision, DSM-IV-TR (American Psychiatric Association 2000),

Extended discussion of the topics in this chapter may be found in Beach SRH, Wamboldt MZ, Kaslow NJ, et al.: "Describing Relationship Problems in DSM-V: Toward Better Guidance for Research and Clinical Practice." *Journal of Family Psychology* (in press).

and highlight deficiencies. Third, we briefly abstract material from the other chapters in this volume to provide a foundation for a new approach to including relational processes in DSM-V. Finally, we discuss potential concerns about the inclusion of relational processes in DSM-V and offer recommendations.

Integration of Relational Processes Into the Dialogue

The dynamic interplay between basic description, bench science, clinical trials, and bedside application is an important source of clinical innovation but one that has been largely absent in the study of relationship influences on mental health. The insularity of research programs that approach relationship phenomena from different levels of analysis is particularly problematic in the context of attempts to characterize the types of relationships that influence mental health or efforts to identify key relational processes related to behavior disorders and mental health. In that context, it is especially important that relationship research be able to interface with research on fundamental processes implicated in behavior disorders and mental health.

An initial step in the direction of reducing insularity was initiated by program staff at the National Institute of Mental Health (NIMH) when they convened a cross-cutting discussion of relationships and relational processes relevant to mental health (Close Relationships Workshop 2001). The success of that meeting inspired the Fetzer Institute to continue supporting progress in this direction. In the spirit of that initial meeting, the Fetzer Institute, in collaboration with NIMH, sponsored "Relational Processes in Mental Health: From Neuroscience to Assessment and Intervention (And Back Again)," a meeting focused on identification of connections between different levels of analysis and the implication of those connections for understanding the effects of relationships on mental health outcomes. The goal was to identify a body of research and create a network that would foster continued progress in the area. In addition, by characterizing relationship problems from multiple levels of analyses, it was hoped that the importance of relationship research in understanding etiology, maintenance, or remediation of mental disorders might be better highlighted. A unifying theme of the conference was that dialogue among researchers should lead to practical implications for improved diagnosis, intervention, and patient care.

To illustrate the potential of a bench-to-bedside dialogue, this volume begins with several chapters that describe links between relational processes and outcomes at the level of genetics, brain function, and biochemistry. Subsequent contributions build on this foundation by examining relational processes related to mental health outcomes in community, treatment, and prevention samples. The final chapters describe a consensus view of researchers from all levels of analysis regarding the necessary research that would further illuminate the role of relational processes in mental health and the best ways to characterize these processes. It is our hope that the resulting body of work 1) illustrates the practical benefits of a bench-to-bedside dialogue, 2) alerts the reader to the limitations inherent in the relationship descriptions currently provided in DSM-IV, and 3) identifies a range of practical options for DSM-V that would allow more adequate inclusion of research on relationships and their connection to behavior disorders and mental health.

Role of Relational Processes in DSM-IV

DSM-IV is limited in its treatment of relational processes and relational disorders. However, the failure of DSM-IV to provide adequate guidance for clinical case management and clinical research does not result from a decision that such processes are unimportant. On the contrary, DSM-IV highlights relational processes in numerous places, including "Other Conditions That May Be a Focus of Clinical Attention" (e.g., partner relational problem, sibling relational problem, parent-child relational problem), Axis IV (e.g., problems with primary support group, problems related to social environment), and the Global Assessment of Functioning (GAF) Scale on Axis V as well as the Global Assessment of Relational Functioning (GARF) Scale in Appendix B. Likewise, considerable effort has been spent in elaborating clinical issues related to some relational problems, such as the discussion of abuse and neglect and other relational problems in Volume III of the *DSM-IV Source Book* (Widiger et al. 1997). There appears to be a widespread consensus that the effects of relationships and relationship events are so central to every aspect of psychopathology and clinical practice that they must be included somewhere in the diagnostic system.

Unfortunately, the descriptions of relational processes provided in DSM-IV do not incorporate advances that have occurred in the empirical science of relationships since DSM-IV was published. In view of the empirical data that have accumulated in the past 15 years, the descriptions of relational context provided by the DSM-IV V codes are overly vague and general. For example, the description of partner relational problems as "a pattern of interaction between spouses or partners characterized by negative communication (e.g., criticism)" (American Psychiatric Association 2000, p. 737) provides so little guidance in determining whether a treatable problem is present that it is an impediment, rather than an aid, to appropriate clinical conceptualization. At a minimum, the descriptions offered by DSM-IV need to be elaborated so they can illuminate important connections between the social environment and particular disorders and provide guidance about the boundary between disorder and normal variations in relationship functioning. In addition, the V codes, problems on Axis IV, and the GAF and GARF scales have been underused by epidemiologists and often are given brief consideration, at best, in basic courses on DSM. Therefore, changes must be made in DSM-V to make the codes and scales clearer, more specific, more reliable, and thus more useful to both researchers and clinicians. At a minimum, it will be important for key findings pertaining to relational processes to be reported in the text descriptions of various disorders.

Key Findings on Relational Processes

Several intriguing findings emerge from the current volume that suggest the need for expansion and revision of the handling of relational processes in DSM-IV and the need for additional attention to relational processes in the background for most disorders. For example, given the astonishing progress made by the Human Genome Project, there is understandably a strong interest in better describing the genetic basis of behavior disorders. However, it appears that adequate description of genetic effects may require good specification of early relationship environment (Reiss and Wamboldt, Chapter 6, this volume). Recent work also shows that the effect of marital satisfaction is a nonshared environmental effect as it relates to depression. Specifically, marital satisfaction is not well modeled as resulting from the same genetic factors that produce the vulnerability for depressive symptoms. Accordingly, it appears that disturbance in intimate adult relationships is important in understanding the etiology and maintenance of depressive symptoms for many individuals, and elucidating its role has the potential to supplement genetically based models (see Reiss and Wamboldt, Chapter 6, this volume; see also Caspi et al. 2000, 2003). As a consequence, better tools for specification of relationship history and current relational processes may prove to be the linchpin of progress in this important area.

The need for better characterization of relational processes in DSM-V is further suggested by the fact that conflict in primary relationships among adults can negatively affect endocrine and immune systems (see Graham et al., Chapter 4, this volume). The potential functional impairment produced by behavior disorders may be increased when they affect primary relationships. In addition, these effects may provide some insights into one of the mechanisms by which relational processes can trigger the onset of some behavior disorders. Likewise, disturbances in primary relationships early in life can change neural systems that control emotional resilience (Suomi 1999; Lim and Young, Chapter 2, this volume), and so create long-term changes in vulnerability (Gallo et al. 2003; Totah and Plotsky, Chapter 3, this volume). As these examples suggest, even from the perspective of understanding the basic neurochemistry of mental health, a diagnostic system that neglects the relational context of disorders is destined to be inadequate—a result that is not surprising given the strong evidence that social bonding (and particularly pair bonding) is manifested biochemically in the brain (see Lim and Young, Chapter 2, this volume), with profound and long-term implications (see Benjamin et al., Chapter 10, this volume). As the data make clear, relationship research should be included in any consideration of etiology and maintenance of major mental illness, even if the discussion is limited to fundamental processes such as genetic effects, effects of gene expression, biochemical effects, and effects related to the stress response.

Also, relationship researchers must overcome their history of insularity and embrace the dialogue that has been encouraged by the NIMH. As the initial chapters in this volume illustrate, bench science has considerable potential to help relationship researchers find exciting new interpretations of their data and to stimulate the development of new hypotheses about the etiological and treatment significance of relational processes, with the potential for promoting rapid clinical advancement. At the same time, there is considerable potential for community-level research on etiology and research on prevention and clinical intervention to inform and influence the direction of basic research. Indeed, recent developments in family-based intervention (McFarlane, Chapter 5, this volume; Sandler et al., Chapter 12, this volume) and enhanced understanding of the key social processes implicated in the etiology and relapse of mental disorder (Brown, Chapter 7, this volume; Hooley et al., Chapter 11, this volume) provide fertile ground for speculating about the fundamental processes that might underlie the substantial effect of relationships on mental health outcomes. Likewise, because relationships often change as a function of psychiatric disturbance (Wamboldt and Wamboldt 2000), and because in some cases relationship difficulties are an integral part of a disorder (e.g., Chatoor et al. 1998; Reid et al. 2002; see also Benjamin et al., Chapter 10, this volume), relationship difficulties often may affect the burden associated with psychiatric impairment (see Whisman, Chapter 14, this volume), as well as the long-term course of some psychiatric illnesses (see Hooley et al., Chapter 11, this volume). These relationship effects may vary depending on cultural context (Bernal et al., Chapter 13, this volume). These research findings can help to guide the focus of research on fundamental processes so as to direct them toward those macro- and microprocesses most likely to influence clinical management and practice.

Research on etiology can help inform research on prevention and clinical intervention, and the reverse can also occur. For example, serious marital[1] dissatisfaction predicts increased risk for a major depressive episode in the subsequent year, even after investigators control for history of depression or comorbidity (see Whisman, Chapter 14, this volume), and both marital conflict and physical abuse predict subsequent increases in depressive symptoms among women (Beach et al.

---

[1]Most of the research on effects of adult intimate relationships has focused on married, heterosexual couples. It is likely, however, that other close relationships have the potential to produce similar effects under some circumstances. In particular, it may be that persons in long-term committed gay and lesbian relationships or cohabiting heterosexual persons have an effect on each other that is similar to the effect married, heterosexual couples have on each other. Accordingly, the use of the term *married couple* is meant to reflect the preponderance of data and not to exclude other types of dyads prematurely.

2004). Likewise, the effect of humiliating marital events on depression has been shown to be substantial (Cano and O'Leary 2000; Kendler et al. 2003). Similarly, alcoholic patients whose spouses are highly negative and critical are more likely to relapse, and also drink on a greater percentage of days, in the year following treatment of alcoholism than are patients whose spouses engage in low levels of negative behaviors (O'Farrell and Fals-Stewart 2003). In a similar manner, critical and hostile attitudes toward mentally ill family members are reliably associated with higher rates of relapse in people with schizophrenia (see Hooley et al., Chapter 11; McFarlane, Chapter 5, this volume). Therefore, disturbances in adult intimate relationships may be an important target for intervention in several behavior disorders, creating a strong need for more precise descriptions and better coverage of key relational processes in DSM-V.

Practical Implications of Current Data for Enhanced Relational Descriptions

Close relationships, such as those in families, appear important for mental health outcomes whether the focus is the basic psychopathology of mental disorders (Reiss and Wamboldt, Chapter 6, this volume), factors influencing maintenance and relapse of disorder (Brown, Chapter 7, this volume; Hooley et al., Chapter 11, this volume), sources of burden for family members (Whisman, Chapter 14, this volume), guiding family-based intervention (McFarlane, Chapter 5, this volume), interventions that deal with the consequences of family processes (Sandler et al., Chapter 12, this volume), or broader cultural issues (Bernal et al., Chapter 13, this volume). Intimate adult relationships (e.g., Brown, Chapter 7, this volume; Graham et al., Chapter 4, this volume; Hooley et al., Chapter 11, this volume) and parenting relationships (e.g., Caspi et al. 2003; Totah and Plotsky, Chapter 3, this volume) are particularly powerful in their effects on psychopathology. Thus, sound measurement of problematic intimate partner and parenting relationships may be particularly important in guiding future research and intervention. Indeed, the salience of family relationships and family events may arise because humans are "hard-wired" to respond to certain types of relationship events (Insel and Young 2001; Young et al. 2003; see also Lim and Young, Chapter 2, this volume), suggesting that these relationships may require special descriptive attention in a revised DSM.

The brief review of the literature provided earlier suggests that in addition to the customary focus on relational problems or disorders such as "marital problem" or "abuse," DSM-V may need to identify relationships that are nonpathological under most circumstances but that can become pathological in the context of some or all psychiatric disorders. This suggests the need for a distinction between relational disorders and relational risk factors. The latter would be a relatively new DSM category and so might require new approaches in the document to facilitate its inclusion. Likewise, some relational processes, such as partner confirmation (i.e., the partner's role in basic self-confirmation processes), may have a clearly established role for only one disorder, whereas other relational processes, such as marital discord, may have implications for many disorders. This suggests the need for a distinction between relational processes with general effects and those with specific effects. We elaborate these two basic distinctions in the following subsections.

RELATIONAL DISORDERS VERSUS RELATIONAL RISK FACTORS

Some relationship problems, such as those identified in the current V codes, produce clinically recognizable sets of symptoms, are associated with distress and interference with personal functioning, and could be a focus of clinical attention in the absence of any other disorder. Conversely, other relationship problems may be of clinical interest because they can be risk factors for negative outcomes in the context of an ongoing psychiatric disorder or increase risk for relapse of that disorder, even though they are not disorders in themselves, do not typically interfere with personal functioning in themselves, and typically would not be the focus of clinical intervention in the absence of any other disorder. For example, expressed emotion (EE) defines a cluster of beliefs and behaviors, with criticism a salient component of the cluster, that are not routinely associated with distress or functional impairment in the absence of a coexisting psychiatric diagnosis but may be associated with problematic outcomes when psychiatric conditions are present. These types of relational processes are not currently highlighted in DSM-IV. Accordingly, the revision should allow for a distinction between relational disorders, which are already included in the form of V codes, and relational risk factors, which are not currently included and would be noteworthy only when they occur in the context of a psychiatric disorder.

GENERAL VERSUS SPECIFIC EFFECTS OF RELATIONAL PROCESSES

It is also important to distinguish between relationship problems, such as marital or couple discord or high EE, that may have strong consequences for maintenance or progression of several disorders (e.g., mood disorders; schizophrenia and other psychotic disorders; substance-related disorders; alcohol-related disorders; disorders usually first diagnosed in infancy, childhood, or adolescence) and relationship problems that have been shown to have an effect only in the context of a particular disorder, such as partner confirmation processes in depression, or that may play a particularly salient role in the context of a particular psychiatric disorder, such as intrusive feeding behavior in the context of feeding disorder of infancy. For practical reasons of efficiency, these different types of relational processes may require somewhat different treatment in DSM. General relational processes could be described readily and efficiently without reference to other mental or physical disorders and so could be described in their own section or on their own axis, assuming a multiaxial system in DSM-V. This would allow general treatment guidelines and case identification methods to be explicated in an efficient manner conducive to both scientific communication and clinical utility. Specific relationship processes, such as anxious, intrusive behavior during feeding, that may be of great importance in one disorder (e.g., feeding disorder of infancy) but of limited relevance for other disorders would be more efficiently described in the context of that particular disorder. Rather than such descriptions being separated in their own section, they would be more useful if tied closely to the specific disorders, suggesting the value of descriptions that are embedded in the text of the disorder or are reflected in modifier codes for that particular disorder. At a minimum, the variability in the types of relational processes that may be important suggests that a comprehensive diagnostic system may need to use more than one approach to describe key relational processes and disorders.

Four basic categories of relational processes potentially requiring different treatment emerge from the above distinctions:

1. Disordered and general relational processes such as abuse or marital discord (i.e., the relational disorders currently described in the V codes)
2. Nondisordered and general relational processes such as high EE or conflict avoidance in marriage (i.e., relational processes not currently included in DSM-IV that affect treatment and research for many disorders)
3. Disordered and specific relational processes such as intrusive feeding in the context of feeding disorder of infancy or problematic parenting in the context of conduct disorder (i.e., disordered relational behavior that is a component of some psychiatric disorders and that affects treatment and research for particular disorders)
4. Nondisordered and specific relational processes such as partner verification in depression or low parental monitoring in teenage drug use (i.e., relational processes that affect treatment and research for particular disorders)

Each of these four categories may require a different type of characterization within DSM, and in some cases, it may be appropriate to use or consider using more than one approach to capture important relational processes.

Sorting Relational Processes Into Four Categories

In all cases, we propose that a relational process should be considered nondisordered until it has been clearly shown to create distress, has not been responsive to self-repair processes, and reflects behavior that is not merely a response to the aberrant behavior of one individual. Accordingly, an empirical criterion would separate nondisordered from disordered behavior and protect against stigmatizing family members who are merely different or reacting to the difficult circumstances imposed by psychiatric disorder in a loved one. Likewise, we propose that relational processes should be considered specific until clearly shown to have implications for multiple forms of psychopathology. That is, an empirical criterion would separate general from specific relational processes. Thus, as new relational processes were considered for inclusion in DSM, there would be a well defined set of defaults and a clear set of empirical hurdles to be overcome prior to inclusion in each category. We illustrate the way in which each type of relational process might be included in DSM-V.

DISORDERED AND GENERAL RELATIONAL DISORDERS

Relational disorders are already identified as V codes in DSM-IV. Of central importance for DSM-V is that the indicator set for each of these disorders be more clearly specified. Given the accumulation of data over the past 20 years, specification of reliable and valid indicators should be possible for each of the current V codes. The circumstances under which these disorders should be a focus of clinical attention also may be an appropriate target for clarification in DSM-V. That is, it may be possible to provide guidance about the threshold for considering a problem an important target for direct clinical attention rather than merely a background variable to consider in treatment planning. The clinical utility of these descriptions might be further enhanced by creating a separate "relational disorders" category that could underscore the importance of continued research on these problems and facilitate the provision of guidance for clinical intervention. More detailed criteria sets for the relational disorders have been proposed previously, with good convergence across prior efforts (First et al. 2002). The following example of parent-child problems illustrates the initial steps in the process of developing criterion sets for a relational disorder on the basis of the empirical literature. The empirical literature pertaining to each proposed relational disorder would have to be reviewed to develop criteria appropriate to that disorder.

Illustrative Example: Parent-Child Conflict Disorder

Although diagnostic criteria have not been proposed, a large empirical literature on parenting identifies potential indicators of parent-child conflict disorder. Parents experiencing depression and substance abuse are at elevated risk for parent-child conflict disorder (Cummings et al. 2001; Goodman and Gotlib 1999). Parent-child conflict disorder is also characterized by several reliable indicators, including developmentally unrealistic expectations, negative misperception of child behaviors (Wahler and Sansbury 1990), negative attributional style with regard to the child (Baden and Howe 1992), and overreactive anger and child discipline (Slep and O'Leary 1998), as well as inconsistent discipline, low supervision, and rigidity. At the same time, child behavior associated with parent-child conflict disorder may include high levels of noncompliance, disapproval, and negativism. Accordingly, it should be possible to develop an empirically grounded set of criteria that capture the shift from nondisordered, transient conflict between parents and children to the type of parent-child conflict that warrants clinical attention. In addition, it should be possible to define subcategories or additional categories that capture additional problematic features such as violence directed toward the child, neglect of the child, or sexual abuse of the child (see Heyman and Slep, in press). However, because appropriate parenting changes across the life span, it may be necessary to specify different indicators for children of different ages.

NONDISORDERED AND GENERAL RELATIONAL PROCESSES ON A SEPARATE AXIS

The importance of nondisordered and general relational processes, such as EE or conflict avoidance in marriage, could be highlighted by creating a separate axis for the description of relational context. In this way, important contextual processes could be better specified, epidemiologists could be encouraged to examine the prevalence and incidence of important aspects of relational context in the general population, and clinical decision making could be better informed. Creating a separate axis would help maintain the distinction between relationship problems that are contextual (i.e., that are important because they increase the probability of symptomatic exacerbation or relapse of an illness despite not being disorders themselves) and relationship problems that are disorders (i.e., that cause distress and morbidity regardless of the presence of other illnesses).

Illustrative Example: Expressed Emotion

An example of an empirically grounded and clinically relevant relationship process that is, nonetheless, not a disorder is provided in the EE literature. EE is a clinically noteworthy process indexed by expressed attitudes toward the identified patient that lends itself to reliable, dimensional assessment. High levels of EE are relatively benign in many family contexts and in others may be elicited by the presence of physical and mental health problems. For example, chronic health conditions in childhood may set the stage for maladaptive changes in family functioning that would not have been manifested if the illness had never occurred (Gustafsson et al. 1994). Likewise, parents or partners of the severely mentally ill may find themselves confronted with situations for which they are poorly prepared, and as a result, their behavior may change in problematic ways (Hooley and Gotlib 2000), leading to high EE. Or, confronted with unusual behavior, family members may misapply strategies that would have been relatively benign in the absence of severe mental illness in a family member, again resulting in high EE. Accordingly, high EE is not appropriately conceptualized as a relational disorder. Nonetheless, high EE has important implications for treatment.

As with the relational disorders, a substantial empirical literature guides the assessment of EE and links ratings of EE to treatment decision making (Hooley and Parker, in press). The best-established measurement approach is the well-validated, semistructured interview known as the Camberwell Family Interview (Leff and Vaughn 1985), conducted with key relatives, typically parents or a spouse, without the patient being present. Ratings on the five dimensions of criticism, hostility, emotional overinvolvement, warmth, and positive remarks allow family members to be classified as high or low in EE. Threshold criteria may be adjusted for different psychiatric problems based on empirical findings. For example, in the case of schizophrenia, a family member making six or more critical remarks would be classified as high in EE (see Hooley et al., Chapter 11, this volume).

DISORDERED AND SPECIFIC RELATIONAL PROCESSES

Not all important relational processes have sufficiently general effects to warrant their inclusion in a "relational disorders" category or on a "relational context" axis. Nonetheless, disorder-specific relational processes may prove to be critical for understanding particular disorders or for distinguishing functionally distinct types of disorder. Accordingly, a third proposal for enhancing the description of relational processes in DSM-V would incorporate a reference to the presence or absence of disorder-specific relational processes with relational specifiers. Specifiers are most often used within DSM to describe significant aspects of the course of the disorder or to highlight prominent symptomatology. However, specifiers also can be used to indicate associated behavior patterns of clinical interest. Because the potential relevance of relational specifiers may be seen clearly in the context of disorders of infancy and childhood, we use feeding disorder of infancy to illustrate the potential advantages of using relational specifiers to incorporate relationship information into DSM-V diagnoses. In the case of feeding disorder of infancy, specifiers might be used to subtype a disorder and so provide more appropriate treatment.

Illustrative Example: Relational Specifiers—
Feeding Disorder of Infancy

DSM-IV (American Psychiatric Association 1994) introduced feeding disorder of infancy or early childhood but made no effort to distinguish among various important subtypes. Preliminary evidence suggests, however, that several important variants present themselves in early childhood. For example, children may refuse to eat subsequent to a serious trauma involving the upper gastrointestinal tract, or their food refusal may reflect the interaction of their own temperament and an anxious, intrusive feeding style on the part of their principal caregiver. These two subtypes may have different patterns of dysfunction and respond to different types of intervention. Feeding disorders secondary to trauma indicate the child's high level of anxiety and difficulty in swallowing early in an episode of feeding, whereas disorders associated with relationship difficulties show conflict between the infant and caregiver during attempted feeding and food refusal by the child. Accordingly, focused attention on explicating relational characteristics of the feeding process could play a pivotal role in enhancing diagnosis and treatment.

Illustrative Example: Elaborate Embedded Criteria— Conduct Disorder

In some cases, the importance of behavior patterns of interest might be better captured by elaborating them as part of the symptom criteria for a particular disorder. Indeed, in some cases, an entire category of disorder has prominent relational characteristics, but these have been omitted or downplayed in the diagnostic criteria for the disorder. Accordingly, an additional proposal for making relational processes more salient would involve better highlighting relational elements that are currently implicit in existing disorders. Current diagnostic criteria for conduct disorder, for example, make no mention of the parent-child relationship. However, the relational problems in this disorder may be so central to its maintenance, if not its etiology, that effective treatment may be impossible without recognizing and delineating the relational aspects of the disorder. Elaborating the embedded relational criteria may be critical for enhancing our understanding of treatment response and relapse. We examine conduct disorder as an example of the value of elaborating embedded relational criteria.

Research on conduct disorders provides ample foundation for including relational patterns in the diagnostic criteria. For example, a coercive, hostile, punitive parenting style is associated with a markedly increased risk for conduct disorder and antisocial behavior (Loeber and Stouthamer-Loeber 1986; Patterson and Forgatch 1995). Although this may reflect a shared genetic makeup contributing to coercive behavior in the parent and antisocial behavior in the child (Reiss et al. 2000), there is little doubt that the interaction pattern is integral to the disorder. Observational data indicate that the parent's desperate effort to control a child who is essentially socially unskilled consists of threats, scolding, and demands (Stoolmiller et al. 1997) that are temporarily effective at best. The child's response to the parent's coercive behavior is in the form of aggressive behaviors, leading the parent to stop demanding the child's compliance temporarily. This sequence of events constitutes a spiral of negative reinforcement for both parent and child that occurs time and again, maintaining, and perhaps escalating, the child's antisocial behavior and the parent's ineffective response. In addition, interrupting the relational pattern is an efficacious treatment for childhood conduct disorders, although the results for adolescents are less certain (Kazdin 1998), and no other approach to treating these disorders has compiled an equally impressive scientific record.

Inclusion of relational characteristics as part of the diagnostic criteria for conduct disorder may be the most appropriate way to recognize the central role of these characteristics in the psychopathology of the disorder as well as their central role in treatment. Although the example above is focused on conduct disorder, it seems clear that many other disorders may be amenable to similar analyses and might benefit from elaboration of the embedded or implicit relational problems that are characteristic of the disorder.

NONDISORDERED AND SPECIFIC RELATIONAL PROCESSES

Presumably, some relational processes are of importance for one disorder but are not yet known to be of general importance or may have negative consequences only in the context of a specific disorder. We briefly examined the case of partner confirmation processes in depression earlier in this chapter. In such cases, it might be most efficient to elaborate the importance of the process in the text. That is, as the text is revised to reflect new findings related to particular disorders, an effort could be made to systematically include the empirical literature linking particular relational processes, whether nondisordered or disordered, to etiology, maintenance, relapse, or burden of the disorder.

Thus, the four different types of relational processes suggest five different ways that DSM-V could be improved relative to DSM-IV:

1. Develop clear criteria for the relational disorders currently described in the V codes, and perhaps create a "relational disorders" category on Axis I.
2. Develop an axis devoted to relational context within the multiaxial system with clear criteria for assessing empirically supported contextual processes that might be the target of clinical intervention, including both family and multisystem contexts.
3. Use relational specifier codes to indicate important disorder-specific relational processes.
4. Elaborate relationship criteria for existing disorders when appropriate.
5. Elaborate in the text the description of relational processes associated with the disorder.

For each of these options, enhancing the current descriptive system could help stimulate new research, guide the integration of applied and basic research findings, and help guide improved clinical services. A solid empirical foundation exists to guide assessment in a few of these areas, and each of the types of relational processes could have several well-supported candidates before the DSM-V revision process is concluded.

Enhancing Clinical Decision Making

Even with changes that highlight specific relational disorders and relationship dimensions with particular clinical relevance, incorporating relational context into treatment planning likely will be challenging. In particular, relational processes are themselves often embedded in larger systems, requiring attention to a multisystemic perspective for the prevention or treatment of many disorders (e.g., Kotchick et al. 2001). It may be useful, therefore, to provide a guide to thinking about disorders in a relationship context either as an appendix to DSM-V or in a companion volume. In this way, an extended discussion of the issues pertinent to assessing and using information about family and the broader social context that may affect relational processes could be included. This would supplement the multiaxial diagnostic system by addressing difficulties in applying the diagnostic system in the context of ongoing relationship problems or broader systemic difficulties.

A guide to relational formulations and social context would suggest that it is important to take into account an individual's primary social group and to describe how it is relevant to clinical care. Areas to be highlighted might include level of family conflict about the disorder, family view of the source and likely course of the illness, family view of the patient and the patient's potential for improvement, family view of treatment and treating agencies, family strengths and sources of support, and family sense of caregiver burden. In addition, this material might address neighborhood effects that have been shown to influence outcomes of interest (e.g., Cutrona et al. 2005). Accordingly, if guidelines for a relational formulation are provided, several issues related to the need for increased specificity of description, the role of the family in treatment implementation and long-term adherence, and the role of the family as a source of both social stress and social support could be addressed. If a companion volume were provided, these general guidelines could be further elaborated with respect to particular mental disorders and the relational processes that have emerged as most central to case management. The inclusion of guidelines for a relational formulation is in keeping with DSM-IV's inclusion of guidelines for a cultural formulation.

Concerns About Inclusion of Relational Problems in DSM-IV

CAN WE MAKE RELIABLE AND VALID JUDGMENTS ABOUT RELATIONSHIP PROBLEMS?

Current definitions of relationship problems in DSM-IV do not allow for reliable or valid assessments of relationship problems. This has slowed research and forced clinicians to rely on idiosyncratic or intuitive approaches. Provision of explicit, data-based criteria for relational disorders, relational context, relational specifiers, and embedded relational diagnostic criteria should help correct this problem. For example, Heyman and Slep (in press) have shown that even nonclinicians can make reliable judgments about partner and child maltreatment when the criteria are well explicated. Nonetheless, considerable research will be necessary to establish the clinical utility of particular sets of relational criteria (see Brown, Chapter 7, this volume; Heyman and Smith Slep, Chapter 9, this volume; Hooley et al., Chapter 11, this volume).

WILL ELABORATION OF RELATIONSHIP PROBLEMS SEPARATE PSYCHIATRY FROM MEDICAL SCIENCE?

The importance of relational disorders and relational context is not limited to psychiatric disorders. These processes are also implicated in a wide range of specific disorders across all branches of medical science. Accordingly, better specification of these processes in DSM-V will make psychiatry more relevant and provide enhanced connections to other branches of medical science. Many disease management strategies for chronic medical illnesses include an assessment of family factors and/or an intervention with families, indicating widespread acceptance of the relevance of relationships for management of physical illness.

WILL GREATER ATTENTION TO RELATIONSHIP PROBLEMS UNDERCUT PARITY FOR MENTAL DISORDERS?

Because neither relational disorders nor relational risk factors are likely to be defined as "individual mental disorders," greater attention to relational context probably would not influence the discussion of reimbursement parity. Elaboration of embedded relational criteria and identification of appropriate opportunities for the use of relational specifiers should be neutral with regard to prevalence and so would be expected to have no effect on the discussion of reimbursement parity. Conversely, to the extent that greater attention to relational context improves efficiency and effectiveness of treatment, or leads to reductions in residual impairment, there may be an indirect, positive effect on this discussion.

Conclusion and Recommendations

A diagnostic system that provides guidance regarding when to provide treatment for relationship difficulties and when to use relationship-oriented interventions to enhance outcomes would have great clinical benefit. A substantial body of basic research shows that the relational context of disorder is consequential for etiology and treatment decision making. The need to make better provisions for the description of relational context is most obvious when disorders of childhood are the focus of attention. However, the effect of relational context on a wide range of outcomes from childhood through adulthood and into aging populations suggests the need to provide relational diagnoses for adult-adult relationships and possibly for child-child relationships as well. At a minimum, it will be important to define relational disorders, relational risk factors, relationship patterns of clinical interest in specific disorders, and embedded relational characteristics with greater precision than is possible within the current diagnostic framework.

The chapters in the current volume illustrate the study of relationships at multiple levels of analysis and the convergence that occurs when these multiple levels are considered simultaneously. As can be seen in the chapters of this volume, we are on the cusp of an exciting era of relationship-focused translational research in which various levels of analysis can be combined to be mutually informative. This should produce rapid progress in understanding the connection between relationships and mental health and produce concomitant advances in both clinical intervention and case management. Relationship problems are inextricably connected to individual mental health problems, changes in fundamental biological processes, and individual developmental outcomes. As a consequence, a diagnostic system that fails to offer guidance with regard to relationship problems will be unable to use a consistent and clinically relevant literature, leading to impoverished clinical decision making and an impoverished understanding of mental health problems.

The conclusion that emerges from consideration of the remaining chapters in this volume is that sufficient literature already exists to show a profound connection between mental health and relational processes. When one looks across levels of analysis and begins a dialogue among researchers who approach the connection between relational processes and mental health outcomes in different ways, the connections become even more striking and more compelling. At the same time, to translate the science of relationships into practical application requires ongoing dialogue among researchers at all levels of analysis. This dialogue is also ideal for identifying the priority areas that must be addressed prior to the DSM revision process if that revision is to be informed by the best available data (see Miklowitz et al., Chapter 15, this volume).

References

American Psychiatric Association: Diagnostic and Statistical Manual of Mental Disorders, 4th Edition. Washington, DC, American Psychiatric Association, 1994

American Psychiatric Association: Diagnostic and Statistical Manual of Mental Disorders, 4th Edition, Text Revision. Washington, DC, American Psychiatric Association, 2000

Baden AD, Howe GW: Mothers' attributions and expectancies regarding their conduct-disordered children. J Abnorm Child Psychol 20:467–485, 1992

Beach SRH, Kim S, Cercone-Keeney J, et al: Physical aggression and depression: gender asymmetry in effects? J Soc Pers Relat 21:341–360, 2004

Cano A, O'Leary KD: Infidelity and separations precipitate major depressive episodes and symptoms of nonspecific depression and anxiety. J Consult Clin Psychol 68:774–781, 2000

Caspi A, Taylor A, Moffitt TE, et al: Neighborhood deprivation affects children's mental health: environmental risks identified in a genetic design. Psychol Sci 11:338–342, 2000

Caspi A, Sugden K, Moffitt TE, et al: Influence of life stress on depression: moderation by a polymorphism in the 5-HTT gene. Science 301:386–389, 2003

Chatoor I, Hirsch R, Ganiban J, et al: Diagnosing infantile anorexia: the observation of mother-infant interactions. J Am Acad Child Adolesc Psychiatry 37:959–967, 1998

Close relationships: basic science and clinical translation. A National Institute of Mental Health Workshop, Bethesda, MD, July 30–31, 2001

Cummings EM, DeArth-Pendley GDR, Schudlich T, et al: Parental depression and family functioning: toward a process-oriented model of children's adjustment, in Marital and Family Processes in Depression: A Scientific Foundation for Clinical Practice. Edited by Beach SRH. Washington, DC, American Psychological Association, 2001, pp 89–110

Cutrona CE, Russell DW, Brown PA, et al: Neighborhood context, personality, and stressful life events as predictors of depression among African America women. J Abnorm Psychol 114:3–15, 2005

First MB, Bell CC, Cuthburt B, et al: Personality disorders and relational disorders: a research agenda for addressing crucial gaps in DSM, in A Research Agenda for DSM-V. Edited by Kupfer DJ, First MB, Regier DA. Washington, DC, American Psychiatric Association, 2002, pp 123–199

Gallo LC, Troxel WM, Matthews KA, et al: Marital status and quality in middle-aged women: associations with levels and trajectories of cardiovascular risk factors. Health Psychol 22:453–463, 2003

Goodman SH, Gotlib IH: Risk for psychopathology in the children of depressed mothers: a developmental model for understanding mechanisms of transmission. Psychol Rev 106:458–490, 1999

Gustafsson PA, Bjorksten B, Kjellman NI: Family dysfunction in asthma: a prospective study of illness development. J Pediatr 125:493–498, 1994

Heyman RE, Slep AMS: Creating and field-testing diagnostic criteria for partner and child maltreatment. J Fam Psychol (in press)

Hooley JM, Gotlib IH: A diathesis-stress conceptualization of expressed emotion and clinical outcome. Applied and Preventive Psychology 9:135–151, 2000

Hooley JM, Parker HA: Measuring expressed emotion: an evaluation of the short cuts. J Fam Psychol (in press)

Insel TR, Young LJ: The neurobiology of attachment. Nat Rev Neurosci 2:129–136, 2001

Kazdin AE: Psychosocial treatments for conduct disorder in children, in A Guide to Treatments That Work. Edited by Nathan PEG, Jack M. London, England, Oxford University Press, 1998, pp 65–89

Kendler KS, Hettema JM, Butera F, et al: Life event dimensions of loss, humiliation, entrapment, and danger in the prediction of onsets of major depression and generalized anxiety. Arch Gen Psychiatry 60:789–796, 2003

Kotchick BA, Shaffer A, Forehand R, et al: Adolescent sexual risk behavior: a multi-system perspective. Clin Psychol Rev 21:493–519, 2001

Leff JP, Vaughn CE: Expressed Emotion in Families. New York, Guilford, 1985

Loeber R, Stouthamer-Loeber M: Family factors as correlates and predictors of juvenile conduct problems and delinquency. Crime and Justice—A Review of Research 7:129–149, 1986

O'Farrell TJ, Fals-Stewart W: Alcohol abuse. J Marital Fam Ther 29:121–146, 2003

Patterson GR, Forgatch MS: Predicting future clinical adjustment from treatment outcome and process variables. Psychol Assess 7:275–285, 1995

Reid JB, Patterson GR, Snyder J: Antisocial Behavior in Children and Adolescents: A Developmental Analysis and Model for Intervention. Washington, DC, American Psychological Association, 2002

Reiss D, Plomin R, Neiderhiser JM, et al: The Relationship Code: Deciphering Genetic and Social Patterns in Adolescent Development. Cambridge, MA, Harvard University Press, 2000

Slep AM, O'Leary SG: The effects of maternal attributions on parenting: an experimental analysis. J Fam Psychol 12:234–243, 1998

Stoolmiller M, Patterson GR, Snyder J: Parental discipline and child antisocial behavior: a contingency-based theory and some methodological refinements. Psychological Inquiry 8:223–229, 1997

Suomi SJ: Developmental trajectories, early experiences, and community consequences: lessons from studies with rhesus monkeys, in Developmental Health and the Wealth of Nations: Social, Biological, and Educational Dynamics. Edited by Keating DP, Hertzman C. New York, Guilford, 1999, pp 185–200

Wahler RG, Sansbury LE: The monitoring skills of troubled mothers: their problems in defining child deviance. J Abnorm Child Psychol 18:577–589, 1990

Wamboldt MZ, Wamboldt FS: Role of the family in the onset and outcome of childhood disorders: selected research findings. J Am Acad Child Adolesc Psychiatry 39:1212–1219, 2000

Widiger TA, Frances AJ, Pincus HA, et al (eds): DSM-IV Sourcebook, Vol 3. Washington, DC, American Psychiatric Association, 1997

Young LJ, Francis DD, Insel TR: The Biochemistry of Family Commitment and Youth Competence: Lessons From Furry Mammals (Working Paper 76-18). New York, Institute for American Values, 2003

PART I

BIOLOGICAL UNDERPINNINGS

CHAPTER 2

NEUROBIOLOGY OF THE SOCIAL BRAIN

Lessons From Animal Models About Social Relationships

Miranda M. Lim, Ph.D.
Larry J. Young, Ph.D.

Social relationships form the foundation of human societies. Both the complex and the enduring qualities of human social relationships are definitive hallmarks that distinguish humans from most other animals. However, glaringly little research exists on the biological mechanisms underlying the formation and maintenance of social relationships. Aside from a handful of postmortem studies and functional imaging approaches, it has been extremely difficult to examine the neurobiology of social behavior in humans. Fortunately, several animal models provide insight into the underpinnings of how the brain controls social relationships. Although the research in this field is far from complete, these animal models can serve to complement existing data on typical human social behavior, as well as in cases of pathological sociality, such as in autism spectrum disorders, schizophrenia, Turner's syndrome, Williams syndrome, and social phobias.

The formation and maintenance of social relationships is a complex process that likely involves several levels of information processing in the brain. A simplified conceptual framework may be used as a general heuristic in understanding the

This research was supported by NIH MH 65050 (M.M.L.), MH 56897 and MH 64692 (L.J.Y.), NSF STC IBN-9876754, and the Yerkes Center Grant RR00165.

role of the brain and biology in social behavior. At the most basic level—social recognition—an individual needs to be able to recognize and remember other individuals before forming the social relationship. The next level—social motivation—includes desire of the individual to engage in social relationships with other individuals. The third level—social approach—necessitates definitive contact with other individuals. The fourth level—social bonding—establishes the formation of an enduring, reciprocal social relationship. Each of these conceptual levels engages different brain regions and neural circuits. Thus, neuropathology can occur at any level of this framework, with the resulting phenotype being a global impairment in the development of social relationships. The neural circuits underlying the "social brain" are multilevel and complex and likely involve fine coordination of multiple brain regions. In this chapter, we discuss the biological and clinical aspects of these four levels.

Social Recognition

Social recognition of other individuals is normally a fundamental behavior in all animal species. Whether this important behavior is related to kin and gender recognition, incest avoidance, or mothers' recognition of their young, it contributes to the survival and fitness of an individual within a species. The neurobiological mechanisms underlying this behavior are likely highly conserved across animals and typically begin with sensory processing (usually visual or olfactory) of the characteristics of the other individual and progress to short- or long-term memory, or recognition.

In humans, social recognition is primarily visual in nature, and selective lesions in a single brain region—the fusiform gyrus—can abolish the ability to recognize faces (a condition known as *prosopagnosia*) (Barton et al. 2002). Other evidence has proposed a role for the fusiform gyrus in the structural, static properties of faces, in contrast to adjacent areas of the temporal lobe, the superior temporal gyrus and sulcus, for processing dynamic configurations of faces such as facial expressions (Haxby et al. 2000). A recent functional magnetic resonance imaging (fMRI) study on brain activation, in which subjects watched animated geometric shapes interacting in either a "social" or a "random" fashion, identified a neural circuit for how the brain responds while attributing social interaction to abstract images. These studies identified a "social circuit" comprising the fusiform gyrus, superior temporal sulcus, amygdala, and prefrontal cortex (Castelli et al. 2002). This social circuit for face recognition and processing is generally consistent with what has been reported from studies in nonhuman primates, which are also heavily dependent on the visual system to recognize faces (Perrett et al. 1982, 1985; Stefanacci and Amaral 2000).

Patients with profound dysfunction in social relationships, such as in autism, schizophrenia, and Turner's syndrome, may have deficits in the cognitive processing of faces and facial cues; therefore, their impairments in forming social relationships might stem from a more fundamental problem with social recognition. Although individuals with autism appear to identify faces normally at a basic object level (i.e., when asked to identify a face from a set of basic objects), they do show impairments when asked to match unfamiliar faces on tests such as the Benton Face Recognition Test (Barton 2003; S. Davies et al. 1994; Szatmari et al. 1990). Additional studies also have reported deficits in perceiving facial expression, age, and sex (Hobson 1987; Tantam et al. 1989). It has been reported that patients with schizophrenia also have deficits in face recognition (Archer et al. 1992; Harrington et al. 1989). Recently, several studies found that the size of the fusiform gyrus is significantly reduced in patients with schizophrenia, and the degree of reduction in fusiform gyrus size is significantly correlated with the degree of deficit in face recognition (C. U. Lee et al. 2002; Onitsuka et al. 2003). Moreover, patients with Turner's syndrome, who coincidentally carry 200 times the risk of autism, also have robust deficits in face recognition and in perceiving fearful facial expressions (Lawrence et al. 2003; Skuse et al. 2003). Williams syndrome patients, who present the other extreme in social relationships and are hypersociable, also show anomalous gaze and face processing because of poor visuospatial abilities (Mobbs et al. 2004; Reiss et al. 2004).

In rodents, olfaction appears to be more important for social recognition, and of particular importance is the vomeronasal organ system, which projects to the accessory olfactory bulb to detect pheromones. Mutant mice lacking the gene for trp2, which is a cation channel exclusively expressed in the vomeronasal organ, have profound deficits in the social recognition of gender (Stowers et al. 2002). In contrast to the visual system, olfactory projections in the brain do not synapse within the fusiform gyrus and superior temporal sulcus, but instead are routed through the piriform cortex. However, it appears that these two sensory systems do eventually converge at a more downstream site, the amygdala. The amygdala has been implicated in the processing of social emotions and memory (Adolphs 2003). In rodents, we have been able to study the connections from the olfactory system to more downstream sites such as the amygdala, lateral septum, and cortex and their respective involvements in social recognition. Social recognition in rodents is easily quantifiable in the laboratory and can be assessed by measuring the duration of social investigation during subsequent exposures to the same individual. This behavioral assay is based on the phenomenon that rodents investigate novel items (or individuals) for a longer time than they do familiar items (or individuals). Thus, if a rodent recognizes a familiar individual, it will spend significantly less time investigating that individual with subsequent exposures (Winslow 2003).

Early studies beginning nearly 20 years ago first implicated the neuropeptide oxytocin in memory and social recognition in rodents (Dantzer et al. 1987; Popik et al. 1992). Transgenic mice that lack the oxytocin gene, and therefore do not produce the oxytocin peptide, are unable to recognize familiar individuals despite repeated exposures (Choleris et al. 2003; Ferguson et al. 2000). This inability is not due to a generalized deficit in olfaction or learning and memory, because these mice can habituate to a nonsocial scent and perform normally on spatial memory tasks (Choleris et al. 2003; Ferguson et al. 2000). The profound social deficits of the oxytocin knockout mice can be restored by a single injection of oxytocin into the lateral ventricles of the brain just prior to the initial encounter with a conspecific (Ferguson et al. 2001).

To investigate the neural circuits of social recognition modulated by oxytocin in the knockout mice, Ferguson et al. (2001) examined a neural marker of brain activation in the olfactory processing circuit during a social encounter, comparing mutant with wild-type mice. Wild-type mice showed brain activation in the olfactory bulbs, piriform cortex, and amygdala during the 90-second social encounter. In contrast, oxytocin knockout mice showed neural activity in only the olfactory bulbs and piriform cortex but not in the amygdala . Furthermore, known downstream targets of the amygdala, such as the bed nucleus of the stria terminalis and the medial preoptic area, were also absent of activity in the knockout mice compared with wild-type mice. Intriguingly, the knockout mice showed a massive activation of other brain regions, such as the cortex and hippocampus, that was absent in the wild-type mice (Ferguson et al. 2001). These results led to the discovery that microinjections of oxytocin specifically into the amygdala could rescue social recognition deficits in the oxtyocin knockout mice (Ferguson et al. 2001). Thus, in mice, oxytocin acts at the amygdala during a social encounter for the normal processing of social information, leading to intact social recognition. In the absence of oxytocin, social information appears to be processed by alternative neural circuits, such as cortical and hippocampal regions.

Alternative neural processing also appears to occur in patients with autism during processing of social cues, and this is evident from several neuroimaging studies. When viewing images of human faces, autistic patients show decreased amygdala and fusiform gyrus activation and increased cortical activation compared with nonautistic subjects (Critchley et al. 2000; Pierce et al. 2001; Schultz et al. 2000). When asked to interpret emotions by judging expression from another person's eyes, persons with autism failed to show amygdala activation seen in nonautistic subjects (Baron-Cohen et al. 1999). This is strikingly reminiscent of the findings reported in the oxytocin knockout mice, which also showed absent amygdala activation and recruitment of cortical areas (Ferguson et al. 2001). Preliminary studies in patients with schizophrenia suggested that schizophrenia might also entail differences in neural processing of social cues; a recent fMRI study showed that schizophrenia patients had significantly exaggerated amygdala activation when asked to judge the emotional intensity of faces compared with nonschizophrenic subjects (Kosaka et al. 2002). In patients with Turner's syndrome, structural studies show that the size of the amygdala is enlarged compared with healthy subjects (Good et al. 2003), and it has been suggested that anomalous modulation of cortical circuits is involved in face processing by the "hyperreactive" amygdala (Skuse et al. 2003). Patients with Williams syndrome, who are hypersociable and therefore could be considered on the opposite end of the social relationship spectrum, also have been reported to have amygdala abnormalities in volume and in gray matter density, among abnormalities in other brain regions (Mobbs et al. 2004; Reiss et al. 2004).

Together, both rodent and human studies suggest that the amygdala may be a prime candidate for dysregulation in psychiatric disorders of dysfunctional social relationships. In both visual and olfactory social recognition, it appears that the relevant neural circuits eventually converge downstream at the amygdala to regulate the processing of facial or social cues. These findings in rodent models and in human patients show that common elements in dysfunctional social behavior, such as alternative social processing, can be closely modeled.

Social Motivation

Once an individual successfully engages in social recognition, he or she then must be motivated to seek contact with the other individual before a social relationship can progress. This phenomenon of social motivation is lacking in higher-functioning patients with autism, who clearly can recognize faces but still have deficits in forming social relationships because of their lack of desire to be social (Lord et al. 2000; Pierce et al. 2004). The lack of social motivation in persons with autism has been well documented: socially intended behaviors are less frequent, less self-initiated, and less complex in children with autism (Ruble 2001). Social motivation also may be primarily impaired in patients with schizophrenia, which might manifest as negative symptoms such as apathy and social withdrawal. In Turner's syndrome, only one-third of patients show severe deficits in emotional perception and social memory, whereas the other two-thirds have functioning that is within low to normal limits, with a clear bimodal distribution of ability (Skuse et al. 2003). However, most Turner's syndrome patients still have difficulties in forming social relationships despite low to normal emotional perception; thus, they may have primary deficits in social motivation (Mazzocco et al. 1998; McCauley et al. 2001). On the opposite end of the spectrum, patients with Williams syndrome were shown to have hypersociability, to the point of dysfunctional social relationships: patients had behavioral and emotional difficulties, were overfriendly and socially disinhibited, and had high levels of anxiety and distractibility (M. Davies et al. 1998; Doyle et al. 2004).

The neurobiology of social motivation can be studied in a handful of animal models, usually by measuring the amount of social contact, or affiliation, of the test animal with a conspecific. Interestingly, across rodent and nonhuman primate species, the neuropeptides oxytocin and vasopressin appear to be involved in affiliative behavior. Affiliation between adult rats can be increased by the chronic infusion of oxytocin directly into the brain (Witt et al. 1992). Among voles, vasopressin infusions increase social interaction behavior in the highly social prairie vole but not in the asocial montane vole (Young et al. 1999). This difference in behavioral response to vasopressin appears to be a result of species differences in the vasopressin receptor expression pattern in the brain, because transgenic mice that express the vasopressin receptor in a pattern similar to that of the prairie vole, but not normal mice, also show a similar increase in social contact after vasopressin treatment. Artificially elevating vasopressin receptors in the brain with viral vector gene transfer also increases social contact between adult rats (Landgraf et al. 2003) and between adult male and juvenile prairie voles (Pitkow et al. 2001). In nonhuman primates, two macaque species with natural species differences in affiliative behavior exist. The naturally gregarious and affiliative bonnet monkey has increased levels of cerebrospinal fluid (CSF) oxytocin compared with the relatively asocial pigtail macaque (Rosenblum et al. 2002).

Notably, a recent study examining the therapeutic value of oxytocin in autism reported that intravenous oxytocin infusion reduced repetitive behaviors in adults with autism and Asperger's syndrome, perhaps freeing the potential of these patients for more social interactions (Hollander et al. 2003). However, much is still lacking in conclusively substantiating a role for oxytocin and vasopressin in human social motivation.

Social Approach

An individual may have intact social recognition and social motivation but lack the ability to approach another individual. This is apparent in social phobias, in which patients appear to be conflicted about social approach. These patients often report that they want to seek social contact but that they are afraid to do so because they are anxious about how they will be perceived (Stein 1998).

A few animal models exist that can inform the neurobiology of social approach and avoidance, including social defeat in hamsters, dominance hierarchy establishment in rats, and social interactions in nonhuman primates. The social defeat model involves placing a male hamster in the cage of an aggressive resident, during which the hamster is defeated. This conditioned social defeat leads to long-lasting changes in the social behavior of the hamster, including inappropriate submissive displays and avoidance of contact with other animals (Potegal et al. 1993). Pharmacological manipulations of the acquisition and expression of conditioned defeat in hamsters have identified a critical role for the amygdala (Jasnow and Huhman 2001; Jasnow et al. 2004). Another study that examined the establishment of dominance hierarchies in rats that used a seminaturalistic burrow system also found amygdala involvement (Albeck et al. 1997). Social anxiety also can be modeled by testing social interactions in rats and by pharmacologically dissociating social anxiety from other nonsocial forms of anxiety. For example, serotonin$_{1A}$ (5-HT$_{1A}$) agonists injected into the amygdala significantly increased social anxiety (as measured by decreased time spent engaged in social interaction) but had no effect on general anxiety (as measured by time spent in the open arms of the elevated plus maze) (Gonzalez et al. 1996). Conversely, injection of the benzodiazepine receptor agonist midazolam into the amygdala resulted in a significant decrease in social anxiety, with no effect on the elevated plus maze (Gonzalez et al. 1996). Neonatal lesions of the amygdala in rhesus macaques caused a selective deficit for fearfulness during dyadic social interactions, as opposed to novel inanimate objects such as rubber snakes, suggesting a separate role for the amygdala in mediating social fear (Prather et al. 2001). Taken together, results from these diverse animal models strongly suggest a cross-species role for the amygdala in the modulation of social anxiety.

In human patients with social anxiety disorder, many studies also have implicated amygdala dysfunction. The first fMRI study showed selective activation of the amygdala in patients with social phobia compared with control subjects while they viewed pictures of faces (Birbaumer et al. 1998). Another experiment used functional positron emission tomography (PET) in these patients and found that subjective feelings of fear and distress were significantly correlated with regional cerebral blood flow in the amygdala during anxiety provocation (Fredrikson and Furmark 2003). Even more interesting is that treatment with cognitive-behavioral therapy and selective serotonin reuptake inhibitors (SSRIs) resulted in a return of amygdala activation to baseline (Fredrikson and Furmark 2003). As in rodent models of social anxiety implicating a role for 5-HT_{1A} and benzodiazepine receptors in the social aspect of anxiety, patients with social phobia appear to show an enhanced sensitivity of postsynaptic 5-HT_{1A} receptors, as reflected by increased anxiety and hormonal responses to serotonergic probes (reviewed in Aouizerate et al. 2004). To date, SSRIs are considered the first-line pharmacotherapy for social phobia, and benzodiazepines also have been proposed because of their relatively rapid onset of action (within 2 weeks of treatment) (Davidson 2004; Van Ameringen et al. 2003).

The hypersociability and social disinhibition seen in patients with Williams syndrome suggests that this disorder and social anxiety disorder lie on opposite ends of a spectrum. Unfortunately, very few studies have examined the neurobiological correlates of hypersociability in patients with Williams syndrome; such studies would go far in piecing together the contrasting story for social approach.

Social Bonding

Once an individual has surpassed the first three levels (social recognition, motivation, approach), the stage is set for the last step in social relationship formation: social bonding. Social bonding can be viewed as the culmination of all the previous social interactions. There are two excellent animal models of social bonding. The first examines the neural substrates of the mother-infant bond and infant-mother bond in rodents, and the second examines social bond formation between adult mates in the monogamous prairie vole.

The desire of the mother rat to seek contact with her pups is deeply rooted and is neurally controlled by several neurotransmitter systems in the brain, including dopamine and oxytocin. Recent research has shown that mother rats will bar press for access to pups and also will prefer a cage associated with pups over a cage associated with cocaine (A. Lee et al. 1999; Mattson et al. 2001). Exposure to pups increases dopamine release in the nucleus accumbens, a region involved in the mesolimbic reward pathway that is associated with drugs of abuse (Hansen et al. 1993). Lesions or injections of dopamine antagonist into the nucleus accumbens inhibit motivational components of maternal behavior but not more reflexive aspects such as nursing (Hansen et al. 1991; Keer and Stern 1999). Oxytocin infusion into the preoptic area induces a rapid onset of maternal behavior in virgin female rats (Pedersen et al. 1982); oxytocin-sensitive neurons in the preoptic area are known to project to the nucleus accumbens (Stack et al. 2002). These experiments suggest that reward systems in the brain are necessary for maternal motivation, strikingly analogous to reward research on feeding, sex, and drugs of abuse.

The infant-mother bond is similarly deep-rooted and also likely involves reward mechanisms (Nelson and Panksepp 1998). A recent report examining the endogenous opioid system in mice reported that mutant pups lacking the mu opioid receptor gene lacked the ability to form social attachments with their mothers, as evidenced by their lack of separation distress and lack of preference for their mothers' cues (Moles et al. 2004). A similar phenomenon also has been observed in oxytocin knockout mouse pups (A. Fusaro and L. Young, unpublished data, November 2001).

Pair bond formation is another avenue with which to study the neurobiology of social motivation. The monogamous prairie vole (*Microtus ochrogaster*) forms selective, enduring pair bonds between adult mates that can last the lifetime of the individual (Getz et al. 1981). These partner preferences are dependent on the release of dopamine, oxytocin, and vasopressin into reward regions of the brain (Aragona et al. 2003; Lim and Young 2004; Young et al. 2001). The prairie vole model of social attachment is complemented by the natural comparison of another vole species, the promiscuous meadow vole (*Microtus pennsylvanicus*). Meadow voles are solitary, do not appear to form social attachments and social bonding, and often abandon their young after just 2 weeks of care (Gruder-Adams and Getz 1985). Both vole species have similar levels of oxytocin and vasopressin in the brain, but the respective receptors, OTR and V1aR, are concentrated in reward regions in the prairie vole but not in the meadow vole (Lim et al. 2004a; Young and Wang 2004). It is hypothesized that the activation of OTR and V1aR in these reward regions provides the social motivation for pair bond formation in the monogamous vole species.

A direct test of this hypothesis was performed recently. Artificial elevation of V1aR in a reward region previously lacking V1aR in the promiscuous meadow vole was found to induce pair bond formation in this species (Lim et al. 2004b). Much as in monogamous prairie voles, pair bond formation in these transgenic meadow voles was dependent on dopamine neurotransmission (Lim et al. 2004b). Thus, the formation of social preferences in voles is likely a result of the interaction of V1aR and dopamine in reward regions of the brain. This phenomenon is strikingly analogous to the formation of conditioned place preferences in the drug literature, which also depends on dopamine neurotransmission in the mesolimbic reward pathway. However, with the formation of conditioned *social* preferences, "social" molecules such as oxytocin and vasopressin can modulate the function of preexisting reward pathways.

Experimental evidence in humans supports the finding in voles that reward circuits may be involved in the neurobiology of social motivation and attachment. One fMRI study examined brain activation in people while viewing photographs of a person with whom the subject reported being deeply in love. The authors observed brain activation in regions that was remarkably similar to those seen in other studies after consumption of cocaine, including dopamine reward circuits (Bartels and Zeki 2000; Breiter et al. 1997). Another fMRI experiment found that even simply viewing beautiful faces has reward value and activates the nucleus accumbens (Aharon et al. 2001), indicating that positive salient social stimuli (in this case, visual) can activate reward areas. Recent fMRI studies found that mothers viewing videos of their own infants showed significant brain activation in the prefrontal cortex (also involved in reward) compared with control subjects (Bartels and Zeki 2004; Ranote et al. 2004).

Do neurobiological correlates support the disruption in social motivation in patients with autism, schizophrenia, Turner's syndrome, and Williams syndrome? Given the roles of oxytocin, vasopressin, opioids, and dopamine in social attachment in rodent models, one might expect to find abnormalities in these neurotransmitters in patients with dysfunctional social relationships. Several studies in human patient populations do in fact support this hypothesis. One study found that children with autism had significantly lower levels of plasma oxytocin as compared with age-matched nonautistic subjects, although this study is awaiting replication in other autistic populations (Modahl et al. 1998). Another recent study reported that intravenous oxytocin infusion reduced repetitive behaviors in adults with autism and Asperger's syndrome (Hollander et al. 2003). Experiments examining the enzymes that posttranslationally process oxytocin, such as the proconvertase family (PC2 and PC5), have found that patients with autism may have abnormalities in converting the prohormone form of oxytocin to the functional form (Gabreels et al. 1998; Green et al. 2001). Notably, the gene *PC2* (20p11) is proximal to the oxytocin gene (20p13), and deficits in oxytocin processing could result from mutations in the 20p11–13 region affecting both PC2 and oxytocin itself (Green et al. 2001).

Alterations in the vasopressin system also may potentially be associated with autism in humans. The vasopressin gene is closely linked to the oxytocin gene (both are located on 20p11–12); conceivably, a single critically placed mutation could influence the expression of both peptides (Fields et al. 2003). The prairie vole model of social attachment implicates V1aR activation in the brain during the formation of social bonds, and genetic polymorphisms exist in the V1aR gene promoter between vole species that are associated with species differences in the ability to form pair bonds (Hammock and Young 2002; Young et al. 1999). Monogamous vole species contain a microsatellite expansion in the promoter of *V1aR* that is thought to regulate *V1aR* expression in the brain, thus leading to differences in social behavior (Hammock and Young 2004; Hammock et al. 2005).

Interestingly, the human V1aR gene has similar repetitive microsatellite elements in the promoter region, with polymorphisms in the number of tandem repeats. Up to 16 different allelic forms at one microsatellite locus exist in the human population, and one of these alleles has been linked to autism via transmission disequilibrium analysis in two independent studies, although a functional variant still needs to be identified before making a definitive link with autism (Kim et al. 2002; Wassink et al. 2004). However, to date, no consistent neurochemical, neurophysiological, or neuroanatomical abnormality has been observed across all patients with autism, and clinical heterogeneity of the disorder poses a monumental challenge to both scientists and clinicians.

Alterations in the dopaminergic and opioidergic systems are less clear in patients with autism. Panksepp and colleagues have proposed since 1979 that autism could arise secondary to "opioid peptide excess," and indeed, two independent reports thereafter found elevated opioid concentrations in the urine of autistic children (Panksepp et al. 1979; see also Alcorn et al. 2004; Reichelt et al. 1981). However, subsequent studies were not able to replicate these findings (Hunter et al. 2003; Pavone et al. 1997). Biological measures of dopaminergic system hypoactivity have been linked to social anxiety disorder, trait detachment, and general deficits in reward and incentive function but not yet to autism per se (reviewed in Schneier et al. 2002).

Oxytocin, vasopressin, opioids, and dopamine have not been demonstrated to have as direct a role in the pathophysiology of other disorders of social motivation such as schizophrenia, Turner's syndrome, and Williams syndrome. Only one previous report found that patients with schizophrenia have increased basal oxytocinergic and decreased vasopressinergic functions (Legros 1992; Legros and Ansseau 1992), but other studies have reported no differences in CSF levels of oxytocin or vasopressin (Beckmann et al. 1985; Glovinsky et al. 1994). However, one experiment showed that administration of synthetic vasopressin (desamino-D-arginine vasopressin; DDAVP) induced a significant improvement in negative symptomatology, including social withdrawal (Brambilla et al. 1989). Pharmacological agents affecting dopamine neurotransmission have long been used to treat schizophrenia; however, little is known about dopamine effects on social motivation per se. One hypothesis is that reduced dopaminergic tone in the prefrontal cortex can cause negative symptoms of schizophrenia such as apathy and social withdrawal (reviewed in Heinz 2002).

Overall, social bonding is a neurobiological phenomenon that can be closely modeled with animal models of social attachment. Both human and animal studies on social bonding have revealed a role for various neurotransmitters (oxytocin, vasopressin, and dopamine) in reward regions of the brain. However, much work still needs to be done to connect this theory with disorders of social bonding.

Conclusion

Social relationships can be viewed heuristically as being composed of four serial components: social recognition, social motivation, social approach, and social bonding. Separate neurobiological mechanisms can be attributed to each of the four levels, and discovery of these mechanisms is complemented by specific animal models. The development and maintenance of social relationships are not only proximately important for functioning in society but also ultimately relevant to fitness. A recent study of baboons in Kenya showed that female baboons who were significantly more social had greater infant survival than did their less social counterparts (Silk et al. 2003). Social relationships are also important for health. Prospective studies consistently show increased risk of death among people with lower quantity and quality of social relationships, and social isolation is a major risk factor for mortality in both people and animal models (House et al. 1988). The factors affecting the development and maintenance of social relationships, as well as the neurobiological mechanisms through which social relationships affect health and fitness, remain to be determined. A better understanding of the neurobiology of the social brain can potentially inform treatment of pathological social behavior as seen in autism, schizophrenia, Turner's syndrome, Williams syndrome, and social phobia.

References

Adolphs R: Cognitive neuroscience of human social behaviour. Nat Rev Neurosci 4:165–178, 2003

Aharon I, Etcoff N, Ariely D, et al: Beautiful faces have variable reward value: fMRI and behavioral evidence. Neuron 32:537–551, 2001

Albeck DS, McKittrick CR, Blanchard DC, et al: Chronic social stress alters levels of corticotropin-releasing factor and arginine vasopressin mRNA in rat brain. J Neurosci 17:4895–4903, 1997

Alcorn A, Berney T, Bretherton K, et al: Urinary compounds in autism. J Intellect Disabil Res 48:274–278, 2004

Aouizerate B, Martin-Guehl C, Tignol J: [Neurobiology and pharmacotherapy of social phobia]. Encephale 30:301–313, 2004

Aragona BJ, Liu Y, Curtis JT, et al: A critical role for nucleus accumbens dopamine in partner-preference formation in male prairie voles. J Neurosci 23:3483–3490, 2003

Archer J, Hay DC, Young AW: Face processing in psychiatric conditions. Br J Clin Psychol 31 (Pt 1):45–61, 1992

Baron-Cohen S, Ring HA, Wheelwright S, et al: Social intelligence in the normal and autistic brain: an fMRI study. Eur J Neurosci 11:1891–1898, 1999

Bartels A, Zeki S: The neural basis of romantic love. Neuroreport 11:3829–3834, 2000

Bartels A, Zeki S: The neural correlates of maternal and romantic love. Neuroimage 21:1155–1166, 2004

Barton JJ: Disorders of face perception and recognition. Neurol Clin 21:521–548, 2003

Barton JJ, Press DZ, Keenan JP, et al: Lesions of the fusiform face area impair perception of facial configuration in prosopagnosia. Neurology 58:71–78, 2002

Beckmann H, Lang RE, Gattaz WF: Vasopressin–oxytocin in cerebrospinal fluid of schizophrenic patients and normal controls. Psychoneuroendocrinology 10:187–191, 1985

Birbaumer N, Grodd W, Diedrich O, et al: fMRI reveals amygdala activation to human faces in social phobics. Neuroreport 9:1223–1226, 1998

Brambilla F, Bondiolotti GP, Maggioni M, et al: Vasopressin (DDAVP) therapy in chronic schizophrenia: effects on negative symptoms and memory. Neuropsychobiology 20:113–119, 1989

Breiter HC, Gollub RL, Weisskoff RM, et al: Acute effects of cocaine on human brain activity and emotion. Neuron 19:591–611, 1997

Castelli F, Frith C, Happe F, et al: Autism, Asperger syndrome and brain mechanisms for the attribution of mental states to animated shapes. Brain 125:1839–1849, 2002

Choleris E, Gustafsson JA, Korach KS, et al: An estrogen-dependent four-gene micronet regulating social recognition: a study with oxytocin and estrogen receptor-α and -β knockout mice. Proc Natl Acad Sci U S A 100:6192–6197, 2003

Critchley HD, Daly EM, Bullmore ET, et al: The functional neuroanatomy of social behaviour: changes in cerebral blood flow when people with autistic disorder process facial expressions. Brain 123 (Pt 11):2203–2212, 2000

Dantzer R, Bluthe RM, Koob GF, et al: Modulation of social memory in male rats by neurohypophyseal peptides. Psychopharmacology (Berl) 91:363–368, 1987

Davidson JR: Use of benzodiazepines in social anxiety disorder, generalized anxiety disorder, and posttraumatic stress disorder. J Clin Psychiatry 65 (suppl 5):29–33, 2004

Davies M, Udwin O, Howlin P: Adults with Williams syndrome: preliminary study of social, emotional and behavioural difficulties. Br J Psychiatry 172:273–276, 1998

Davies S, Bishop D, Manstead AS, et al: Face perception in children with autism and Asperger's syndrome. J Child Psychol Psychiatry 35:1033–1057, 1994

Doyle TF, Bellugi U, Korenberg JR, et al: "Everybody in the world is my friend" hypersociability in young children with Williams syndrome. Am J Med Genet A 124:263–273, 2004

Ferguson JN, Aldag JM, Insel TR, et al: Oxytocin in the medial amygdala is essential for social recognition in the mouse. J Neurosci 21:8278–8285, 2001

Ferguson JN, Young LJ, Hearn EF, et al: Social amnesia in mice lacking the oxytocin gene. Nat Genet 25:284–288, 2000

Fields RL, House SB, Gainer H: Regulatory domains in the intergenic region of the oxytocin and vasopressin genes that control their hypothalamus-specific expression in vitro. J Neurosci 23:7801–7809, 2003

Fredrikson M, Furmark T: Amygdaloid regional cerebral blood flow and subjective fear during symptom provocation in anxiety disorders. Ann N Y Acad Sci 985:341–347, 2003

Gabreels BA, Swaab DF, de Kleijn DP, et al: The vasopressin precursor is not processed in the hypothalamus of Wolfram syndrome patients with diabetes insipidus: evidence for the involvement of PC2 and 7B2. J Clin Endocrinol Metab 83:4026–4033, 1998

Getz LL, Carter CS, Gavish L: The mating system of the prairie vole *Microtus ochragaster:* field and laboratory evidence for pair-bonding. Behav Ecol Sociobiol 8:189–194, 1981

Glovinsky D, Kalogeras KT, Kirch DG, et al: Cerebrospinal fluid oxytocin concentration in schizophrenic patients does not differ from control subjects and is not changed by neuroleptic medication. Schizophr Res 11:273–276, 1994

Gonzalez LE, Andrews N, File SE: 5-HT1A and benzodiazepine receptors in the basolateral amygdala modulate anxiety in the social interaction test, but not in the elevated plus-maze. Brain Res 732:145–153, 1996

Good CD, Lawrence K, Thomas NS, et al: Dosage-sensitive X-linked locus influences the development of amygdala and orbitofrontal cortex, and fear recognition in humans. Brain 126:2431–2446, 2003

Green L, Fein D, Modahl C, et al: Oxytocin and autistic disorder: alterations in peptide forms. Biol Psychiatry 50:609–613, 2001

Gruder-Adams S, Getz LL: Comparison of the mating system and paternal behavior in Microtus ochragaster and M. pennsylvanicus. J Mammal 66:165–167, 1985

Hammock EAD, Young LJ: Variation in the vasopressin V1a receptor promoter and expression: implications for inter- and intraspecific variation in social behaviour. Eur J Neurosci 16:399–402, 2002

Hammock EA, Young LJ: Functional microsatellite polymorphism associated with divergent social structure in vole species. Mol Biol Evol 21:1057–1063, 2004

Hammock EA, Lim MM, Nair HP, et al: Association of vasopressin 1a receptor levels with a regulatory microsatellite and behavior. Genes Brain Behav 4:289–301, 2005

Hansen S, Harthon C, Wallin E, et al: The effects of 6-OHDA-induced dopamine depletions in the ventral or dorsal striatum on maternal and sexual behavior in the female rat. Pharmacol Biochem Behav 39:71–77, 1991

Hansen S, Bergvall AH, Nyiredi S: Interaction with pups enhances dopamine release in the ventral striatum of maternal rats: a microdialysis study. Pharmacol Biochem Behav 45:673–676, 1993

Harrington A, Oepen G, Spitzer M: Disordered recognition and perception of human faces in acute schizophrenia and experimental psychosis. Compr Psychiatry 30:376–384, 1989

Haxby JV, Hoffman EA, Gobbini MI: The distributed human neural system for face perception. Trends Cogn Sci 4:223–233, 2000

Heinz A: Dopaminergic dysfunction in alcoholism and schizophrenia—psychopathological and behavioral correlates. Eur Psychiatry 17:9–16, 2002

Hobson RP: The autistic child's recognition of age- and sex-related characteristics of people. J Autism Dev Disord 17:63–79, 1987

Hollander E, Novotny S, Hanratty M, et al: Oxytocin infusion reduces repetitive behaviors in adults with autistic and Asperger's disorders. Neuropsychopharmacology 28:193–198, 2003

House JS, Landis KR, Umberson D: Social relationships and health. Science 241:540–545, 1988

Hunter LC, O'Hare A, Herron WJ, et al: Opioid peptides and dipeptidyl peptidase in autism. Dev Med Child Neurol 45:121–128, 2003

Jasnow AM, Huhman KL: Activation of GABA(A) receptors in the amygdala blocks the acquisition and expression of conditioned defeat in Syrian hamsters. Brain Res 920:142–150, 2001

Jasnow AM, Davis M, Huhman KL: Involvement of central amygdalar and bed nucleus of the stria terminalis corticotropin-releasing factor in behavioral responses to social defeat. Behav Neurosci 118:1052–1061, 2004

Keer SE, Stern JM: Dopamine receptor blockade in the nucleus accumbens inhibits maternal retrieval and licking, but enhances nursing behavior in lactating rats. Physiol Behav 67:659–669, 1999

Kim SJ, Young LJ, Gonen D, et al: Transmission disequilibrium testing of arginine vasopressin receptor 1A (AVPR1A) polymorphisms in autism. Mol Psychiatry 7:503–507, 2002

Kosaka H, Omori M, Murata T, et al: Differential amygdala response during facial recognition in patients with schizophrenia: an fMRI study. Schizophr Res 57:87–95, 2002

Landgraf R, Frank E, Aldag JM, et al: Viral vector-mediated gene transfer of the vole V1a vasopressin receptor in the rat septum: improved social discrimination and active social behaviour. Eur J Neurosci 18:403–411, 2003

Lawrence K, Kuntsi J, Coleman M, et al: Face and emotion recognition deficits in Turner syndrome: a possible role for X-linked genes in amygdala development. Neuropsychology 17:39–49, 2003

Lee A, Clancy S, Fleming AS: Mother rats bar-press for pups: effects of lesions of the mpoa and limbic sites on maternal behavior and operant responding for pup-reinforcement [corrected and republished in Behav Brain Res 108:215–231, 2000]. Behav Brain Res 100:15–31, 1999

Lee CU, Shenton ME, Salisbury DF, et al: Fusiform gyrus volume reduction in first-episode schizophrenia: a magnetic resonance imaging study. Arch Gen Psychiatry 59:775–781, 2002

Legros JJ: Neurohypophyseal peptides and psychopathology. Horm Res 37 (suppl 3):16–21, 1992

Legros JJ, Ansseau M: Neurohypophyseal peptides and psychopathology. Prog Brain Res 93:455–460, discussion 461, 1992

Lim MM, Young LJ: Vasopressin-dependent neural circuits underlying pair bond formation in the monogamous prairie vole. Neuroscience 125:35–45, 2004

Lim MM, Murphy AZ, Young LJ: Ventral striatopallidal oxytocin and vasopressin V1a receptors in the monogamous prairie vole (Microtus ochrogaster). J Comp Neurol 468:555–570, 2004a

Lim MM, Wang Z, Olazabal DE, et al: Enhanced partner preference in a promiscuous species by manipulating the expression of a single gene. Nature 429:754–757, 2004b

Lord C, Cook EH, Leventhal BL, et al: Autism spectrum disorders. Neuron 28:355–363, 2000

Mattson BJ, Williams S, Rosenblatt JS, et al: Comparison of two positive reinforcing stimuli: pups and cocaine throughout the postpartum period. Behav Neurosci 115:683–694, 2001

Mazzocco MM, Baumgardner T, Freund LS, et al: Social functioning among girls with fragile X or Turner syndrome and their sisters. J Autism Dev Disord 28:509–517, 1998

McCauley E, Feuillan P, Kushner H, et al: Psychosocial development in adolescents with Turner syndrome. J Dev Behav Pediatr 22:360–365, 2001

Mobbs D, Garrett AS, Menon V, et al: Anomalous brain activation during face and gaze processing in Williams syndrome. Neurology 62:2070–2076, 2004

Modahl C, Green L, Fein D, et al: Plasma oxytocin levels in autistic children. Biol Psychiatry 43:270–277, 1998

Moles A, Kieffer BL, D'Amato FR: Deficit in attachment behavior in mice lacking the mu-opioid receptor gene. Science 304:1983–1986, 2004

Nelson EE, Panksepp J: Brain substrates of infant-mother attachment: contributions of opioids, oxytocin, and norepinephrine. Neurosci Biobehav Rev 22:437–452, 1998

Onitsuka T, Shenton ME, Kasai K, et al: Fusiform gyrus volume reduction and facial recognition in chronic schizophrenia. Arch Gen Psychiatry 60:349–355, 2003

Panksepp J, Najam N, Soares F: Morphine reduces social cohesion in rats. Pharm Biochem Behav 11:131–134, 1979

Pavone L, Fiumara A, Bottaro G, et al: Autism and celiac disease: failure to validate the hypothesis that a link might exist. Biol Psychiatry 42:72–75, 1997

Pedersen CA, Ascher JA, Monroe YL, et al: Oxytocin induces maternal behavior in virgin female rats. Science 216:648–650, 1982

Perrett DI, Rolls ET, Caan W: Visual neurones responsive to faces in the monkey temporal cortex. Exp Brain Res 47:329–342, 1982

Perrett DI, Smith PA, Potter DD, et al: Visual cells in the temporal cortex sensitive to face view and gaze direction. Proc R Soc Lond B Biol Sci 223:293–317, 1985

Pierce K, Muller RA, Ambrose J, et al: Face processing occurs outside the fusiform 'face area' in autism: evidence from functional MRI. Brain 124:2059–2073, 2001

Pierce K, Haist F, Sedaghat F, et al: The brain response to personally familiar faces in autism: findings of fusiform activity and beyond. Brain 127:2703–2716, 2004

Pitkow LJ, Sharer CA, Ren X, et al: Facilitation of affiliation and pair-bond formation by vasopressin receptor gene transfer into the ventral forebrain of a monogamous vole. J Neurosci 21:7392–7396, 2001

Popik P, Vetulani J, van Ree JM: Low doses of oxytocin facilitate social recognition in rats. Psychopharmacology (Berl) 106:71–74, 1992

Potegal M, Huhman K, Moore T, et al: Conditioned defeat in the Syrian golden hamster (Mesocricetus auratus). Behav Neural Biol 60:93–102, 1993

Prather MD, Lavenex P, Mauldin-Jourdain ML, et al: Increased social fear and decreased fear of objects in monkeys with neonatal amygdala lesions. Neuroscience 106:653–658, 2001

Ranote S, Elliott R, Abel KM, et al: The neural basis of maternal responsiveness to infants: an fMRI study. Neuroreport 15:1825–1829, 2004

Reichelt KL, Hole K, Hamberger A, et al: Biologically active peptide-containing fractions in schizophrenia and childhood autism. Adv Biochem Psychopharmacol 28:627–643, 1981

Reiss AL, Eckert MA, Rose FE, et al: An experiment of nature: brain anatomy parallels cognition and behavior in Williams syndrome. J Neurosci 24:5009–5015, 2004

Rosenblum LA, Smith EL, Altemus M, et al: Differing concentrations of corticotropin-releasing factor and oxytocin in the cerebrospinal fluid of bonnet and pigtail macaques. Psychoneuroendocrinology 27:651–660, 2002

Ruble LA: Analysis of social interactions as goal-directed behaviors in children with autism. J Autism Dev Disord 31:471–482, 2001

Schneier FR, Blanco C, Antia SX, et al: The social anxiety spectrum. Psychiatr Clin North Am 25:757–774, 2002

Schultz RT, Gauthier I, Klin A, et al: Abnormal ventral temporal cortical activity during face discrimination among individuals with autism and Asperger syndrome. Arch Gen Psychiatry 57:331–340, 2000

Silk JB, Alberts SC, Altmann J: Social bonds of female baboons enhance infant survival. Science 302:1231–1234, 2003

Skuse D, Morris J, Lawrence K: The amygdala and development of the social brain. Ann N Y Acad Sci 1008:91–101, 2003

Stack EC, Balakrishnan R, Numan MJ, et al: A functional neuroanatomical investigation of the role of the medial preoptic area in neural circuits regulating maternal behavior. Behav Brain Res 131:17–36, 2002

Stefanacci L, Amaral DG: Topographic organization of cortical inputs to the lateral nucleus of the macaque monkey amygdala: a retrograde tracing study. J Comp Neurol 421:52–79, 2000

Stein MB: Neurobiological perspectives on social phobia: from affiliation to zoology. Biol Psychiatry 44:1277–1285, 1998

Stowers L, Holy TE, Meister M, et al: Loss of sex discrimination and male-male aggression in mice deficient for TRP2. Science 295:1493–1500, 2002

Szatmari P, Tuff L, Finlayson MA, et al: Asperger's syndrome and autism: neurocognitive aspects. J Am Acad Child Adolesc Psychiatry 29:130–136, 1990

Tantam D, Monaghan L, Nicholson H, et al: Autistic children's ability to interpret faces: a research note. J Child Psychol Psychiatry 30:623–630, 1989

Van Ameringen M, Allgulander C, Bandelow B, et al: WCA recommendations for the long-term treatment of social phobia. CNS Spectr 8 (8 suppl 1):40–52, 2003

Wassink TH, Piven J, Vieland VJ, et al: Examination of AVPR1a as an autism susceptibility gene. Mol Psychiatry 9:968–972, 2004

Winslow JT: Mouse social recognition and preference, in Current Protocols in Neuroscience. Edited by Crawley JN, Gerfen CR, Rogawski MA, et al. New York, Wiley, 2003, pp 8.16.1–8.16.16

Witt DM, Winslow JT, Insel TR: Enhanced social interactions in rats following chronic, centrally infused oxytocin. Pharmacol Biochem Behav 43:855–861, 1992

Young LJ, Wang Z: The neurobiology of pair bonding. Nat Neurosci 7:1048–1054, 2004

Young LJ, Nilsen R, Waymire KG, et al: Increased affiliative response to vasopressin in mice expressing the V1a receptor from a monogamous vole. Nature 400:766–768, 1999

Young LJ, Lim MM, Gingrich B, et al: Cellular mechanisms of social attachment. Horm Behav 40:133–138, 2001

CHAPTER 3

REFINING THE CATEGORICAL LANDSCAPE OF THE DSM

Role of Animal Models

Nelson K. B. Totah, B.S.
Paul M. Plotsky, Ph.D.

Considerable evidence indicates that the brain's fundamental nature is already being constructed in the prenatal environment of the mother's uterus. Moreover, during neonatal, postnatal, and adult life, genes and environment interact to produce an individual's unique developmental trajectory. A genetic abnormality or an environmental alteration can perturb this trajectory and, potentially, produce psychopathology. In this chapter, we examine the categorical organization of DSM-IV-TR (American Psychiatric Association 2000) in light of the fact that individuals are unique products of gene–environment interaction. Reconceptualization of the DSM classifications can inform how clinicians diagnose and effectively treat disorders. Specifically, we review how animal models of early life experience can elucidate what DSM-IV-TR classifies as mood disorders.

Mental disorders can be viewed as being on a spectrum, with some patients having comorbid disorders such as depression and anxiety. Generally, this may be because brain regions with reported structural or physiological anomalies in many mental diseases (e.g., schizophrenia, autism, depression) show substantial anatom-

This research was supported by the National Institute of Mental Health–funded Silvio O. Conte Center for the Neuroscience of Mental Disease (MH58922) and by grants MH50113, MH62577, and MH065046.

TABLE 3–1.   Two hypothetical patients with an affirmative diagnosis of major depressive disorder

Patient 1	Patient 2
1. Sadness and depressed mood	1. Anhedonia
2. Hypersomnia	2. Insomnia
3. Increased locomotor activity	3. Reduced locomotor activity
4. Weight loss	4. Weight loss
5. Difficulty concentrating	5. Feelings of worthlessness or guilt

Note. The table presents the different symptoms of two hypothetical patients who would meet the DSM-IV-TR criteria for major depressive disorder.
Source.   Adapted from Halbreich 2006.

ical overlap (e.g., prefrontal cortex, cingulate cortex, hippocampus, amygdala). Some patients also have irregular symptoms; for instance, a patient could have hypomania in addition to unipolar depression. Table 3–1 shows a hypothetical case in which two patients would receive diagnoses of the same disease but would have varying symptoms. This difference may occur because the unique developmental trajectory of an individual's brain can cause widespread alterations that lead to variability in the phenotype of a disease between individuals.

Variability in the symptoms of mood disorders also can be found in animal models. For instance, different strains of rats have different behavioral phenotypes in response to the same early life experience. The different phenotypes of various rat genotypes to the same experience can be graphically represented by "norms of reaction" graphs (Fuller et al. 2005). In a recent study, Nair et al. (2005) showed that rats have individual variation in their response to the stressor of social isolation. Additionally, the authors found that vulnerability to stress is encoded by the gene expression pattern of multiple neuropeptide receptor systems that are specific to that individual animal. This profound study illustrated that genes interact with the prenatal and postnatal environment to program a specific landscape of receptors—a developmental trajectory—that defines stress vulnerability, stress resilience, and potential for psychopathology for that individual.

Examination of posttraumatic stress disorder (PTSD) epidemiological data provides yet another example of patients having different disease phenotypes after similar experience. Only a portion of a traumatized population will show signs and symptoms of PTSD (Breslau et al. 1991; Helzer et al. 1987; Resnick et al. 1993; Yehuda and McFarlane 1995). Why are some people resilient to stress and subsequent psychopathology but not others? In the context of early life experience, we think that resilience to stress results from the variability surrounding basic developmental trajectories. Resilience is commonly referred to as the absence of disease; however, the absence of disease better characterizes the normal state of an organism.

Thus, resilience may be represented as the portion of a population that is a standard deviation from the mean normative phenotype on a curve reflecting genes and experience. Accordingly, the population with vulnerability to stress may be represented as a standard deviation on the other side of the mean. The reason that some people lie outside of the mean—that some are vulnerable and some are resilient to stress—is rooted in the developmental trajectory of the developing brain.

Role of Animal Models in Understanding Developmental Trajectories

Animal models can help us understand the phenotypic results of alterations in genes and environment. Consequently, animal studies may lead to an improved ability to group patients with the same developmental trajectory into a classification of psychopathology. Importantly, the human, rat, and nonhuman primate brains have all evolved from common ancestors; thus, the human mind can be studied in the context of its evolutionary precursors. Although it would be presumptuous to assume that animal models can ever fully replicate the multiple dimensions of human diseases, they can model various aspects of mood disorder symptomatology, as well as alterations of underlying neurophysiology. DSM can be used as a starting point, along with close observations of patients and postmortem data, to begin to approximate comprehensive models of mental disorders.

Animal Models of Early Life Experience

The models used in our laboratory focus on improving our understanding of the role of gene–environment interactions in the developmental trajectory of the brain and how mental disorders arise in individuals with particular trajectories. Central to the work of the laboratory is the idea that early life stress interacting with as-yet-unidentified genotypic features may alter stress-sensitive neurocircuits at a fundamental level. The resultant changes render certain individuals more vulnerable to stress and subsequent psychopathology. Genes and epigenetic factors contribute significantly to cognition and behavior, and then cognition and behavior influence both gene expression and neural connectivity through learning. Enriched environments and social support can use this plasticity to buffer against or possibly mitigate the neural changes caused by an early adverse environment (Figure 3–1). We are using rat and nonhuman primate models to investigate early life environmental contributions to disease, define critical neural development periods, determine the importance of the nature of adverse experience, link genetic polymorphisms to vulnerability to early adverse experience, and develop effective interventions for use at prenatal, neonatal, and postnatal periods.

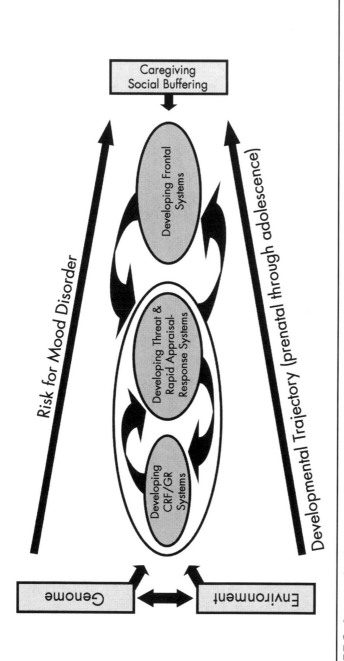

FIGURE 3–1. Graphical representation of gene–environment interaction leading to a unique developmental trajectory.

Note. Caregiver and social interaction and the environment tune the corticotropin-releasing factor (CRF) system, which interacts with other neurotransmitter systems and frontal brain areas. GR=glucocorticoid receptor.

Source. Adapted from M. Gunnar, "Early Adverse Experience, Stress Neurobiology, and Prevention Science Network," unpublished manuscript.

Stress Neurobiology

Before a detailed discussion of the animal models, we briefly review stress neurophysiology (see Vazquez 1998 for an extensive review). The major stress response measured is the hormonal output of the limbic-hypothalamic-pituitary-adrenal axis (Figure 3–2). The axis has numerous connections with forebrain areas, which link stress with behavior and cognitive changes. Information is processed and funneled into the paraventricular nucleus of the hypothalamus, a bilateral medial structure situated at the ventral base of the brain around the third ventricle, in which neurons produce corticotropin-releasing factor (CRF) and arginine vasopressin (which is involved in water regulation). CRF is synthesized in the somas and transported to the median eminence, where, in response to physiological and psychological stressors, it is released into the hypophyseal portal blood circulation (a specialized circulatory system feeding the pituitary). Receptors for CRF on cells of the anterior pituitary are then stimulated to release adrenocorticotropic hormone (ACTH) into the bloodstream. Peripherally circulating ACTH acts on the cortical cells of the adrenal glands and causes synthesis and release of glucocorticoids: corticosterone in rodents and cortisol in primates (CORT). A major action of glucocorticoids is to mobilize energy resources in response to stress. Furthermore, glucocorticoids bind to intercellular receptors and act as transcriptional regulators of gene expression. The stress response is deactivated by various physiological mechanisms that operate on different temporal scales, one of which is glucocorticoid-mediated feedback at the level of the pituitary and the hypothalamus.

Human Mood Disorder Risk Factors

In humans, the risk factors associated with depression include a family history of depression, certain genetic polymorphisms, prior personal episodes of depression, a history of anxiety disorders, female gender, and a stressful or an adverse environment (e.g., bereavement, severe financial loss, violence, rape). However, a profound link exists between stress in early life—such as the loss of a parent, the lack of parental warmth, or abuse—and risk of depression in adulthood. Unfortunately, the rate of childhood abuse and neglect internationally and in the United States is disturbingly high and may be underreported. In 2003, U.S. Child Protective Services substantiated approximately 906,000 cases of abuse. About 61% of the reported abuse was in the form of neglect, about 19% was in the form of physical abuse, and another 10% was related to sexual abuse. The majority of the abuse occurred in children aged birth to 3 years (U.S. Department of Health and Human Services 2005).

Early life stress in the form of childhood abuse or neglect is a pervasive social problem that is frequently associated with long-term psychiatric sequelae (Hor-

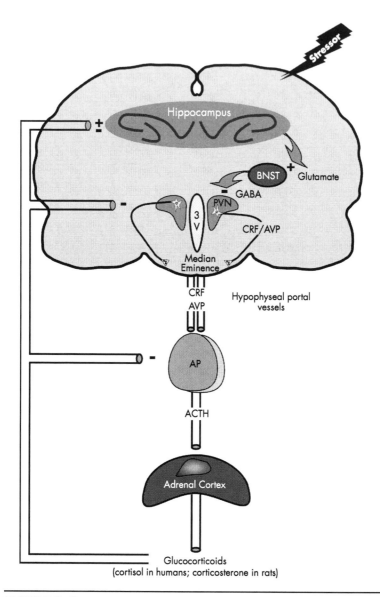

FIGURE 3–2. Overview of the limbic-hypothalamic-pituitary-adrenal axis and the stress response.

Note. 3V = third ventricle; ACTH = adrenocorticotropic hormone; AP = anterior pituitary; AVP = arginine vasopressin; BNST = bed nucleus of the stria terminalis; CRF = corticotropin-releasing factor; GABA = γ-aminobutyric acid; PVN = paraventricular nucleus of the hypothalamus.

witz et al. 2001; MacMillan et al. 2001). Childhood sexual abuse is associated with an increased risk of depression, anxiety, and suicide (Brown et al. 1999; McCauley et al. 1997). McCauley et al. (1997) reported the results of 424 respondents who reported childhood or adolescent physical or sexual abuse out of almost 2,000 individuals polled. Females with a history of early life stress had an increase in physical symptoms and higher scores for depression, anxiety, somatization, and interpersonal sensitivity. They also had an increased prevalence of drug abuse, including alcohol abuse; numerous suicide attempts; and an increased incidence of actual psychiatric admissions. A wealth of evidence now links childhood adversity with vulnerability to mood disorders (Heim et al. 2004; Penza et al. 2003). Although genetic background is a contributing factor, a significant environmental influence is also apparent (Kendler et al. 2002).

Animal Models of Physiological and Behavior Changes in Humans

The behavior and physiological changes induced by early life stress and observed in humans with depression can be assessed and explored in animal models. According to DSM-IV-TR, a diagnosis of depression requires at least a 2-week duration of prolonged impairment in social or other important life functioning. In nonhuman primates and rodents, we can assess alterations in social functioning. Also needed for an affirmative diagnosis is sadness or anhedonia; anhedonia can be studied in animals through numerous methods. Other symptoms that can contribute to a diagnosis of depression are a significant change in weight or appetite, changes in sleep microarchitecture, changes in locomotor activity, fatigue, altered cognitive abilities, and feelings of worthlessness or inappropriate guilt and suicidal ideation. All of these symptoms (except feelings of worthlessness or guilt and suicidal ideation) can be examined with clarity in animal models. However, it is important to recognize that humans and other animals have different developmental trajectories depending on their species. These species-specific differences are important considerations when animal models are used as avenues for future research.

Physiological changes in depressed humans and in response to early life stress also can be assessed in animal models. Numerous studies have implicated CRF and stress neurocircuitry in the pathophysiology of mood disorders as well as in the expression of depression- and anxiety-like behaviors in animals. Considerable evidence supports the hypothesis that the effects of early life stress may be mediated by an upregulation of CRF in hypothalamic and extrahypothalamic stress neurocircuits (Kaufman et al. 2000). Childhood abuse and severity of depression and PTSD have been positively correlated with increased net ACTH and CORT responses to psychological stressors (Heim et al. 2000). Moreover, humans with PTSD, depression, and panic disorder overproduce and hypersecrete CRF (Bremner et al.

1997; Forman et al. 1994; Heim and Nemeroff 2001). Both CRF peptide and CRF messenger RNA (mRNA) in the paraventricular nucleus are increased in depressed patients (Nemeroff et al. 1988, 1991; Raadsheer et al. 1995). Importantly, the persistent CRF pathway changes observed in humans can be reproduced in animal models of early life stress.

The importance of early life experience in the shaping of the brain cannot be espoused enough. Because an organism requires increased parental investment for maturation and protection, the infant learns from the caregiver a sense of environmental predictability and controllability. Proximity, body contact, feeding, and eye contact are vehicles for the transmission of social and cultural information needed to survive throughout life. In a chaotic caregiving situation, the developmental trajectory of an individual is altered because brain circuits will be optimized to deal with a chaotic world with less predictability. The delicate balance of genes and environment in brain circuit connectivity is then perturbed and must settle on a new state that is prone to psychopathology. It cannot be denied that we are products of our past. Animal models of early life experience serve as probes into how an individual's past shapes his or her brain, creating a varying array of vulnerable individuals, resilient individuals, and individuals who lie within the spectrum of disorder and normalcy. Our inability to escape the impact of the past is conveyed quite eloquently by American author F. Scott Fitzgerald (1925, p. 115) in *The Great Gatsby*: "So we beat on, boats against the current, borne back ceaselessly into the past."

Rat Models of Early Life Experience: The Maternal Separation Paradigm

Our laboratory uses a rat model of maternal separation to examine the effects of genotype and early life stress on adulthood vulnerability to stress and psychopathology. Experimental animals (termed *HMS180*) are handled and separated from the dam for 180 minutes daily from postnatal day 2 through postnatal day 14. Two other groups serve as controls: rats in the HMS15 group are handled and separated from the dam for 15 minutes daily during the same period, and rats in the animal facility–reared group are given twice-weekly cage changes and not disturbed. All groups receive routine care from postnatal day 14 to postnatal day 21 and are then weaned from the dam. Testing and intervention occur at postnatal day 60 and later.

ALTERED MATERNAL BEHAVIOR AND IMMUNE CHALLENGE: A FIRST ADVERSE LIFE EVENT?

One of the most noticeable changes for the HMS180 animals is that the frequency of maternal behavior is altered. Maternal caregiving and maternal contact are markedly decreased as measured by licking, various nursing positions, carrying, and the dam's time away from the pups. Levine (2001) has shown that as these changes in maternal behavior are taking place, both basal levels and stress-induced levels of CORT begin to increase by postnatal day 7 and continue through postnatal day 11. Furthermore, in adulthood, plasma concentrations of ACTH and CORT in response to an air puff startle are still significantly higher and decrease at a slower rate than in control rats. Similarly, human adults with major depressive disorder (MDD) who experienced early life abuse have a larger-magnitude and longer-lasting CORT response to a stressor than was seen in control subjects (Heim et al. 2000). In a related observation, 6-month-old human infants of mothers with MDD during pregnancy and postpartum had a significantly greater CORT release in response to a stressor in comparison to infants of mothers with MDD but no current symptoms and mothers without MDD. Furthermore, as observed in HMS180 rat pups, the level of CORT after insult not only is higher in magnitude but also does not decrease quickly (Z. N. Stowe et al., unpublished observation, February 2004).

In a related line of work, the laboratory has shown the validity of a subclinical immune system challenge as a potentially maladaptive early life stressor (P. M. Plotsky, preliminary data, 2002). Each cage rack in animal housing has a sentinel rat, which is a normal adult male rat that is taken for pathology screening every 2–3 months. If a pregnant dam were on a rack with a sentinel positive for parvovirus and pinworm, the HMS180 offspring of that dam would have the increased ACTH and CORT magnitude and duration in response to an air puff startle. However, HMS180 pups whose dams were on a rack with a negative sentinel did not have an altered ACTH and CORT response after maternal separation. None of the pups or their dams showed any overt sickness behavior or other symptoms. Exposure of the mother to subthreshold immune challenge may sensitize the fetal brain so that an early life stressor, such as maternal separation, may result in an accentuated stress response. Humans probably have many undiagnosed or unnoticed infections and immune activations that could affect the stress circuitry of the fetal brain. This is particularly important to consider in lower-socioeconomic communities in which access to medical care is not always available during pregnancy. Altered maternal physiology (during pregnancy) or altered maternal behavior (postpartum) may serve as a first adverse life event for these infants, helping to tune the brain for a stressful life.

IMPORTANCE OF CRITICAL DEVELOPMENTAL PERIODS

The maternal separation model has shown that during critical developmental periods, adverse experience has the most intense effect on adulthood physiobehavioral phenotype. In comparison to animal facility–reared rat pups, HMS180 rats separated from their dam from postnatal days 2 to 4, postnatal days 2 to 8, and post-

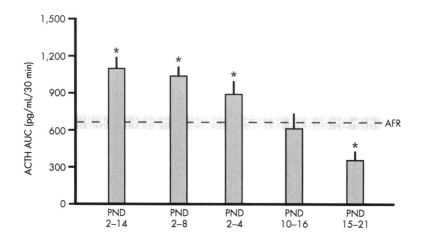

FIGURE 3–3.   Effect of maternal separation stress depends on the timing of the insult during developmentally critical periods.

Note.   Depending on time of maternal separation stress, adult HMS180 rats can exhibit a potentiated ($P<0.001$), equivalent, or suppressed ($P<0.001$) stress response in comparison to AFR control rats. The stress response is measured in pg/mL of mean ACTH (adrenocorticotropic hormone) release over 30 minutes. AFR=animal facility–reared; PND=postnatal day.

natal days 2 to 14 had, as expected, a significantly higher ACTH response to an air puff startle (Figure 3–3). However, HMS180 rats that were separated from their dams only from postnatal days 10 to 16 did not have altered stress neurophysiology. Moreover, HMS180 pups separated from postnatal days 15 to 21 actually had a hypoactive ACTH response to stress in comparison to animal facility–reared pups (P.M. Plotsky et al., manuscript in preparation, March 2003). There may be critical time periods during which the exact same caregiver interaction or environmental events have opposite effects on gene expression and circuit-level neuroplasticity.

EARLY LIFE STRESS-INDUCED ALTERATIONS

Corticotropin-Releasing Factor System

Overview of the CRF system.   The rat maternal separation model of early life stress has identified many physiological changes that occur throughout frontal, limbic, and brain stem areas affecting behavior and cognition. Many of the changes involve CRF release and CRF receptor distribution throughout the brain. In adult HMS180 animals, the basal CRF content of the median eminence is doubled in comparison to that of control rats, as expected considering the increased ACTH and CORT responses to stressors in those animals. Furthermore, hypophyseal portal dissections indicated hypersecretion of CRF into the portal vasculature of HMS180 animals. In response, CRF type 1 receptors in the anterior pituitary downregulate (i.e., decrease in number). These data correlate with the clinical observation that a blunted ACTH release to exogenous CRF challenge occurs in some patients with MDD. The same changes have been observed in nonhuman primates, except that both CRF type 1 and type 2 receptors are downregulated.

Moving dorsally from the hypothalamus, we reach the hippocampus, a structure involved in deactivating the neuroendocrine stress response (see Figure 3–1). Early life stress has an effect on the balance of the glucocorticoid receptor (GR) system of the hippocampus. The two subtypes of corticoid receptors are glucocorticoid and mineralocorticoid; they are set in a balance to regulate release of CRF from the hypothalamus. Mineralocorticoid receptors (MRs) have a high affinity for CORT but are saturated quickly. They are likely involved in tonic regulation of basal levels of ACTH and CORT release in a diurnal rhythm. GRs, on the contrary, have a low affinity for CORT but a high capacity. In a stress response in which CORT-mediated negative feedback floods the hippocampus, MRs become saturated, which forces the GRs to take over and return the neuroendocrine response to homeostasis.

In HMS180 animals, MRs are upregulated such that the MR-to-GR ratio in HMS180 rats is significantly greater than in HMS15 rats (Figure 3–4). Recall that HMS180 animals have a suppressed and flattened diurnal CORT rhythm as well as prolonged deactivation of the stress response. Alterations in the balance of MRs and GRs may contribute to the observed hormonal alterations. GR mRNA expression is also altered in the prefrontal cortex, which may have effects not only on the neuroendocrine alterations in depression but also on the cognitive deficits observed in the disease.

Effects of CRF system dysfunction.   CRF is distributed extremely widely throughout the central nervous system, especially in the central nucleus of the amygdala, the bed nucleus of the stria terminalis, the locus coeruleus peribrachial region, the hippocampus, and interneurons in the cortex (Reul and Holsboer 2002). A simple hypothesis is that CRF is a key mediator of the neuroendocrine, behavioral, emotional, and cognitive responses to stress. Early life stress–induced dysfunction of the CRF system may lead to the myriad symptoms observed in mood disorders. However, differing developmental trajectories can cause the same CRF system changes that produce different symptoms in different patients.

Early life stress has persistent effects throughout the lives of HMS180 rats, including increased hypothalamic-pituitary-adrenal (HPA) axis sensitivity to psychological stressors, dysfunction of HPA axis regulation, enhanced anxiety-like behavior, increased preference for ethanol, and anhedonia-like behavior (Caldji et al. 2000; Huot et al. 2001; Ladd et al. 2000; Liu et al. 2000; Plotsky and Meaney

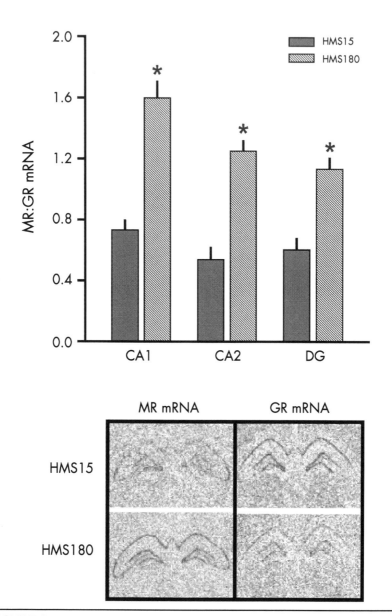

FIGURE 3–4. The hippocampal glucocorticoid receptor (GR) system is imbalanced in HMS180 rats.

(Top) In HMS180 rats, MRs are upregulated, leading to significantly higher MR-to-GR ratio compared with HMS15 rats ($P<0.05$). Alterations to MR-to-GR ratio may contribute to alterations in HMS180 stress hormone responses. DG=dentate gyrus; MR= mineralocorticoid receptor. (Bottom) In situ picture of corticoid receptor mRNA in HMS180 and HMS15 rats. *Source.* Adapted from Ladd et al. 2004.

1993). The observed anxiety, anhedonia, and drug-seeking behavior alterations may be attributed to hyperactivity of CRF in brain areas mediating emotion and cognition; CRF mRNA expression and peptide production are significantly increased in the locus coeruleus, bed nucleus of stria terminalis, central nucleus of the amygdala, and paraventricular nucleus of the hypothalamus of HMS180 rats (Plotsky et al. 2005). Similar changes occur in nonhuman primates reared by mothers exposed to unpredictable conditions with respect to food access, which resulted in diminished perception of security and reduced maternal care of infants (Coplan et al. 1996; Rosenblum et al. 2001).

It is difficult to determine the exact contributions of CRF upregulation in specific brain regions and developmental periods to the adulthood physiobehavioral phenotype. Therefore, we are using a lentivirus-mediated CRF gene transfer technique that allows us to examine the contribution of CRF change in a particular brain region at a specific postnatal time in relation to adulthood phenotype (N.K.B. Totah, H.P. Nair, L.J. Young, et al., manuscript in preparation, May 2005). This technique will allow us to manipulate CRF production spatially and temporally in a neonatal rat brain to refine the role of specific brain regions and time points in the adulthood phenotype of maternally separated rats.

Other Neurotransmitter Systems

Extensive early life stress–induced changes in other neurotransmitter systems occur, some of which are mediated by changes in the CRF system. In the HMS180 rats, alterations span systems of neurotransmitters, including norepinephrine (NE), inhibitory γ-aminobutyric acid (GABA), dopamine (DA), and serotonin (5-HT). George Koob (1999) proposed a feed-forward, excitatory circuit, which links corticolimbic CRF changes with the noradrenergic system. The locus coeruleus noradrenergic neurons supply two-thirds of the NE in the forebrain. The CRF-NE-CRF feed-forward loop between forebrain and brain stem is involved in regulation of vigilance and attention, regulation of anxiety and fear, and integration of endocrine and autonomic nervous system functioning. In HMS180 rats, amplitude of stimulus-induced locus coeruleus activity is increased, and NE biosynthesis and release are greater; furthermore, the autoinhibitory system that deactivates the locus coeruleus is attenuated in HMS180 animals (P.M. Plotsky et al., unpublished observation, May 2002). Tyrosine hydroxylase (the biosynthetic precursor of NE) mRNA in the locus coeruleus is increased, as is local NE secretion in the terminal fields of locus coeruleus neurons in the hippocampus, prefrontal cortex, amygdala, and hypothalamus (P.M. Plotsky et al., unpublished observation, January 2003). The dysfunction of CRF systems is a fundamental method by which diffuse forebrain NE content, as well as the content of other neurotransmitters, may be altered.

Evidence also shows other transmitter system alterations. In the dorsal raphe, 5-HT_{1B} receptor mRNA is increased; however, no other consistent changes are seen in the serotonergic system of maternally separated rats (Neumaier et al.

2002). Caldji et al. (2000) has shown that $GABA_A$ receptor binding in the prefrontal cortex, basolateral amygdala, and locus coeruleus is decreased. Moreover, the subunit structure of the $GABA_A$ receptor is changed such that it lacks the endogenous benzodiazepine binding element. Lastly, DA transporter binding in the nucleus accumbens is reduced in HMS180 rats (Meaney et al. 2002).

Morphological Alterations

Hippocampal morphology changes.

Shifting away from CRF and other neuropharmacological alterations, there appear to be morphological alterations in animals subjected to early life stress. Robert Sapolsky proposed a hypothesis by which glucocorticoids released during stress damage the hippocampus, such that structural alterations accompany depression, PTSD, and abuse (Lee et al. 2002). In collaboration with Elizabeth Gould at Princeton University, our laboratory has shown that hippocampal alterations do occur, but they may not be lasting. On postnatal days 4 through 6, HMS180 rats were administered bromodeoxyuridine (BrdU), which labels dividing neurons. BrdU was administered in drinking water after the pups were returned to their dam so that no new handling or stress was introduced. After weaning, at postnatal day 21, brains were collected and cells were costained for BrdU and a neuronal marker. In comparison to HMS15 rats, the HMS180 group had a 50% decrease in the number of neurons in the dentate gyrus of the hippocampus. However, in adult animals, no significant difference was seen (P.M. Plotsky et al., unpublished data, April 2003).

Dendritic branch complexity changes.

An increased level of glucocorticoids is known to decrease dendritic branch plasticity in the hippocampus of adult animals (Figure 3–5). It may be speculated that if the increase were to occur over a period during which axons from other areas were seeking their hippocampal targets, then, in the long term, synaptic input density would decrease in the hippocampus. In the laboratory, we used electron microscopy to show that, relative to animal facility–reared rats, HMS180 rats had a significant decrease in synaptic density (P.M. Plotsky et al., unpublished observation, August 2004). Chronic stress also decreases dendritic spine density in the rat medial prefrontal cortex (Radley et al. 2006), which may relate to deficits involving affect and executive control in patients with stress-related mental disorders. Stress is thereby placed in a position to alter information processing at the synaptic level, which could have effects on learning, sensory experience, emotional processing, and numerous other activities. We are currently investigating alterations in the number of dendritic spines in these animals. Patients with depression have brain-derived neurotrophic factor (BDNF) polymorphisms; BDNF is involved in synaptic plasticity and repair in the dentate gyrus and frontal cortex. In HMS180 animals, hippocampal and frontal cortical BDNF mRNA is reduced in comparison to animal facility–reared and HMS15 animals. Furthermore, this effect can be reversed by concurrent treatment with antidepressants (P.M.

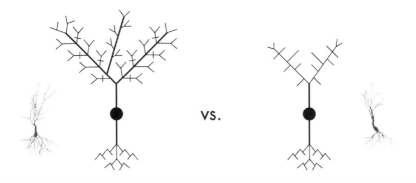

FIGURE 3–5. Effect of early life environment on dendritic complexity in the prefrontal cortex and hippocampus in HMS180 rats.

Note. This schematic of two actual traces shows the decreased dendritic branching in HMS180 rats, which is accompanied by decreased synaptic density.

Plotsky et al., unpublished observation, January 2004). More empirical work is needed before stress, depression, and morphological alterations are understood.

Behavioral Alterations

Many behavior changes also occur in adult rats that were maternally separated. Both emergence tests (such as elevated plus maze) and nonemergence tests (such as acoustic startle) have found increased anxiety-like behavior. The laboratory also has investigated anhedonia, a major symptom of depression. Rats were implanted with an intracranial self-stimulation electrode in the medial forebrain bundle (self-stimulation in the medial forebrain bundle is a measure of reward-seeking behavior and anhedonia). HMS180 rats would not learn to self-stimulate at a high stable rate, and some would stimulate at about 10-fold less than other groups, indicating general anhedonia. However, when animals were primed by increasing the current delivered for two sessions and then returned to the normal current load, they were able to stimulate at a high and stable level (Watts et al. 2005). The reason that priming helped the rats attain stable responding is not yet understood. The laboratory also has examined responding for sucrose pellets in non-food-deprived animals (Watts et al. 2004). The rats are trained to a "fixed ratio" schedule in which they receive a pellet for each bar press (i.e., FR1). On the FR1 schedule, HMS15 and HMS180 rats had no differences in responding. When the rats had to work harder for a reward on an FR2 schedule (two bar presses are needed to receive a pellet), the HMS180 rats seemed to lose interest in bar pressing or eating the pellets. With an FR4 schedule, an even greater separation was seen in the performance of the groups. We think that the HMS180 rats have anhedonia, or at least a degree of hypohedonia.

The laboratory also has shown that HMS180 rats prefer ethanol, which is normally avoided as an aversive stimulus. Animals were presented with a two-bottle home cage choice test. One bottle contained 0.2% saccharine, and another bottle contained 0.2% saccharine with 10% ethanol. The animal facility–reared and HMS15 rats did not like the smell or taste of the ethanol bottle and avoided it. However, with no training, the HMS180 rats imbibed a large amount of ethanol. Furthermore, when a stressor (a randomly occurring fire bell and strobe light) was added, the animal facility–reared and HMS15 rats had a slight increase in ethanol intake, whereas the HMS180 rats had a two- to threefold increase in intake and became physically dependent on ethanol.

In summary, many of the behavior changes observed in HMS180 rats resemble the changes observed in humans with depression. Besides anxiety-like behavior, anhedonia, and ethanol preference, the HMS180 rats showed increased cocaine locomotor sensitization at low doses. Alterations also occur in sleep microarchitecture; in particular, the latency to the first rapid eye movement (REM) sleep episode is reduced, and the frequency of REM episodes is increased. Many of these changes are analogous to those observed in humans with depression.

Effect of the Prenatal Environment

In addition to neonatal and postnatal alterations, the prenatal environmental conditions in which the fetus develops can have effects on adulthood physiobehavioral phenotype. Maternal hormonal conditions preimplantation can have an effect on a human offspring's stress neurophysiology and vulnerability to mood disorders (De Kloet et al. 2005). Prenatal glucocorticoid manipulation is also known to have a profound effect on human offspring (Owens et al. 2005). Maternal behavioral and cognitive characteristics, as well as the physiological changes that accompany those characteristics, are capable of fetal programming. The effect of maternal stress on the developing fetus may occur via CORT transmission through the placental barrier (Van den Bergh 2005). The effect of prenatal environment on adult phenotype and the clinical interventions that may occur during this period are an avenue for future investigation.

Genetic Polymorphisms, Early Life Environment, and Vulnerability to Stress

OVERALL ALTERATIONS IN GENE EXPRESSION

It is important to consider prenatal, neonatal, and postnatal environmental conditions in terms of the genetic coding that they interact with. We are examining the overall alterations in gene expression that take place in specific brain regions altered in our rat models. We have used gene chips to look at regions microdissected from eight rat pups from different litters, at different ages, and from maternal separation experimental and control groups. One interesting change was that DNA methyltransferase was altered in the hippocampus and the prefrontal cortex of HMS180 rats (P.M. Plotsky et al., unpublished observation, October 2003). Weaver et al. (2004) found that offspring of mothers giving appropriate maternal care (high levels of licking, grooming, and arched-back nursing), compared with offspring of mothers providing less care, have differences in methylation of the GR gene, which influences the expression of the gene and production of GRs. Furthermore, the authors showed that the effect persisted into adulthood but could be reversed with cross-fostering the pup to a normal mother. In our gene chip analysis, we found increased expression of zinc finger protein in the hippocampus and prefrontal cortex of HMS180 rats. Activity levels of BDNF and nerve growth factor IA are also decreased in the hippocampus and prefrontal cortex. The GABAergic system is altered, with GAD-65 (which is involved in the synthesis of GABA) being decreased in the locus coeruleus, amygdala, and bed nucleus of stria terminalis. Also, CART (cocaine amphetamine related transcript) gene expression is decreased in the locus coeruleus and peribrachial nucleus, which may be involved in the anhedonia and hypohedonia that we have observed in the HMS180 rats.

SEROTONIN TRANSPORTER POLYMORPHISMS

A growing field of literature establishes an association between serotonin transporter (5-HTT) polymorphisms, vulnerability to stress in an early life environment, and adulthood psychopathology (Caspi et al. 2003; Champoux et al. 2002; Holden 2003). The two 5-HTT promoter alleles are long (l) and short (s). Animals that are homogeneous for the long allele (ll) have more resilience to stress and subsequent pathology, whereas those that are homogeneous for the short allele (ss) are vulnerable to psychopathology. Work by Mar Sanchez has established an interaction between early abuse, gender, and 5-HTT genotype in rhesus macaques (M.M. Sanchez, unpublished observation, March 2005). Initial studies have shown that alteration of normal basal CORT levels depends on 5-HTT genotype; however, this dependence exists in males who were subjected to early life stress and females who were not subjected to early life stress.

Studies examining the genetic polymorphisms that interact with stress during early development to produce adulthood phenotype are forthcoming. At this time, these genetic polymorphisms are largely unknown. However, as indicated by our microdissection studies, the genetic factors are likely to be wide-ranging, given the extensive effects of early life experience on brain neurophysiology and morphology. Animal models of early life development will help provide insight into the genetic boundaries that constrain the path generated by early life experience.

Interventions at Prenatal, Neonatal, and Postnatal Time Periods

Although animal models are helping to clarify the gene–environment interactions that lead to psychopathology, the practical concern is whether we can prevent or reverse the way that genes and environment wire the brain. Can we shift a vulnerable person toward resilience to stress?

One method is simply to improve parenting. Cross-fostering studies have shown that this method can ameliorate the effect of maternal separation and altered maternal care. Postnatal enrichment also can have a favorable effect; however, it does not normalize gene expression changes. Of course, instead of changing the mother through cross-fostering, we can also leave the infant with his or her mother but alter the care that the mother provides for the offspring. By treating the dam with a short-lasting benzodiazepine anxiolytic during the separation period, we can prevent the changes in maternal behavior and the effects on the offspring that those behaviors may mediate. The same effect can be achieved by giving a CRF type 1 receptor antagonist to the mother; however, with both benzodiazepine and CRF antagonists, discontinuing the treatment allows the animals to revert back to a pathological state. Finally, it would be immensely helpful to be able to intervene pharmacologically during the neonatal and early postnatal ages to prevent the brain being locked into a pathological state. In fact, paroxetine, a serotonin reuptake inhibitor, administered by Alzet minipump (DURECT Corporation, Cupertino, CA) for 28 days in rats can completely normalize the abnormally increased CRF mRNA expression in the paraventricular nucleus of the HMS180 rats (P.M. Plotsky, unpublished observation, February 2005).

Clearly, understanding ways to intervene and provide treatment for mood disorders is a key aim of our work. Animal models can help improve our understanding of the etiology of mood disorders.

Developmental Trajectories and a Novel Understanding of Psychopathology

The global conclusion from the studies reviewed is that the timing of environmental insult or enrichment interacts with genes during sensitive periods for the organization of neural systems. Proper organization of the nervous system requires that experience alter gene expression as well as morphological features such as dendritic complexity. Thus, genes and environment interact during early life to produce a neural developmental trajectory for an individual. The widespread changes that occur in many brain areas—such as major changes to the CRF system—can produce a common disease (e.g., depression) across many individuals. However, because of the unique developmental trajectory that emerges from the complexity of neural organization and gene–environment interaction, some variability from the common theme occurs, leading to disease symptoms specific to a patient.

Understanding the mechanisms underlying the formation of developmental trajectories will help improve how DSM organizes and classifies mental disorders and will aid in the treatment of comorbid disorders. The current categorical organization of DSM-IV-TR has effects on misdiagnosis, assessment, and treatment. Bipolar disorders are often misdiagnosed as unipolar depression or bipolar I disorder (Judd and Akiskal 2003); however, the antidepressants administered to these patients may worsen their bipolar disorder (Ghaemi et al. 2000). Furthermore, assessing depression with the Mood Disorder Questionnaire has variable sensitivity across the bipolar spectrum (Miller et al. 2004). Additionally, the comorbidity of anxiety and depression can lead to difficulty in determining appropriate pharmacological intervention (Moller 2002). Indeed, defining mood disorders on a spectrum may clarify our neurobiological understanding of anxiety and depression rather than cloud it (Shear et al. 2002).

Of central importance is that many of the behavior, cognitive, and physiological changes that occur in mood disorders can be modeled in animals. Thus, animal models can help us understand how the same environmental and genetic alterations interact with a developmental trajectory to produce common ground between different diseases and variability between individuals with the same disease. Different pathologies of the mind may have similar environmental and genetic roots that allow them to converge on related neural circuitry, such that the pathologies are often comorbid and fall on a spectrum of similarity. Progress in understanding human mental illness relies not only on understanding the general workings of the human brain across a population but also on understanding the developmental trajectory that produces the unique brain of the individual.

References

American Psychiatric Association: Diagnostic and Statistical Manual of Mental Disorders, 4th Edition, Text Revision. Washington, DC, American Psychiatric Association, 2000

Bremner JD, Licinio J, Darnell A, et al: Elevated CSF corticotropin-releasing factor concentrations in posttraumatic stress disorder. Am J Psychiatry 154:624–629, 1997

Breslau N, Davis GC, Andreski P, et al: Traumatic events and posttraumatic stress disorder in an urban population of young adults. Arch Gen Psychiatry 48:216–222, 1991

Brown J, Cohen P, Johnson JG, et al: Childhood abuse and neglect: specificity of effects on adolescent and young adult depression and suicidality. J Am Acad Child Adolesc Psychiatry 38:1490–1496, 1999

Caldji C, Francis D, Sharma S, et al: The effects of early rearing environment on the development of GABAA and central benzodiazepine receptor levels and novelty-induced fearfulness in the rat. Neuropsychopharmacology 22:219–229, 2000

Caspi A, Sugden K, Moffitt TE, et al: Influence of life stress on depression: moderation by a polymorphism in the 5-HTT gene. Science 301:386–389, 2003

Champoux M, Bennett A, Shannon C, et al: Serotonin transporter gene polymorphism, differential early rearing, and behavior in rhesus monkey neonates. Mol Psychiatry 7:1058–1063, 2002

Coplan JD, Andrews MW, Rosenblum LA, et al: Persistent elevations of cerebrospinal fluid concentrations of corticotropin-releasing factor in adult nonhuman primates exposed to early life stressors: implications for the pathophysiology of mood and anxiety disorders. Proc Natl Acad Sci U S A 93:1619–1623, 1996

De Kloet ER, Sibug RM, Helmerhorst FM, et al: Stress, genes and the mechanism of programming the brain for later life. Neurosci Biobehav Rev 29:271–281, 2005

Fitzgerald FS: The Great Gatsby. New York, Grosset & Dunlap, 1925

Forman SD, Bissette G, Yao J, et al: Cerebrospinal fluid corticotropin-releasing factor increases following haloperidol withdrawal in chronic schizophrenia. Schizophr Res 12:43–51, 1994

Fuller T, Sarkar S, Crews D: The use of norms of reaction to analyze genotypic and environmental influences on behavior in mice and rats. Neurosci Biobehav Rev 29:445–456, 2005

Ghaemi SN, Boiman EE, Goodwin FK: Diagnosing bipolar disorder and the effect of antidepressants: a naturalistic study. J Clin Psychiatry 61:804–808; quiz 809, 2000

Halbreich U: Major depression is not a diagnosis, it is a departure point to differential diagnosis—clinical and hormonal considerations (A commentary and elaboration on Antonejevic's paper). Psychoneuroendocrinology 31:16–22, 2006

Heim C, Nemeroff CB: The role of childhood trauma in the neurobiology of mood and anxiety disorders: preclinical and clinical studies. Biol Psychiatry 49:1023–1039, 2001

Heim C, Newport DJ, Heit S, et al: Pituitary-adrenal and autonomic responses to stress in women after sexual and physical abuse in childhood. JAMA 284:592–597, 2000

Heim C, Plotsky PM, Nemeroff CB: Importance of studying the contributions of early adverse experience to neurobiological findings in depression. Neuropsychopharmacology 29:641–648, 2004

Helzer JE, Robins LN, McEvoy L: Post-traumatic stress disorder in the general population: findings of the Epidemiologic Catchment Area survey. N Engl J Med 317:1630–1634, 1987

Holden C: Behavioral genetics: getting the short end of the allele. Science 301:291–293, 2003

Horwitz AV, Widom CS, McLaughlin J, et al: The impact of childhood abuse and neglect on adult mental health: a prospective study. J Health Soc Behav 42:184–201, 2001

Huot RL, Thrivikraman KV, Meaney MJ, et al: Development of adult ethanol preference and anxiety as a consequence of neonatal maternal separation in Long Evans rats and reversal with antidepressant treatment. Psychopharmacology (Berl) 158:366–373, 2001

Judd LL, Akiskal HS: The prevalence and disability of bipolar spectrum disorders in the US population: re-analysis of the ECA database taking into account subthreshold cases. J Affect Disord 73:123–131, 2003

Kaufman J, Plotsky PM, Nemeroff CB, et al: Effects of early adverse experiences on brain structure and function: clinical implications. Biol Psychiatry 48:778–790, 2000

Kendler KS, Gardner CO, Prescott CA: Toward a comprehensive developmental model for major depression in women. Am J Psychiatry 159:1133–1145, 2002

Koob GF: Corticotropin-releasing factor, norepinephrine, and stress. Biol Psychiatry 46:1167–1180, 1999

Ladd CO, Huot RL, Thrivikraman KV, et al: Long-term behavioral and neuroendocrine adaptations to adverse early experience. Prog Brain Res 122:81–103, 2000

Ladd CO, Huot RL, Thrivikraman KV, et al: Long-term adaptations in glucocorticoid receptor and mineralocorticoid receptor mRNA and negative feedback on the hypothalamo-pituitary-adrenal axis following neonatal maternal separation. Biol Psychiatry 55:367–375, 2004

Lee AL, Ogle WO, Sapolsky RM: Stress and depression: possible links to neuron death in the hippocampus. Bipolar Disord 4:117–128, 2002

Levine S: Primary social relationships influence the development of the hypothalamic–pituitary–adrenal axis in the rat. Physiol Behav 73:255–260, 2001

Liu D, Caldji C, Sharma S, et al: Influence of neonatal rearing conditions on stress-induced adrenocorticotropin responses and norepinephrine release in the hypothalamic paraventricular nucleus. J Neuroendocrinol 12:5–12, 2000

MacMillan HL, Fleming JE, Streiner DL, et al: Childhood abuse and lifetime psychopathology in a community sample. Am J Psychiatry 158:1878–1883, 2001

McCauley J, Kern DE, Kolodner K, et al: Clinical characteristics of women with a history of childhood abuse: unhealed wounds. JAMA 277:1362–1368, 1997

Meaney MJ, Brake W, Gratton A: Environmental regulation of the development of mesolimbic dopamine systems: a neurobiological mechanism for vulnerability to drug abuse? Psychoneuroendocrinology 27:127–138, 2002

Miller CJ, Klugman J, Berv DA, et al: Sensitivity and specificity of the Mood Disorder Questionnaire for detecting bipolar disorder. J Affect Disord 81:167–171, 2004

Moller HJ: Anxiety associated with comorbid depression. J Clin Psychiatry 63 (suppl 14):22–26, 2002

Nair HP, Gutman AR, Davis M, et al: Central oxytocin, vasopressin, and corticotropin-releasing factor receptor densities in the basal forebrain predict isolation potentiated startle in rats. J Neurosci 25:11479–11488, 2005

Nemeroff CB, Owens MJ, Bissette G, et al: Reduced corticotropin releasing factor binding sites in the frontal cortex of suicide victims. Arch Gen Psychiatry 45:577–579, 1988

Nemeroff CB, Bissette G, Akil H, et al: Neuropeptide concentrations in the cerebrospinal fluid of depressed patients treated with electroconvulsive therapy: corticotrophin-releasing factor, beta-endorphin and somatostatin. Br J Psychiatry 158:59–63, 1991

Neumaier JF, Edwards E, Plotsky PM: 5-HT(1B) mRNA regulation in two animal models of altered stress reactivity. Biol Psychiatry 51:902–908, 2002

Owen D, Andrews MH, Matthews SG: Maternal adversity, glucocorticoids and programming of neuroendocrine function and behaviour. Neurosci Biobehav Rev 29:209–226, 2005

Penza KM, Heim C, Nemeroff CB: Neurobiological effects of childhood abuse: implications for the pathophysiology of depression and anxiety. Arch Women Ment Health 6:15–22, 2003

Plotsky PM, Meaney MJ: Early, postnatal experience alters hypothalamic corticotropin-releasing factor (CRF) mRNA, median eminence CRF content and stress-induced release in adult rats. Brain Res Mol Brain Res 18:195–200, 1993

Plotsky PM, Thrivikraman KV, Nemeroff CB, et al: Long-term consequences of neonatal rearing on central corticotropin-releasing factor systems in adult male rat offspring. Neuropsychopharmacology 30:2192–2204, 2005

Raadsheer FC, van Heerikhuize JJ, Lucassen PJ, et al: Corticotropin-releasing hormone mRNA levels in the paraventricular nucleus of patients with Alzheimer's disease and depression. Am J Psychiatry 152:1372–1376, 1995

Radley JJ, Rocher AB, Miller M, et al: Repeated stress induces dendritic spine loss in the rat medial prefrontal cortex. Cereb Cortex 16:313–320, 2006

Resnick HS, Kilpatrick DG, Dansky BS, et al: Prevalence of civilian trauma and posttraumatic stress disorder in a representative national sample of women. J Consult Clin Psychol 61:984–991, 1993

Reul JM, Holsboer F: Corticotropin-releasing factor receptors 1 and 2 in anxiety and depression. Curr Opin Pharmacol 2:23–33, 2002

Rosenblum LA, Forger C, Noland S, et al: Response of adolescent bonnet macaques to an acute fear stimulus as a function of early rearing conditions. Dev Psychobiol 39:40–45, 2001

Shear MK, Cassano GB, Frank E, et al: The panic-agoraphobic spectrum: development, description, and clinical significance. Psychiatr Clin North Am 25:739–756, 2002

U.S. Department of Health and Human Services, Children's Bureau: Child Maltreatment 2003. Washington, DC, U.S. Government Printing Office, 2005

Van der Bergh BRH, Mulder EJH, Mennes M, et al: Antenatal maternal anxiety and stress and the neurobehavioral development of the fetus and child: links and possible mechanism. Neurosci Biobehav Rev 29:237–258, 2005

Vazquez DM: Stress and the developing limbic-hypothalamic-pituitary-adrenal axis. Psychoneuroendocrinology 23:663–700, 1998

Watts KD, Plotsky PM, Neill DB: Neonatal maternal separation in rats affects reward responding for sucrose, in Abstracts of the 34th Annual Meeting of the Society for Neuroscience, San Diego, CA, October 23–27, 2004, Abstract 571.17

Watts KD, Plotsky PM, Neill DB: Deficits in intracranial self-stimulation reward from neonatal maternal separation in rats, in Abstracts of the 35th Annual Meeting of the Society for Neuroscience, Washington, DC, November 12–16, 2005, Abstract 58.12

Weaver IC, Cervoni N, Champagne FA, et al: Epigenetic programming by maternal behavior. Nat Neurosci 7:847–854, 2004

Yehuda R, McFarlane AC: Conflict between current knowledge about posttraumatic stress disorder and its original conceptual basis. Am J Psychiatry 152:1705–1713, 1995

CHAPTER 4

MARRIAGE, HEALTH, AND IMMUNE FUNCTION

Jennifer E. Graham, Ph.D.
Lisa M. Christian, M.A.
Janice K. Kiecolt-Glaser, Ph.D.

Marital relationships are strongly related to many aspects of physical health (Burman and Margolin 1992; Kiecolt-Glaser and Newton 2001). Not only are married individuals healthier than single, divorced or separated, and widowed individuals after income and age are controlled (Johnson et al. 2000; Verbrugge 1979), but also marital status has substantial predictive power for mortality from a range of chronic and acute conditions (Johnson et al. 2000; Verbrugge 1979). Compared with other social relationships, marital relationships tend to have a greater effect on an individual's emotional and physical well-being (Glenn and Weaver 1981). Indeed, a meta-analysis of autonomic, endocrine, and immune data suggested that family relationships, including marriage, are particularly important (Uchino et al. 1996).

Several pathways have been proposed by which marriage can affect an individual's health (Burman and Margolin 1992; Kiecolt-Glaser and Newton 2001), many of which are bidirectional. Although selection undoubtedly plays a role, with healthier individuals more likely to marry and to stay married, the association between physical health and marriage remains after adjustment for selection effects (Wu et al. 2003). Stress and social support are widely acknowledged to play a major role in accounting for both protective and deleterious correlates of marital status and quality (Burman and Margolin 1992; Graham et al., in press), with rel-

Work on this chapter was supported by grants T32AI55411, AG16321, DE13749, M01-RR-0034, and CA16058 from the National Institutes of Health.

atively direct mechanisms via physiological responses to stress (Umberson 1992) in addition to more indirect effects related to individual cognitions, affect, coping, and health behaviors (e.g., diet, sleep, exercise, and medication adherence).

In this chapter, we focus on key findings linking marriage, immune function, and overall health. Throughout, we highlight the role of depression, as well as gender and other individual differences, such as trait hostility. The role of stress, social support, and coping mechanisms is also addressed. The current chapter is not exhaustive, but rather provides an overview of the importance of relationship factors. Another goal of this chapter is to encourage discussion and research on practical considerations related to diagnosis and intervention, such as the need for better characterization of relational processes in DSM.

Biological Outcomes of Interest

NEUROENDOCRINE MEASURES OF STRESS

Although marriage is typically considered to be beneficial or protective, marital conflict can function as both an acute stressor (e.g., a solitary argument) and a chronic stressor (e.g., daily arguments for years). Such stress is associated with changes in endocrine functioning, which can affect the immune system indirectly (Ader et al. 1991; Malarkey et al. 1994). Two pathways are key to maintaining homeostasis during stress: the hypothalamic-pituitary-adrenal (HPA) axis and the sympathetic-adrenal-medullary (SAM) system. Activation of these axes results in the release of stress hormones, including cortisol, and the catecholamines epinephrine and norepinephrine (Groth et al. 2000). Both cortisol and catecholamines are believed to play a significant role in the development of disease under conditions of chronic stress (S. Cohen et al. 1995).

IMMUNE MEASURES

The immune system can be divided conceptually into natural (innate) and specific (adaptive) immunity. *Natural immunity* is a vital and almost immediate response to foreign invaders (e.g., bacteria and certain viruses) but one that is general and nonspecific to pathogens. The key elements of natural immunity are neutrophils, macrophages, natural killer (NK) cells, and complement proteins. In contrast to natural immunity, *specific immunity* takes several days to engage but—once activated—is more efficient and effective than natural immunity. The main cell type is the lymphocyte, which includes T cells and B cells. Two of the primary populations of T cells are CD4 (helper) and CD8 (cytotoxic) cells; CD4 cells are further subdivided into either T_H1 (T-helper-1) or T_H2 (T-helper-2) subtypes, which are associated with different functional properties and produce different cytokines.

Cytokines, which are produced by macrophages and other cells in addition to lymphocytes, are soluble proteins involved in communication between cells. Cytokines are a vital part of the immune system and are involved in adaptive response to immune challenge, including site-specific inflammation, fever, and improved wound healing (Rabin 1999). However, psychological stress also appears to stimulate cytokine production, and chronically elevated amounts of certain cytokines are implicated in morbidity and mortality, especially in older adults. For example, increased levels of proinflammatory cytokines, such as interleukin 6 (IL-6), are associated with a variety of diseases, including cardiovascular disease, arthritis, type 2 diabetes, and certain cancers (Kiecolt-Glaser et al. 2003b). IL-6 also triggers the increase of C-reactive protein (CRP), a general marker of inflammation associated with increased risk for myocardial infarction (Ridker et al. 2000).

Quantifiable measures related to immune function can be obtained in several ways. Enumerative assays quantify cell numbers or percentages because both the number of cells (e.g., an absolute count of the number of NK cells) and the relative balance of different cells (e.g., the ratio of T_H1-type cells to T_H2-type cells) are relevant to the overall function of the immune system. In contrast, functional assays assess performance of particular cells, typically in vitro. Both enumerative and functional assays are influenced by acute stress, but chronic and severe stress responses in humans tend to be more strongly and reliably associated with functional assays (Kiecolt-Glaser and Glaser 1995). Examples of functional assays commonly used in psychological research with humans are the ability of NK cells to lyse (i.e., destroy) tumor cells and the ability of lymphocytes to proliferate when stimulated with mitogens. Other assays include antibody responses to viruses and antibody and T-cell responses to vaccines. The amount of antibody or cytokine protein can be measured in vitro after stimulation of cells or in vivo (e.g., amount of a particular cytokine in the circulating blood).

Marriage and Immune Function

MARITAL RELATIONSHIPS AND GENERAL HEALTH

According to a large review of U.S. federal health data, married people have the lowest rates of disability due to chronic conditions (Verbrugge 1979). In terms of both acute and chronic conditions, separated and divorced individuals appear least healthy, followed by widowed, and then single individuals (Verbrugge 1979). In addition, the risk of mortality from a variety of conditions is typically lower among the married than among the unmarried in a wide range of populations and after adjustment for income and biomedical risk factors (Goodwin et al. 1987; Gordon and Rosenthal 1995; Johnson et al. 2000). Null findings are rare and typically have occurred in contexts in which the marital relationship is not as central to support provision, such as among first-generation immigrants or residents of small, rural communities (Burman and Margolin 1992; House et al. 1988).

In general, the effect of marital status on both mortality and morbidity is substantially stronger for men than for women (Kiecolt-Glaser and Newton 2001). For example, nonmarried women have a 50% greater risk of mortality than do otherwise comparable married women, compared with a 250% greater risk for nonmarried compared with married men (C.E. Ross et al. 1990). The increased risk of mortality associated with marital disruption is also often stronger for men (Kiecolt-Glaser and Newton 2001). Indeed, a particularly well-controlled and comprehensive study found that survivin g one's spouse led to increased risk of mortality among men but not among women over a 10-year period (Helsing et al. 1981).

Several plausible explanations exist for why marriage confers greater health benefits to men than to women. First, wives tend to influence their spouses to improve health behaviors to a greater extent than do husbands (Umberson 1992). Second, many married women do a greater percentage of housework and child care, with a particularly adverse effect on marital satisfaction for women with egalitarian ideals, and evidence indicates that such factors are associated with adverse cardiovascular and catecholamine responses (for a review, see Kiecolt-Glaser and Newton 2001). Women who become married are also more likely to cease employment, which may result in the loss of that social network (Johnson et al. 2000).

Although being married confers health benefits, on average, the mere existence of a close relationship is not enough to be protective. Indeed, poor marital quality is strongly associated with worse health (Kiecolt-Glaser and Newton 2001). For example, in a population-based, prospective follow-up study conducted in Stockholm, Sweden, of women with coronary heart disease, marital stress worsened the prognosis 2.9-fold for recurrent coronary events (Orth-Gomer et al. 2000). Among patients with congestive heart failure, marital quality predicted 4-year survival as well as illness severity (Coyne et al. 2001). Similarly, greater dyadic conflict was associated with a 46% higher relative death risk among female hemodialysis patients (Kimmel et al. 2000).

Although men appear to benefit more from being married overall, the weight of evidence suggests that women suffer more from poor marital quality. For example, in a large sample randomly selected from members of a health maintenance organization, companionship in marriage and equality in decision making were associated with a lower risk of death over 15 years among women but not among men (Hibbard and Pope 1993). Similarly, in another large study, women who reported that they had considerable conflicts with their husbands and who also reported work conflict had a 2.54-fold risk of work-related disability related to a variety of health problems in the ensuing 6 years; neither work nor marital conflict was a risk factor for men (Appelberg et al. 1996). Women and men may respond differently to marital quality for various reasons (for a comprehensive review, see Kiecolt-Glaser and Newton 2001). One difference of note is that women's self-representations tend to be characterized by greater relational interdependence (Cross and Madson 1997). In addition, women tend to spend more time thinking about marital events than do men (Burnett 1987; M. Ross and Holmberg 1990). For these reasons, conflictual marriages may dampen the benefits of being married more for women than for men.

MARITAL STATUS AND IMMUNE FUNCTION

Several of the first studies of marriage and immune function were designed in part to explain the particularly strong association between marital disruption and health. One study found that married women had better immune function than did comparable recently separated or divorced women (Kiecolt-Glaser et al. 1987), with the latter showing higher antibody titers in response to in vitro stimulation with Epstein-Barr virus (EBV) and lower percentages of NK cells (Kiecolt-Glaser et al. 1987). These effects were not explained by differences in drug or alcohol use, diet, or sleep. Similar results were found with men: divorced or separated men showed higher antibody titers to two herpesviruses, indicating poorer immune system control over viral latency (Kiecolt-Glaser et al. 1988).

Several studies have shown dysregulation of immune function following the death of a spouse (Bartrop et al. 1977), mirroring data showing increased mortality among bereaved individuals. Although most studies linking bereavement and specific immune measures have been of older women, the association between bereavement and health in younger individuals is likely to be even stronger. Younger people are at greater risk for both mortality and morbidity from spousal bereavement than are older individuals (for a review, see Schulz and Rau 1985), perhaps because of differences in their expectations of the preparedness of their social networks to provide support following this event. Depressive symptoms common among the bereaved may play a substantial role in the association between bereavement and immunity: more severe depressive symptoms among bereaved women are associated with a less adaptive pattern of immune response (Irwin et al. 1987). Thus, depressive symptoms may mediate immune responses to bereavement. However, other explanations for such associations are also possible, including third variables, such as genetics, that might influence both depressive and immune responses to stress.

MARITAL QUALITY AND IMMUNE FUNCTION

In the last 10 years or so, research on the effect of marital factors on immune function has focused on aspects of relationship quality rather than marital status. One commonly used indicator of marital quality is self-reported satisfaction with marriage. In the studies described earlier comparing married men and women with separated or divorced individuals, lower marital satisfaction was associated with several indicators of poorer immune function (Kiecolt-Glaser et al. 1987, 1988). Again, depression seems to play a role; poorer marital quality was related to greater depression, which also was associated with poorer immune function (Kiecolt-Glaser et al. 1988). Because these studies were retrospective, they did not examine depression as a mediator of a causal relation, and more recent studies have not tested this hypothesis to our knowledge. In the next section in this chapter, we review more fully other literature relevant to the possible role of depression.

In addition to self-report measures of marital satisfaction, marital quality has increasingly been assessed by observing behavior during couples' interactions. Although several studies have explored positive interactions (such as support provision and general positive behavior), hostile behaviors (such as interrupting and criticizing) appear to be more predictive of physiological outcomes. Hostile behaviors during marital discussions are associated with adverse changes in blood pressure, endocrine levels, and immune responses (Ewart et al. 1991; Kiecolt-Glaser et al. 1993; Malarkey et al. 1994). For example, in a sample of healthy newlywed couples with high marital satisfaction overall, subjects who showed more negative or hostile behavior during a 30-minute discussion of marital problems had greater decrements over 24 hours on four immune measures as compared with other subjects (Kiecolt-Glaser et al. 1993).

Such findings have been replicated with a variety of populations and by several different laboratories. In addition to our newlywed sample, for example, older couples also showed endocrine and immune dysregulation following marital conflict discussion (Kiecolt-Glaser et al. 1997); both men and women who showed more negative behavior had the poorest immunological responses across three assays. In another marital interaction study, wives responded to a 45-minute conflictive discussion task with greater increases in depression, hostility, and systolic blood pressure than did husbands (Mayne et al. 1997). In addition, women's lymphocyte proliferative responses decreased following conflict, whereas men's responses increased (Mayne et al. 1997).

Overall, as with the gender differences in response to marital conflict, the relation between physiological change and negative marital behavior typically has been stronger for women than for men (e.g., Kiecolt-Glaser et al. 1996; Malarkey et al. 1994; Mayne et al. 1997). These differences between wives and husbands do not seem to be a function of gender differences in broader physiological patterns of responding to acute stress (Kiecolt-Glaser and Newton 2001).

Individuals with high levels of trait hostility also were more likely to show greater endocrine and immune responses to marital conflict and only in part because they showed more negative conflict behaviors during marital interactions (Mayne et al. 1997; Newton et al. 1995). Indeed, another study found no significant association between behaviorally coded affect during conflict and cardiovascular, immune, or cortisol data, except among husbands who had high levels of cynical hostility (Miller et al. 1999).

In addition to their relevance to health, these findings have important implications for understanding marital stability. In our study of newlyweds, evidence suggested that stress hormone responses can predict marital satisfaction and divorce. Those with higher levels of stress hormones throughout the day as measured in their first year of marriage (not necessarily stress hormone levels linked to a conflict discussion) were more likely to divorce subsequently (Kiecolt-Glaser et al. 2003a). Moreover, higher stress hormone reactivity in response to the problem-solving discussion was associated with poorer marital satisfaction 10 years later (Kiecolt-Glaser et al. 2003a).

For some individuals, the marital relationship is chronically stressful not because of conflict or hostility per se but because of the health status of the partner. Individuals who are caring for spouses with Alzheimer's and other forms of dementia experience chronic stress, report low levels of social support, and are at elevated risk for depressive symptoms and mood disorders even after the death of their spouse (Esterling et al. 1994). As compared with sociodemographically similar control subjects, caregivers reported more days of infectious illness (Kiecolt-Glaser et al. 1991), had poorer immune responses to virus and vaccine challenges (Glaser et al. 2000; Vedhara et al. 1999), and experienced slower healing of laboratory-induced wounds (Kiecolt-Glaser et al. 1995). In addition, both current and former caregivers showed evidence of dysregulated inflammation. For example, caregivers have poorer NK cell responses to cytokines in vitro (Esterling et al. 1994, 1996), show a substantially greater increase in IL-6 over a 6-year period (Kiecolt-Glaser et al. 2003b), and show a stronger association between pain and CRP (Graham et al. 2005) as compared with noncaregivers. Relational processes appear to play a strong role in the adverse effect of caregiving. Caregivers who are most bothered by dementia-related behaviors of their spouse show the most uniformly negative changes in immune function (Kiecolt-Glaser et al. 1991), and poor NK cell responses among caregivers are associated with less positive social support and less emotional closeness among social contacts (Esterling et al. 1996).

Marriage and Mental Health

Overall, those who are married enjoy better mental health than do those who are not (Kessler and McRae 1984; Pearlin and Johnson 1977; Thoits 1986). Much research has focused specifically on depressive symptoms, which are lower among married people than among unmarried people overall (Wu et al. 2003). Although this association between marriage and better mental health is partially explained by selection effects (Overbeek et al. 2003), a substantial amount appears to be explained by the health advantages of being married (Horowitz et al. 1996; Wu et al. 2003). However, as noted earlier, not all marriages are created equal. Indeed, unmarried people are happier, on average, than those who are unhappily married (Glenn and Weaver 1981). Moreover, among married people, those in less conflictual marriages report greater overall mental health (Berry and Worthington 2001). One study found that those reporting marital discord had a 10-fold increase in risk for depressive symptoms (O'Leary et al. 1994). Similarly, data from a large epidemiological study indicated that unhappy marriages were associated with a 25-fold increase in major depressive disorder over untroubled marriages (Weissman 1987).

The magnitude of the association between marital distress and depressive symptomatology is comparable for women and men (O'Leary et al. 1994). However, a prospective study suggested that poor marital quality is more likely to lead to depression for women than for men (Fincham et al. 1997), and this may partly explain why marital quality tends to have a greater effect on women's physical health and immunity specifically. Marital dissolution is also strongly associated with increases in depression and depressive symptoms for both men and women (Wade and Pevalin 2004). For example, a large longitudinal study of older adults found a ninefold increase in major depression and a fourfold increase in depressive symptoms among the recently bereaved as compared with married individuals (Turvey et al. 1999). A rise in depressive symptoms following bereavement is particularly common among those for whom the loss of the spouse was unexpected (Carnalley et al. 1999) and for whom social support is lacking (Wortman et al. 2004).

The association between marital relationships and depressive symptoms has important implications for physical health. Clinical depression is generally associated with immune dysregulation, as evidenced by several indicators. Importantly, depression can directly increase production of proinflammatory cytokines, including IL-2, IL-6, and tumor necrosis factor–α (for a review, see Kiecolt-Glaser and Glaser 2002), which, when levels are chronically elevated, play a pathogenic role in a range of diseases (Kiecolt-Glaser et al. 2003b). In addition to direct physiological alterations, depression affects health indirectly by influencing health-related behaviors, including alcohol use, sleep, diet, and exercise (Kiecolt-Glaser and Glaser 1988). Depression also affects subjective reports of physical health. After objective indicators of physical health are controlled, those who are depressed tend to report worse perceived current health and greater bodily pain than do those who are not depressed (Wells et al. 1989). This difference may be a reflection of physical symptoms related to depression and/or cognitive differences in how depressed individuals perceive their health (Pinquart 2001). Given that depression affects a variety of health behaviors, physiology, and the subjective experience of health, the association between marriage and depressive symptoms may be a key pathway linking close relationships and health (Kiecolt-Glaser and Newton 2001).

Future Research and Clinical Implications

The institution of marriage and gender roles associated with marriage change over time. Although a majority of U.S. households (52%) are headed by married couples, the number of households headed by couples who cohabit has increased to 5.5 million in 2000 from 3.2 million in 1990 (Simmons and O'Connell 2003). Of these, more than 11% are same-sex couples (Simmons and O'Connell 2003). Both heterosexual and same-sex cohabiting partners represent a largely unstudied population. Data on the mental and physical health effects of cohabitation have been inconsistent. Some studies have found that the self-reported health of cohabitants is better than that of single persons but not as good as that of married individuals (Joung et al. 1995). Recent data suggest that cohabiting partners share most of the physical and psychological advantages of married people, after controlling for income and age (Wu et al. 2003). Research comparing cohabitants with married individuals may be particularly useful in determining precisely what aspects of close relationships are protective for health and immune function.

A growing body of research suggests that psychopharmacological, psychotherapeutic, and behavioral interventions can reduce the effect of stress on immune parameters (Kiecolt-Glaser et al. 2002). The particularly potent effects of marital distress on immune and health outcomes suggest that couple-based interventions targeting relevant aspects of the marital relationship may effectively improve mental and physical health. For example, an intervention targeting marital communication has been shown to reduce cardiovascular responses during a relationship problem discussion in those with hypertension (Ewart et al. 1984). To our knowledge, no similar evidence is available in terms of the effects of such an intervention on immune parameters.

Another important and related element of couples interventions is the degree to which couples discuss their emotional reactions to stress. Disclosure of emotions is related to better-perceived partner responsiveness and, in turn, with the couple's feelings of intimacy (Laurenceau et al. 1998). Consistent mental and physical effects of written emotional disclosure about stressful events have been found in both clinical and nonclinical populations (Pennebaker 1997; Smyth et al. 1999). Preliminary evidence suggests that changes in immune function play a role (Booth and Petrie 2002), whereas changes in health behaviors do not appear to be relevant (Stone et al. 2000). Although most of these interventions have involved nondirected, journal-type writing, preliminary evidence with chronic pain patients suggests that writing in a directed way about angry feelings specifically can be beneficial in terms of pain severity, control over pain, and depression (Graham 2004). Treatment group participants in this study expressed anger in letters, which were often addressed to a spouse. Individual variation in response to any intervention focused on interpersonal processes is likely (Kiecolt-Glaser et al. 2002) and needs particular attention before interventions designed around interactions between couples are implemented in practice.

Given the relation between marital distress, depression, and immune function, marital interventions should include measures of depression to determine whether depressive symptoms mediate effects of improved marital quality on immune function. There is a lack of research assessing the effects on immune function of interventions targeting depression directly, with most psychosocial interventions focused on stress reduction. The potential role of other variables, such as stress responses and genetics, also should be examined. Additional research is needed with older populations, who are at greater risk for morbidity and mortality resulting from dysregulated immune function (Kiecolt-Glaser et al. 2003b). Finally, to the extent that future interventions are successful, assessing their effects on health longitudinally would be ideal.

Chronically ill populations are another important direction for future research, both to determine the effect of psychosocial factors on health and to develop meaningful interventions. Although aspects of marriage have been studied in populations with illnesses of particular immunological relevance—such as rheumatoid arthritis, HIV, mouth ulcers, and certain cancers—little direct evidence links those health outcomes to specific immune parameters (Kiecolt-Glaser and Newton 2001). Marital interaction unquestionably alters symptom expression in some chronic conditions. For example, men and women reporting lower marital quality have increased risk of periodontal disease and dental cavities (Marcenes and Sheiham 1996). Similarly, large prospective epidemiological studies have implicated marital strain as a factor in the development of ulcers (e.g., Levenstein et al. 1999). Thus far, most studies of health populations have not included direct measures of endocrine and/or immune function, which would allow for clearer delineation of mediating factors. However, this direction is promising. For example, interpersonal stress has been linked to both endocrine and immune alterations among those with rheumatoid arthritis, changes that were associated with clinician-rated disease activity as well as self-reported joint tenderness in well-designed prospective studies (Waltz et al. 1998). Similarly, preliminary work indicates that psychological stress predicts NK cell lysis and NK response to cytokine stimulation among cancer patients (Andersen et al. 1998); however, this is only one avenue by which the immune system defends against malignancy, and research with other measures will be valuable.

In addition to studies with clinical populations, further evidence of the clinical relevance of immune alterations will be helpful in understanding the full effect of marital stress. Longitudinal studies reporting that immune dysregulation observed during partner conflict is predictive of morbidity and mortality in the long term are particularly needed. Within short-term research designs, the use of outcomes with clear clinical relevance will strengthen our ability to interpret immunological changes. Wound healing is one such outcome. Recent work from our laboratory on the effects of marital interactions has assessed healing of experimentally induced wounds. Couples who showed consistently higher levels of hostile behavior during both conflictive and supportive interactions healed wounds at 60% of the rate of couples with low levels of hostile behavior (Kiecolt-Glaser et al. 2005). Use of such methodologies provides clinically relevant data over a relatively short time.

Finally, another important area for future research on the association between marital factors and immune function is positive and supportive aspects of relationships (Robles and Kiecolt-Glaser 2003). Although research to date suggests that hostile and negative behavior is more toxic to health than supportive behaviors are beneficial or protective (Kiecolt-Glaser and Newton 2001), the effects of positive marital interactions may be underestimated because the methods used in most research may promote negativity (e.g., by focusing on conflict discussions) and limit opportunities for couples to show supportive behavior. One important question is whether the effect of conflict behaviors is buffered in typically supportive marriages and exacerbated in those in which support is low (Bradbury et al. 1998). Positive support provided by close relationships is associated with more adaptive immune function (Uchino et al. 1996), often apparently by buffering the effects of stress (for a review, see Graham et al., in press). In addition, other well-validated and important measures of marital quality, such as partner closeness, are assessed with pictorial diagrams and unobtrusive reaction time tests (Aron et al. 1992). The health effect of such measures has not been studied at all, to our knowledge, and will make a valuable addition to our understanding of close relationships, immunity, and health.

Conclusion

Immune function appears to play an important role in the association between marital factors and health. Both the state of being married and marital satisfaction are associated with adaptive immune responses and better overall health, whereas marital disruption and hostile marital interactions are associated with dysregulation of immune function according to a range of markers. Although many processes are at work, and these processes are frequently bidirectional, stress appears to play a significant role in accounting for these associations; for example, being happily married likely buffers the effects of life stress, especially for men, but marital conflict is itself a powerful psychosocial stressor, especially for women. Marital conflict appears to be particularly toxic in terms of immune function for those who tend to have frequent and intense hostile reactions to stress. In addition, changes in depression may help account for the association between marital factors and health: as described earlier, marriage, marital disruption, and marital conflict are strongly associated with depressive symptomatology, which is also associated with the dysregulation of immune function both directly via physiological mechanisms and indirectly via health behaviors. Even as societal patterns of marriage change, key partnerships with close others remain and retain the power to affect us negatively and positively. In developing the next edition of DSM, additional consideration of relational risk factors and disorders is warranted. Moreover, greater understanding of the scope, mediating factors, and effect of marriage and close partnerships on health and immunity is essential as we strive to develop targeted interventions to improve both psychological and physical well-being.

References

Ader R, Felten DL, Cohen N (eds): Psychoneuroimmunology. San Diego, CA, Academic Press, 1991

Andersen BL, Farrar WB, Golden-Kreutz D, et al: Stress and immune responses after surgical treatment for regional breast cancer. J Natl Cancer Inst 90:30–36, 1998

Appelberg K, Romanov K, Heikkila K, et al: Interpersonal conflict as a predictor of work disability: a follow-up study of 15,348 Finnish employees. J Psychosom Res 40:157–167, 1996

Aron A, Aron EN, Smollan D: Inclusion of Other in the Self Scale and the structure of interpersonal closeness. J Pers Soc Psychol 63:596–612, 1992

Bartrop R, Luckhurst E, Lazarus L, et al: Depressed lymphocyte function after bereavement. Lancet 1:374–377, 1977

Berry JW, Worthington EL: Forgivingness, relationship quality, stress while imagining relationship events, and physical and mental health. J Counsel Psychol 48:447–455, 2001

Booth RJ, Petrie KJ: Emotional expression and health changes: can we identify biological pathways?, in The Writing Cure: How Expressive Writing Promotes Health and Emotional Well-Being. Edited by Lepore SJ, Smyth JM. Washington, DC, American Psychological Association, 2002, pp 157–175

Bradbury TN, Cohan CL, Karney BR: Optimizing longitudinal research for understanding and preventing marital dysfunction, in The Developmental Course of Marital Dysfunction. Edited by Bradbury TN. New York, Cambridge, 1998, pp 279–311

Burman B, Margolin G: Analysis of the association between marital relationships and health problems: an interactional perspective. Psychol Bull 112:39–63, 1992

Burnett R: Reflections in personal relationships, in Accounting for Relationships: Explanation, Representation, Consciousness. Edited by Burnett R, McGhee P, Clarke D. New York, Methuen, 1987, pp 102–110

Carnalley KB, Wortman CB, Kessler RC: The impact of widowhood on depression: findings from a prospective study. Psychol Med 29:1111–1123, 1999

Cohen S, Kessler R, Gordon LG (eds): Measuring Stress. New York, Oxford University Press, 1995

Coyne JC, Rohrbaugh MJ, Shoham V, et al: Prognostic importance of marital quality for survival of congestive heart failure. Am J Cardiol 88:526–529, 2001

Cross SE, Madson L: Models of the self: self-construals and gender. Psychol Bull 122:5–37, 1997

Esterling BA, Kiecolt-Glaser JK, Bodnar J, et al: Chronic stress, social support, and persistent alterations in the natural killer cell response to cytokines in older adults. Health Psychol 13:291–299, 1994

Esterling BA, Kiecolt-Glaser JK, Glaser R: Psychosocial modulation of cytokine-induced natural killer cell activity in older adults. Psychosom Med 58:264–272, 1996

Ewart CK, Taylor CB, Kraemer HC, et al: Reducing blood pressure reactivity during interpersonal conflict: effects of marital communication training. Behav Res Ther 15:473–484, 1984

Ewart CK, Taylor CB, Kraemer HC, et al: High blood pressure and marital discord: not being nasty matters more than being nice. Health Psychol 10:155–163, 1991

Fincham FD, Beach SRH, Harold GT, et al: Marital satisfaction and depression: different causal relationships for men and women? Psychol Sci 8:351–357, 1997

Glaser R, Sheridan JF, Malarkey WB, et al: Chronic stress modulates the immune response to a pneumococcal pneumonia vaccine. Psychosom Med 62:804–807, 2000

Glenn ND, Weaver CN: The contribution of marital happiness to global happiness. J Marriage Fam 43:161–168, 1981

Goodwin JS, Hunt WC, Key CR, et al: The effect of marital status on stage, treatment, and survival of cancer patients. JAMA 34:20–26, 1987

Gordon HS, Rosenthal GE: Impact of marital status on outcomes in hospitalized patients. Arch Intern Med 155:2465–2471, 1995

Graham JE, Robles TF, Kiecolt-Glaser JK, et al: Hostility and pain are related to inflammation in older adults [Epub ahead of print]. Brain Behav Immun 2005

Graham JE, Christian LM, Kiecolt-Glaser JK: Close relationships and immunity, in Psychoneuroimmunology. Edited by Ader R. Burlington, MA, Elsevier, (in press)

Graham JE: Effects of written constructive anger expression on health and coping in patients with chronic pain. Dissertation Abstracts International 64(9-B) (UMI No 3106517)

Groth T, Fehm-Wolfsdorf G, Hahlweg K: Basic research on the psychobiology of intimate relationships, in The Psychology of Couples and Illness: Theory, Research and Practice. Edited by Schmaling K, Sher TG. Washington, DC, American Psychological Association, 2000, pp 13–42

Helsing K, Szklo M, Comstock G: Factors associated with mortality after widowhood. Am J Public Health 71:802–809, 1981

Hibbard JH, Pope CR: The quality of social roles as predictors of morbidity and mortality. Soc Sci Med 36:217–225, 1993

Horowitz AV, White HR, Howell-White S: Becoming married and mental health: a longitudinal study of a cohort of young adults. J Marriage Fam 58:895–907, 1996

House JS, Landis KR, Umberson D: Social relationships and health. Science 241:540–545, 1988

Irwin M, Daniels M, Bloom ET, et al: Life events, depressive symptoms, and immune function. Am J Psychiatry 144:437–441, 1987

Johnson NJ, Backlund E, Sorlie PD, et al: Marital status and mortality: the National Longitudinal Mortality Study. Ann Epidemiol 10:224–238, 2000

Joung IM, Stronks K, van de Mheen H, et al: Health behaviours explain part of the differences in self reported health associated with partner/marital status in The Netherlands. J Epidemiol Community Health 49:482–488, 1995

Kessler RC, McRae JA: Trends in the relationships of sex and marital status to psychological distress. Res Community Ment Health 4:109–130, 1984

Kiecolt-Glaser JK, Glaser R: Methodological issues in behavioral immunology research with humans. Brain Behav Immun 2:67–78, 1988

Kiecolt-Glaser JK, Glaser R: Measures of immune response, in Measuring Stress. Edited by Cohen S, Kessler R, Gordon LG. New York, Oxford University Press, 1995, pp 213–229

Kiecolt-Glaser JK, Glaser R: Depression and immune function: central pathways to morbidity and mortality. J Psychosom Res 53:873–876, 2002

Kiecolt-Glaser JK, Newton T: Marriage and health: his and hers. Psychol Bull 127:472–503, 2001

Kiecolt-Glaser JK, Fisher LD, Ogrocki P, et al: Marital quality, marital disruption, and immune function. Psychosom Med 49:31–34, 1987

Kiecolt-Glaser JK, Kennedy S, Malkoff S, et al: Marital discord and immunity in males. Psychosom Med 50:213–229, 1988

Kiecolt-Glaser JK, Dura JR, Speicher CE, et al: Spousal caregivers of dementia victims: longitudinal changes in immunity and health. Psychosom Med 53:345–362, 1991

Kiecolt-Glaser JK, Malarkey WB, Chee M, et al: Negative behavior during marital conflict is associated with immunological down-regulation. Psychosom Med 55:395–409, 1993

Kiecolt-Glaser JK, Marucha PT, Malarkey WB, et al: Slowing of wound healing by psychological stress. Lancet 346:1194–1196, 1995

Kiecolt-Glaser JK, Newton T, Cacioppo JT, et al: Marital conflict and endocrine function: are men really more physiologically affected than women? J Consult Clin Psychol 64:324–332, 1996

Kiecolt-Glaser JK, Glaser R, Cacioppo JT, et al: Marital conflict in older adults: endocrinological and immunological correlates. Psychosom Med 59:339–349, 1997

Kiecolt-Glaser JK, McGuire L, Robles TR, et al: Emotions, morbidity, and mortality: new perspectives from psychoneuroimmunology. Annu Rev Psychol 53:83–107, 2002

Kiecolt-Glaser JK, Bane C, Glaser R, et al: Love, marriage, and divorce: newlywed's stress hormones foreshadow relationship changes. J Consult Clin Psychol 71:176–188, 2003a

Kiecolt-Glaser JK, Preacher KJ, MacCallum RC, et al: Chronic stress and age-related increases in the proinflammatory cytokine IL-6. Proc Natl Acad Sci U S A 100:9090–9095, 2003b

Kiecolt-Glaser JK, Loving TJ, Stowell JR, et al: Hostile marital interactions, proinflammatory cytokine production, and wound healing. Arch Gen Psychiatry 62:1377–1384, 2005

Kimmel PL, Peterson RA, Weihs KL, et al: Dyadic relationship conflict, gender, and mortality in urban hemodialysis patients. J Am Soc Nephrol 11:1518–1525, 2000

Laurenceau J, Barrett LF, Pietromonaco PR: Intimacy as an interpersonal process: the importance of self-disclosure, partner disclosure, and perceived partner responsiveness in interpersonal exchanges. J Pers Soc Psychol 74:1238–1251, 1998

Levenstein S, Ackerman S, Kiecolt-Glaser JK, et al: Stress and peptic ulcer disease. JAMA 281:10–11, 1999

Malarkey W, Kiecolt-Glaser JK, Pearl D, et al: Hostile behavior during marital conflict alters pituitary and adrenal hormones. Psychosom Med 56:41–51, 1994

Marcenes W, Sheiham A: The relationship between marital quality and oral health status. Psychol Health 11:357–369, 1996

Mayne TJ, O'Leary A, McCrady B, et al: The differential effects of acute marital distress on emotional, physiological and immune functions in maritally distressed men and women. Psychol Health 12:277–288, 1997

Miller GE, Dopp JM, Myers HF, et al: Psychosocial predictors of natural killer cell mobilization during marital conflict. Health Psychol 18:262–271, 1999

Newton TL, Kiecolt-Glaser JK, Glaser R, et al: Conflict and withdrawal during marital interaction: the roles of hostility and defensiveness. Personality and Social Psychology Bulletin 21:512–524, 1995

O'Leary KD, Christian JL, Mendell NR: A closer look at the link between marital discord and depressive symptomatology. J Soc Clin Psychol 13:33–41, 1994

Orth-Gomer K, Wamala SP, Horsten M, et al: Marital stress worsens prognosis in women with coronary heart disease. JAMA 284:3008–3014, 2000

Overbeek G, Vollegergh W, Engels RCME, et al: Young adults' relationship transitions and the incidence of mental disorders. Soc Psychiatry Psychiatr Epidemiol 38:669–676, 2003

Pearlin LI, Johnson J: Marital status, life strains, and depression. Am Sociol Rev 42:704–715, 1977

Pennebaker JW: Writing about emotional experience as a therapeutic process. Psychol Sci 8:162–166, 1997

Pinquart M: Correlates of subjective health in older adults: a meta-analysis. Psychol Aging 16:414–426, 2001

Rabin BS: Stress, Immune Function, and Health: The Connection. New York, Wiley-Liss, 1999

Ridker PM, Hennekens CH, Buring JE, et al: C-Reactive protein and other markers of inflammation in the prediction of cardiovascular disease in women. N Engl J Med 342:836–843, 2000

Robles TF, Kiecolt-Glaser JK: The physiology of marriage: pathways to health. Physiol Behav 79:409–416, 2003

Ross CE, Mirowsky J, Goldsteen K: The impact of the family on health: the decade in review. J Marriage Fam 52:1059–1078, 1990

Ross M, Holmberg D: Recounting the past: gender differences in the recall of events in the history of a close relationship, in Self-Influence Processes. Edited by Olson JM, Zanna MP. Hillsdale, NJ, Lawrence Erlbaum, 1990, pp 135–152

Schulz R, Rau MT: Social support through the life course, in Social Support and Health. Edited by Cohen S, Syme SL. San Diego, CA, Academic Press, 1985, pp 129–149

Simmons T, O'Connell M: Married-Couple and Unmarried-Partner Households: 2000. Washington, DC, U.S. Census Bureau, 2003

Smyth JM, Stone AA, Hurewitz A, et al: Effects of writing about stressful experiences on symptom reduction in patients with asthma or rheumatoid arthritis. JAMA 281:1304–1309, 1999

Stone AA, Smyth JM, Kaell A, et al: Structured writing about stressful events: exploring potential psychological mediators of positive health effects. Health Psychol 19:619–624, 2000

Thoits P: Multiple identities: examining gender and marital status differences in psychological distress. Am Sociol Rev 51:259–272, 1986

Turvey C, Carney C, Arndt S, et al: Conjugal loss and syndromal depression in a sample of elders aged 70 years or older. Am J Psychiatry 156:1596–1601, 1999

Uchino BN, Cacioppo JT, Kiecolt-Glaser JK: The relationship between social support and physiological processes: a review with emphasis on underlying mechanisms and implications for health. Psychol Bull 119:488–531, 1996

Umberson D: Gender, marital status and the social control of health behavior. Soc Sci Med 24:907–917, 1992

Vedhara K, Cox NKM, Wilcock GK, et al: Chronic stress in elderly carers of dementia patients and antibody response to influenza vaccination. Lancet 353:627–631, 1999

Verbrugge LM: Marital status and health. J Marriage Fam 41:267–285, 1979

Wade TJ, Pevalin DJ: Marital transitions and mental health. J Health Soc Behav 45:155–170, 2004

Waltz M, Kriegel W, Bosch PV: The social environment and health in rheumatoid arthritis: marital quality predicts individual variability in pain severity. Arthritis Care Res 11: 356–374, 1998

Weissman MM: Advances in psychiatric epidemiology: rates and risks for major depression. Am J Public Health 77:445–451, 1987

Wells KB, Stewart A, Hays RD, et al: The functioning and well-being of depressed patients. JAMA 262:914–919, 1989

Wortman CB, Wolff K, Bonanno GA: Loss of an intimate partner through death, in Handbook of Closeness and Intimacy. Edited by Mashek DJ, Aron AP. Mahwah, NJ, Lawrence Erlbaum, 2004, pp 305–320

Wu Z, Penning MJ, Pollard MS, et al: In sickness and in health: does cohabitation count. J Fam Issues 24:811–838, 2003

CHAPTER 5

FAMILY EXPRESSED EMOTION PRIOR TO ONSET OF PSYCHOSIS

William R. McFarlane, M.D.

The diathesis-stress model or vulnerability-stress model provides a widely accepted, empirically supported, and useful framework for describing the relations among provoking agents (stressors), vulnerability (diathesis), and symptom formation and functional outcomes in schizophrenia (Zubin and Spring 1977; Zubin et al. 1992). Similar mechanisms for the transduction of psychosocial stress into the neurobiology of major mood disorders have been proposed (Post 1992). A vulnerable person whose inborn tolerance for stress is incompatible with exposure to either internally or externally generated stimulation may be thrown into a first or a recurring episode of illness. This principle underlies the Biosocial Hypothesis: *Major psychotic disorders are the result of the continual interaction of specific biological disorders of the brain with specific psychosocial and other environmental factors* (McFarlane 2002).

In the context of that model of precipitation of relapse and, possibly, initial episodes of psychosis, one important form of psychosocial stressor is *expressed emotion* (EE). In established and first-episode psychotic and mood disorders, acute episodes have been found to be more frequent and to cause poorer functioning in families in which a relative is critical of the family member with the disorder (Bebbington and Kuipers 1994; Brown et al. 1962; Cook et al. 1989; Hooley and Licht 1997; Hooley et al. 1995; Miklowitz et al. 1988). Rather than being seen as the fault of the relative, current understanding of this phenomenon includes the concept that the individual with these disorders is unusually vulnerable to arousal dyscontrol and cognitive disruption in the face of critical comments and emotional negativity, especially when the criticism carries with it hostility and personal rejection rather than simple irritation (Cook et al. 1989). Continued and ongoing exasperation on the part of close relatives can generate overt anger and frequent eruptions of irritation that probably have the same effects.

Modulation of the effect of EE by another family member appears to be common in clinical observations but has not been conclusively established empirically. Some evidence indicates that emotional overinvolvement leads to relapse and dysfunction via a related pathway (Leff and Vaughn 1985). This effect is seen as mediated instead by transmitted anxiety; intense, frequent interpersonal contacts and interactions; and, over the long term, the disabling effects of overcompensating for the patient's functional impairments. These behaviors on the part of relatives appear to derive from their well-intentioned attempts to assist and support their ill relative in the absence of understanding of, and clear guidance about, the symptomatic and neurological bases of disorders and disabilities (McFarlane 2002). The other major family interactional factor that has been found to be associated with schizophrenic and bipolar disorders is *communication deviance,* a measure of distracted or vague conversational style (Miklowitz et al. 1986, 1991; Wynne 1981; Wynne et al. 1977).

These same family interactional factors—EE and communication deviance— have been found to predict the onset of schizophrenia (Goldstein 1985; Tienari et al. 1994, 2004). Goldstein showed that onset of psychosis in disturbed, but not psychotic, adolescents seeking psychiatric treatment could be predicted by in vivo assessment of negative family affective style (a directly observed form of EE) and difficulties in clarity and structure of communication (communication deviance). It is important to note that subjects in Goldstein's landmark study were already ill enough to be referred and to accept outpatient treatment for a variety of nonpsychotic disorders and problems. Tienari and colleagues (2004) reported that similar family factors (communication, boundary, and critical abnormalities) account for the excess cases of schizophrenia among adopted-away children of Finnish mothers with schizophrenia. Those who developed schizophrenia, followed up through the age at onset and risk, were found almost entirely among those with genetic risk *and* high ratings of family dysfunction. Genetic and family dysfunction were equally predictive of onset, but neither was predictive after the other factor was controlled. Similar high ratings of family dysfunction among those at low genetic risk accounted for no excess likelihood of onset. As the authors suggested, what is inherited is a vulnerability to even minor degrees of family difficulties. Thus, the family interactional predictors of onset can be parsimoniously explained by their interaction with genetic and probably neurodevelopmental factors. These findings emphasize the power of chronic, low-intensity stressors, in contrast to acute life events. These data strongly support the concept that well-defined family factors can predispose to onset of psychosis, but primarily in those who are already having symptoms or who are at high genetic risk.

These family factors have been the target of family psychoeducation, which has been found to have a major and positive effect on EE, relapse rates, and functioning in schizophrenia and bipolar disorder (Dixon et al. 2001; McFarlane et al. 2003). More than 20 controlled trials have shown that whatever effects family members are having on symptoms, relapse risk, and poor functioning in the psychotic and mood disorders can be reversed through education, support, ongoing guidance, behavioral intervention, and treatment collaboration with key family members. The result has been an impressive level of relapse prevention, functional improvement, and improved family well-being that is currently unobtainable with medication treatment alone or with individual supportive or dynamically oriented psychotherapy.

Because the goals for this treatment approach are increasing understanding, coping capacity, and social support for families and patients alike, the outcomes tend to support a more narrow and specific version of the vulnerability stress model: negative family influences are largely the result of the effects on relatives of the disorder and its complex manifestations rather than a trait characteristic of the relatives themselves. This theory—that EE is largely reactive to symptoms and disabilities—has received increasingly strong support from a series of studies that have dissected the directionality and reciprocity of this interactional process. In summary, these studies have prompted a new paradigm: symptoms and subtle negativity on the part of the person with the illness provoke negativity on the part of caregiving and otherwise supportive relatives, but patient negativity is largely a subclinical expression of the disorder itself (Cook et al. 1989; Strachan et al. 1989; Woo et al. 2004). Although these studies involved zero-order correlational analyses, other family interaction studies (Cook and Kenny 2004; Cook et al. 1991), which used more precise modeling techniques, have substantiated the reciprocity in family relationships, including between-spouse (Gottman et al. 1998), parent-child (G.R. Patterson 1976), between-siblings, and transdyadic constellations (Cook and Kenny 2004).

Family interaction has emerged as a predictor of other psychiatric disorders, particularly conduct disorder and antisocial personality disorder in studies by Plomin and Daniels (1987), Reiss (2003), and Reiss et al. (2000). Similar to results in schizophrenia, outcome in these disorders was predicted most strongly by genetic risk for the disorders in the child, negativity expressed by the mother, and characteristics of the father and his relationship to the mother. In these studies as well, the child appears to induce in the mother the very negativity that then strongly predicts later disorder in the child. The confluence of findings in such disparate disorders is remarkable and, in our view, points to a more complex but much more accurate paradigm of onset and risk for psychiatric disorders—mutual influence of genetic and neurodevelopmental characteristics in the child and responsive interpersonal characteristics of the family and others in ongoing proximity.

Systemic Theoretical Model for the Process of Onset in Family

I have previously proposed a model for onset of psychosis that builds on this empirical background (see Figure 5–1) (McFarlane 2001). In this conception, first episodes are induced in biologically vulnerable individuals by 1) major stresses imposed by role transitions and other life events; 2) family negativity, exasperation, overinvolvement, and conflict; 3) social isolation or rejection; 4) separation from family of origin; and 5) stigma. More precisely, the process is initiated by stressors such as entering a new social, vocational, or educational context; social network disruptions; and losses through death or normal developmental milestones. The effect on a genetically or neurodevelopmentally vulnerable youth is the onset of subtle cognitive deficits and very early, minor prodromal symptoms. Family members, particularly parents, begin to notice these changes but may be unable to understand or identify them as symptoms of a psychiatric disorder. As relatives' anxiety and uncertainty increase, the youth's anxiety increases in response, leading to heightened arousal, increasing cognitive disruption, and prodromal psychotic symptoms. This positive feedback cycle continues to intensify until, on the relatives' side, concern leads to increasing frustration and then anger and criticism. On the youth's side, increasing interpersonal intensity and received negativity provoke increasing symptoms, cognitive deterioration, and, in many cases, reciprocal negativity and hostility.

Some empirical support exists for this model. A series of recent studies that used three-dimensional and longitudinal magnetic resonance imaging reported a posterior-to-anterior brain volume reduction in adolescents with childhood-onset schizophrenia, spreading from parietal to prefrontal and superior temporal cortices, that appears to be initiated by environmental factors. Once initiated, the process appears to be under genetic control (Sporn et al. 2003).

In some families, preexisting family conflict or communication and boundary difficulties could initiate the process of onset alone or lower the threshold necessary for external stressors to initiate the process (Tienari et al. 2004). Family communication deviance, a measure of distracted or vague conversational style, has been consistently associated with schizophrenia and bipolar disorder (Miklowitz et al. 1986, 1991; Singer and Wynne 1985). Family communication deviance was the other cofactor in the UCLA prospective long-term outcome study that predicted the onset of schizophrenic psychosis in families of disturbed, but nonpsychotic, adolescents (Goldstein 1985). More recent studies have determined that communication deviance is correlated with cognitive dysfunction in the relatives that is similar to (of the same type but lower severity) that seen in probands with schizophrenia (Wagener et al. 1986). This factor is significant because it suggests that even during the prodromal period, some family members will have difficulty holding a focus of attention. This factor is another example of the "double jeopardy" model: a young person

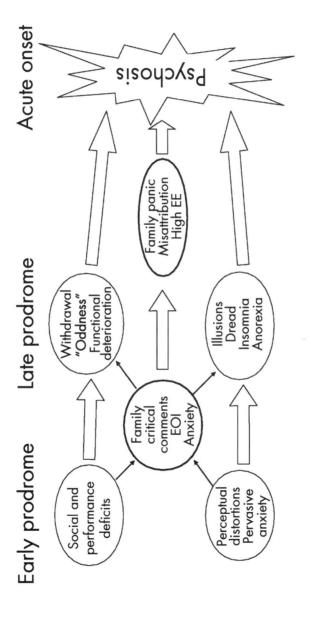

FIGURE 5–1.   Biosocial causal interactions in late schizophrenic prodrome.

Note.   EE = expressed emotion; EOI = emotional overinvolvement.

in the prodromal state may have inborn cognitive and attentional dysfunction exacerbated by family communicational difficulties, which themselves are the result of a heritable diathesis that affects attentional functioning, thought, and communication. Consequently, a child with subtle cognitive deficiencies may learn to converse in a communication milieu that is less able to compensate and correct. Once severe functional and performance deterioration begins, the family may have coping skills that are inadequate to deal with the increasing complexity and anxiety inherent in the situation. These difficulties are not primarily personality defects in the relatives; rather, they are manifestations of the schizophrenic diathesis playing itself out in both the interpersonal and the neurological domains.

Put simply, biology provides the necessary precondition, whereas environmental factors constitute the final common pathway. As shown in the Finnish adoptive study, both genetic and psychosocial causal factors must operate together and are necessary, but they are not individually sufficient in themselves. These psychosocial factors are the proximal causes of relapse in established cases and, I argue here, of the initial psychotic episode. In essence, the first psychotic episode is similar to a relapse, from a causal standpoint: it is better viewed as a new phase of a disease process that is already well under way at a subclinical, but biologically significant, level. Within this framework, the first episode begins when manifestations of accelerating deterioration first emerge, but the beginning of frank psychosis is, for many purposes, best seen as the first relapse. Furthermore, the first episode of a psychotic disorder would be represented by the onset of *any* disease manifestations (i.e., of prodromal positive symptoms, negative symptoms, or new cognitive impairments). This distinction is not trivial within a family context, because we are proposing that, regardless of the subtlety of prodromal symptoms or the requirements for making a DSM-IV (American Psychiatric Association 1994, 2000) diagnosis, family members are reacting to these prodromal symptoms in ways that have a powerful effect on the progression of the disease process itself. Even if only at a preconscious level, family members know that their child or sibling is becoming ill, but with a disease that is difficult in the prodromal phase to specify or understand.

Thus, an empirically derived and parsimonious hypothesis is that a large degree of family "dysfunction" in the prodromal phase is *secondary* to the deterioration that is occurring in the affected young person, even though it is also powerfully interacting with the adolescent's vulnerability to amplify symptoms and other functional sequelae of the accelerating biological process. If this model were the case, the earliest manifestation of EE would be emotional overinvolvement, whereas critical comments would be expected to arise later, most likely during or after onset of frank psychosis. This was the result in a study of first-episode early psychosis, in which families manifested evolution of high emotional overinvolvement to either low EE or high criticism, depending on the degree of perceived loss (P. Patterson et al. 2000). Furthermore, emotional overinvolvement would be expected to be greater in those families in which the young person was experiencing and manifesting greater functional impairments, whereas criticism would be greater in families in which the adolescent's symptoms were manifested as increased negativity, suspiciousness, and hostility. In relation to deterioration in functioning, mothers and fathers would be expected to differ in many families, with the mothers increasingly overinvolved and the fathers possibly more prone to criticism. Indeed, two independent studies have found that at first episode, high EE is predominantly emotional overinvolvement; remarkably, in both samples, 64% of the high-EE relatives manifested high emotional overinvolvement but not criticism (P. Patterson et al. 2000; Stirling et al. 1991). More specifically, EE is a state characteristic arising during the early prodrome in reaction to emerging manifestations of illness; in a minority of families, EE is a stable family trait of all those who develop a psychotic disorder and evident consistently throughout the period prior to onset of prodrome. Furthermore, components of EE—criticism and emotional overinvolvement—arise somewhat independently, beginning with components derivative of fear, anxiety, and natural tendencies toward protectiveness of a child or sibling.

This question was explored in a preliminary analysis of assessments and comparisons of three samples, two composed of patients with well-established schizophrenia or mood disorders (Samples 1 and 2) and another composed of young people determined to be at risk for, but not yet experiencing, psychosis (Sample 3). The samples were assessed at baseline as part of three randomized clinical trials that were testing efficacy of family-oriented psychoeducational treatments. The chronically ill samples (1 and 2) ranged in age from 18 to 55, had involvement of parents, and were participating in clinical trials of an intervention to increase participation in competitive employment among those with an Axis I DSM-IV psychiatric disorder receiving treatment at large community mental health centers. Subjects were clinically stable for at least 6 months. Sample 3 consisted of 35 subjects ages 12–35 and their families participating in a randomized comparative treatment trial testing family intervention to prevent onset of psychosis in youths meeting criteria for being at risk for psychosis according to the Structured Interview for Prodromal Syndromes (McGlashan et al. 2003). Although parents in Samples 1 and 2 had similarly high EE scores, the prodromal patients' parents differed dramatically. Warmth was higher, rejection and fusion were lower, and protectiveness was in the midrange for mothers and lower for fathers. Warmth and rejection scores between established and prodromal samples were all but reciprocals of the other. Highly significant correlations were found between duration of prodrome for protectiveness and a smaller but significant correlation for fusion in mothers but not fathers. The trend was toward increasing rejection with time for mothers.

Conclusion

Rejection, critical comments, and negativity appear to be all but absent in both fathers and mothers of youths found to meet criteria for being in the prodromal or early first-episode phase of a psychotic disorder. This finding contrasts sharply with criticism and rejection levels found in many samples of chronically ill adults assessed in 12 countries and over a period of nearly 40 years (Bebbington and Kuipers 1994). The existing data, although minimal currently, strongly suggest that these differences are fundamental and related to stage and progression of illness. Some confirmation that these differences manifest a progression of EE in response to continuing symptoms across the prodromal phase is found in the correlation of duration with the protectiveness and fusion components of emotional overinvolvement.

The process that emerges from this and previous studies is consistent: relatives tend to respond with negative and increasingly intense emotion and behavior to subtle symptoms and negative expression and behavior on the part of the person either developing or affected by a major psychiatric disorder. The initial response by parents appears to be one of protectiveness and, at least implicitly, anxiety. Parents become more attached and preoccupied, seemingly responding to increasing distress and psychological abnormalities in an adolescent child. As the prodromal period continues and symptoms and functioning worsen, parents begin to manifest more rejection and less warmth. An extrapolation of these data suggests that the end point of high levels of parental rejection, criticism, and hostility occurs after full psychosis develops and the child assumes a more chronic and disabled phase of illness. Further research is needed both to confirm the findings in this study and to fill in the process of progression to elucidate the provoking agents. One study found that criticism and hostility rates rose rapidly in the first few years of the course of illness, peaking at 50% of the sample after 5 years but also reaching 35% within 1–3 years of onset (Hooley and Richters 1995). The rate for those with less than 1 year of illness was 14%. Other studies have noted similar findings, particularly correlation of relatives' criticism and their estimate of time since onset of first evidence of illness (Stirling et al. 1991).

A key implication of these findings is that prevention of psychosis in youths who are genetically or neurodevelopmentally predisposed would be aided by assisting family members to *remain* low in rejection and criticism levels because that component most powerfully predicts relapse and, in our view, initial onset. Clearly, for those families in which criticism is long-standing before onset, perhaps secondary to equally long-standing functional and cognitive deficits of an evolving type II schizophrenic disorder, efforts would be needed to decrease EE. However, in the average situation, the task of family intervention would be to decrease parental anxiety, overprotectiveness, and fusion and to prevent, rather than reduce, rejection and criticism. Furthermore, some types and degrees of protectiveness would be appropriate, if not essential, for safety and well-being; they would be supported. Experience with family psychoeducation in both prodromal and established disorders to date suggests that this task is relatively simpler and more reliably accomplished than reducing EE in families with decades of bad experiences with mental illness and treatment services. Prevention of onset requires "lower doses" of both medication and family psychoeducation to reduce the known provoking factors. From that perspective, the preliminary findings of this study are most promising.

References

American Psychiatric Association: Diagnostic and Statistical Manual of Mental Disorders, 4th Edition. Washington, DC, American Psychiatric Association, 1994

American Psychiatric Association: Diagnostic and Statistical Manual of Mental Disorders, 4th Edition, Text Revision. Washington, DC, American Psychiatric Association, 2000

Bebbington P, Kuipers L: The predictive utility of expressed emotion in schizophrenia: an aggregate analysis. Psychol Med 24:707–718, 1994

Brown GW, Monck EM, Carstairs GM, et al: Influence of family life on the course of schizophrenic illness. Br J Psychiatry 16:55–68, 1962

Cook WL, Kenny DA: Application of the social relations model to family assessment. J Fam Psychol 18:361–371, 2004

Cook WL, Strachan AM, Goldstein MJ, et al: Expressed emotion and reciprocal affective relationships in families of disturbed adolescents. Fam Process 28:337–348, 1989

Cook WL, Kenny DA, Goldstein MJ: Parental affective style risk and the family system: a social relations model analysis. J Abnorm Psychol 100:492–501, 1991

Dixon L, McFarlane WR, Lefley H, et al: Evidence-based practices for services to families of people with psychiatric disabilities. Psychiatr Serv 52:903–910, 2001

Goldstein M: Family factors that antedate the onset of schizophrenia and related disorders: the results of a fifteen year prospective longitudinal study. Acta Psychiatr Scand 71 (suppl 319):7–18, 1985

Gottman JM, Coan J, Carrere S, et al: Predicting marital happiness and stability from new-lywed interactions. J Marriage Fam 60:5–22, 1998

Hooley JM, Licht DM: Expressed emotion and causal attributions in the spouses of depressed patients. J Abnorm Psychol 106:298–306, 1997

Hooley J, Richters JE: Expressed emotion: a developmental perspective, in Emotion, Cognition and Representation. Edited by Cicchetti D, Toth SL. Rochester, NY, University of Rochester Press, 1995, pp 133–166

Hooley JM, Rosen LR, Richters JE: Expressed emotion: toward clarification of a critical construct, in The Behavioral High-Risk Paradigm in Psychopathology. Edited by Miller GA. New York, Springer-Verlag, 1995, pp 88–120

Leff J, Vaughn C: Expressed Emotion in Families: Its Significance for Mental Illness. New York, Guilford, 1985

McFarlane WR: Family based treatment in prodromal and first-episode psychosis, in Early Intervention in Psychotic Disorders. Edited by Miller T. Amsterdam, Kluwer Academic Publishers, 2001, pp 197–230

McFarlane WR: Multifamily Groups in the Treatment of Severe Psychiatric Disorders. New York, Guilford, 2002

McFarlane WR, Dixon L, Lukens E, et al: Family psychoeducation and schizophrenia: a review of the literature. J Marital Fam Ther 29:223–245, 2003

McGlashan TH, Miller TJ, Woods SW, et al: Structured Interview for Prodromal Syndromes. New Haven, CT, Yale School of Medicine, 2003

Miklowitz DJ, Strachan AM, Goldstein MJ, et al: Expressed emotion and communication deviance in the families of schizophrenics. J Abnorm Psychol 95:60–66, 1986

Miklowitz DJ, Goldstein MJ, Nuechterlein KH, et al: Family factors and the course of bipolar affective disorder. Arch Gen Psychiatry 45:225–231, 1988

Miklowitz DJ, Velligan DI, Goldstein MJ, et al: Communication deviance in families of schizophrenic and manic patients. J Abnorm Psychol 100:163–173, 1991

Patterson GR: The aggressive child: victim and architect of a coercive system, in Behavior Modification in Families, I: Theory and Research. Edited by Handy L. New York, Brunner/Mazel, 1976

Patterson P, Birchwood M, Cochrane R: Preventing the entrenchment of high expressed emotion in first episode psychosis: early developmental attachment pathways. Aust N Z J Psychiatry 34(suppl):S191–S197, 2000

Plomin R, Daniels D: Why are children in the same family so different from one another. Behav Brain Sci 10:1–60, 1987

Post RM: Transduction of psychosocial stress into the neurobiology of recurrent affective disorder. Am J Psychiatry 149:999–1010, 1992

Reiss D: Child effects on family systems: behavioral genetic strategies, in Children's Influence on Family Dynamics: The Neglected Side of Family Relationships. Edited by Booth A. Mahwah, NJ, Lawrence Erlbaum Associates, 2003

Reiss D, Neiderhiser JM, Heatherington EM, et al: The Relationship Code: Deciphering Genetic and Social Influences on Adolescent Development. Cambridge, MA, Harvard University Press, 2000, pp 3–25

Singer MT, Wynne LC: Schizophrenics, families and communication disorders, in Research in the Schizophrenic Disorders: The Stanley R. Dean Award Lectures. Edited by Cancro R, Dean SR. New York, Spectrum Publications, 1985, pp 231–247

Sporn AL, Greenstein DK, Gogtay N, et al: Progressive brain volume loss during adolescence in childhood-onset schizophrenia. Am J Psychiatry 160:2181–2189, 2003

Stirling J, Tantam D, Thomas P, et al: Expressed emotion and early onset schizophrenia: a one year follow-up. Psychol Med 21:675–685, 1991

Strachan AM, Feingold D, Goldstein MJ, et al: Is expressed emotion an index of a transactional process? II: patient's coping style. Fam Process 28:169–181, 1989

Tienari P, Wynne LC, Moring J, et al: The Finnish adoptive family study of schizophrenia: implications for family research. Br J Psychiatry 164 (suppl 23):20–26, 1994

Tienari PA, Wynne LC, Sorri A, et al: Genotype-environment interaction in schizophrenia-spectrum disorder. Br J Psychiatry 184:216–222, 2004

Wagener DK, Hogarty GE, Goldstein MJ, et al: Information processing and communication deviance in schizophrenic patients and their mothers. Psychiatry Res 18:365–377, 1986

Woo SM, Goldstein MJ, Nuechterlein KH: Relatives' affective style and the expression of subclinical psychopathology in patients with schizophrenia. Fam Process 43:233–247, 2004

Wynne L: Current concepts about schizophrenics and family relationships. J Nerv Ment Dis 169:82–89, 1981

Wynne LC, Singer MT, Bartko JJ, et al: Schizophrenics and their families: research on parental communication, in Developments in Psychiatry Research. Edited by Tanner JM. London, England, Hodder & Stoughton, 1977, pp 254–286

Zubin J, Spring B: Vulnerability: a new view of schizophrenia. J Abnorm Psychol 86:103–126, 1977

Zubin J, Steinhauer SR, Condray R: Vulnerability to relapse in schizophrenia. Br J Psychiatry 161 (suppl 18):13–18, 1992

CHAPTER 6

GENETIC STRATEGIES FOR DELINEATING RELATIONAL TAXONS

Origins, Outcomes, and Relation to Individual Psychopathology

David Reiss, M.D.
Marianne Z. Wamboldt, M.D.

DSM-IV (American Psychiatric Association 1994) (and its text revision, DSM-IV-TR [American Psychiatric Association 2000]) has become an international standard for psychiatric nosology. The growing success of its evolving taxonomy derives from the breadth of the consensus process used to develop it and its predecessors DSM-III and DSM-III-R (American Psychiatric Association 1980, 1987). It also reflects an increasing body of research on its reliability and validity. However, recent reviews suggest at least three important limitations. First, the current taxonomy is defined only by the behavior, thoughts, and feelings of individuals; it does not reflect distinctive underlying pathogenic mechanisms. Second, it is a limited guide to treatment. Some discriminations are useful for pharmacological treatment, but none provide guidance for psychological treatments. Third, DSM-IV provides no guidance for prevention of disorders. We show that adding data on a patient's relationships can address all three of these limitations. We summarize here data with a surprising tool: behavioral genetics. This tool has been used to link more firmly the DSM taxonomy of individual behavior to pathogenesis, treatment, and prevention. It is equally valid to clarify how including relational data in the taxonomy can advance the same three aims.

Fundamental Strategies for Validating the DSM Taxonomy

Genetic strategies for validating the DSM taxonomy are part of a broader and collective scientific enterprise for validating existing taxons or revising them when required. We review those strategies here, as they have been applied to individual behavior, and summarize the role of genetics for each of them. There are no essential differences in how genetics can be applied to relational data, such as adult-partner or caregiver-child relationships, to help delineate valid and useful taxons.

RELIABILITY

The cornerstone of any strategy for validation is the *reliability* of the assessment of individuals by which they are placed in taxons. Thus, it is important to emphasize that the reliability of portions of the DSM taxonomy for adults has been assessed mostly under rigorously controlled research conditions via carefully structured, standardized diagnostic interviews. Under these conditions, many of DSM-IV's adult taxons have shown adequate interrater reliability (Blais et al. 1999; Hilsenroth et al. 2004; Keller et al. 1995; Todd et al. 2003; Zanarini et al. 2000). Reliability poses a more difficult problem for childhood taxons. Children have developmental limitations on their ability to adequately describe their internal state, on their memory of salient events and sequences, and on their ability to put their own experiences and behaviors in a context of normative behaviors.

VALIDITY

Classificatory Validity

In evaluating the DSM taxonomy, three approaches to *validity* have been used. The first, *classificatory validity* (Robins and Guze 1970), evaluates taxons before a clear cause or pathogenesis for the disorder taxon is understood and relies on straightforward clinical observation: what are the current signs and symptoms of patient suffering, what are the long-term consequences of this suffering, what patterns of behavior typically precede this suffering, and what clinical observations can be made in family members?

In establishing classificatory validity, four questions must be answered. First, can members of the same taxon be readily distinguished from members in descriptively similar taxons? For example, atypical and typical depression can be reliably distinguished by increased appetite, food consumption, and the body mass index in the former. Second, do members of the same taxon have, without treatment, a common fate? For example, Kendler and colleagues (1996) reported that atypical depression tends to recur in the same form in subsequent episodes, whereas the common fate of patients in the endogenous subtype taxon has not fared as well, showing less stability of form across recurrences in contiguous episodes or noncontiguous episodes (Coryell et al. 1994; Young et al. 1987). Third, does a common set of precursors of the taxon exist? Preliminary data suggest that certain temperament and personality features (sensitivity to rejection by others, social phobia, and avoidant personality disorder) coexist with (and may precede) atypical depression in contrast to other subtypes of depression (Alpert et al. 1997; Kendler et al. 1996; Parker et al. 2002). Fourth, can family history also estimate homogeneity of characteristics of individuals assigned to taxons?: bipolar disorder is found with increased frequency in family members of patients with atypical depression (Benazzi 2003), raising the question of whether atypical depression is a variant of bipolar or mood disorders.

Pathogenic Validity

A second approach to assessment of validity is *pathogenic validity*. Do patients in the same taxon share a common etiology for their disorder? Here, studies of pathogenesis and current taxonomy are an ungainly fit. For example, Charney and colleagues (2002) noted the following:

> At the risk of making an overly broad status of neurobiological investigations of the major psychiatric disorders…it can be concluded that the field of psychiatry has thus far failed to identify a single neurobiological phenotypic marker or gene that is useful in making a diagnosis of a major psychiatric disorder or for predicting response to psychopharmacologic treatment. (p. 33)

One productive strain of combined taxonomic and pathogenic research has been to identify more unitary psychological components among the complex, polythetic psychiatric taxons. The hope is that these might be more securely linked to neurobiological systems and become the building block for a more valid taxonomy. These efforts typically go beyond clinical description and involve standardized psychological testing or biological assessments. For example, the well-established Five-Factor Model of personality consists of five continuous dimensions that can make clear distinctions among all 10 DSM-IV personality disorders (B.P. O'Connor and Dyce 1998). As much as the psychological components of personality are precursors to atypical depression, understanding these aspects of personality helps define pathogenesis of atypical depression.

Utilization Validity

A third approach for evaluating taxons may be called *utilization validity*, as outlined by First and colleagues (2004). The fundamental question here is whether use of a taxon leads to measurable improvement in the assessment or treatment of patients within the taxon. One example is bipolar II disorder, a new taxon in DSM-IV. The careful delineation of hypomanic episodes in this disorder has led to revised treatment protocols, which include the addition of mood stabilizers, with beneficial results (Kahn et al. 1996).

Genetic Strategies for Validating and Revising Taxons of Individual Behavior

Two major genetic techniques have been used to validate and revise DSM taxons. The first, *quantitative behavioral genetics,* uses twin and adoption studies to draw inferences about differences among individuals of their entire genome—*genotypic differences.* More recently, several techniques converged in identifying individual differences in biochemical structure of well-identified genes; these differences are termed *polymorphisms* or *alleles,* and the focus of this work is on *allelic differences* among individuals. We illustrate here how each technique has been used to validate or suggest revisions of existing taxons and then, in the final sections, how similar techniques are currently being used with relational data.

GENETIC ANALYSIS OF TAXONS: GENERAL CONCEPTS

Most readers are familiar with how inferences are drawn from twin and adoption data to distinguish genetic influences and environmental influences. For example, if we find that monozygotic (MZ) twins' correlation on a measure of depression is 0.70 and that of dizygotic (DZ) twins is 0.40, we can estimate the heritability of depression at 60% ($2 \times [0.70 - 0.40]$), meaning that—in some way—individual genotypic differences in the population sampled account for 60% of individual differences. We also can estimate sibling-specific environmental influences at 30% ($1.00 - 0.70$); these include experiences that are unique for each sibling as well as measurement error. The remainder of influence must be attributable to environments shared by twins; in this example, and in most studies, it is small: 10%. Reiss et al. (2000) has reviewed comprehensively the many assumptions of these analyses.

   An extension of the behavioral genetic approach enables us to compute the role of genetic and environmental factors in the covariance between two or more variables. For example, to determine how much common or joint genetic influences account for the comorbidity of depression and generalized anxiety disorder (GAD), we would correlate the depression score of one twin with the anxiety score of the cotwin. If these *cross-correlations* were higher for MZ twins than for DZ twins, we would infer that a common set of genes—influencing both depression and anxiety—accounts substantially for their comorbidity. The use of cross-correlations and multivariate genetic analysis has proven an important tool in taxometric analyses (see Reiss et al. 2000 for a complete review of these techniques).

GENETIC ANALYSIS OF TAXONS: CLASSIFICATORY VALIDITY

Behavioral genetic analyses have been used to test the boundaries or discriminability of taxons. For example, Kendler et al. (1995) used multivariate genetic techniques to distinguish among five syndromes in women: phobias, GAD, panic disorders, bulimia, and major depression. With the use of these multivariate methods, they found genetic influences common to phobias, panic disorders, and bulimia and a second set of genetic influences common to GAD and major depression, suggesting that two distinct underlying genetic or neurobiological mechanisms account for five taxonomically distinct disorders (Kendler et al. 1995). Here, a genetic analysis validated some boundaries in the existing taxonomy, particularly the distinctions between phobias and panic disorders on the one hand and generalized anxiety and depression on the other. It also opens the possibility for revising taxon definitions by emphasizing the overlap, for example, between GAD and major depression. However, because these findings provide so little concrete evidence about the specific genetic or neurobiological mechanisms involved in these discriminations, this finding may be thought of as providing more pointed information on the classificatory validity of these taxons.

As we have noted, a critical analysis of common fate is whether patients grouped in a taxonomy on the basis of the manifestations of its initial occurrence have a common fate in the persistence or recurrence of that disorder over time. Kendler et al. (1993b) analyzed the persistence or recurrence of major depressive disorder over a 1-year period in a large sample of female twins in mid adulthood. They found that genetic factors accounted for the entire covariance of depression scores in these women from the first observation to the second. The findings were different for women whose status had changed over time (i.e., women who were not depressed initially but became so or those who were depressed and then recovered). These changes were accounted for by twin-specific environmental influences present at the second time but not at the first time (Kendler et al. 1993b). Indeed, in midlife, the genetic factors do not change at all across a year's span. Genetic analysis here adds to conventional common fate analyses by suggesting that a remarkable stability of an underlying genetic or neurobiological process accounts for the common fate of members of the taxon. Because a finding of this kind strongly encourages a search for this stable process that maintains a well-specified taxon, it argues for keeping the taxon in place while the search is on.

Genetic analyses also help delineate common origins of a taxon. Again, we turn to major depressive disorder and the work of Kendler et al. (1993a), who explored the relation between the personality trait of neuroticism (high emotional reactivity) and subsequent depression. They found that the covariance between the two is attributable almost entirely to genetic factors (Kendler et al. 1993a). A similar finding has been obtained for the covariance of neuroticism and GAD (Hettema et al. 2004). Taken together, these data enhance the descriptive validity of internalizing disorders in adult life: GAD and major depressive disorder share genetic influences that first manifest as neuroticism. However, unspecified environmental influences determine whether this premorbid condition becomes GAD or major depressive disorder.

GENETIC ANALYSIS OF TAXONS: PATHOGENIC VALIDITY

Genetic analyses have begun to delineate suggested revisions of taxons that might yield a clearer picture of pathogenesis. Molecular genetic studies would appear to have particular promise here, particularly if the neuroregulatory function of the genes is well understood and connections are established between that function and problem behavior. For example, executive functioning is impaired in several psychiatric conditions. At its simplest, executive functioning requires individuals to hold in memory a particular stimulus and *delay* a response until a second suitable stimulus appears. Importantly, success in this fundamental psychological task requires adequate levels of dopamine in the dorsolateral prefrontal cortex, and these levels are largely under the control of a single gene, the COMT (catechol-*O*-methyltransferase) gene, with two common variants: one that rapidly metabolizes dopamine and is associated with diminished executive functioning and one that allows for adequate levels of dopamine to accumulate and, as a consequence, is associated with competent executive functioning (Akil et al. 2003; Goldberg et al. 2003; Ono et al. 2004; Rosa et al. 2004; Strobel et al. 2003). Thus, variants of the COMT gene that lead to reduced dopamine in the dorsolateral prefrontal cortex have been associated with vulnerability to schizophrenia, suicide completion in males, and impairments in executive functioning in the velocardiofacial syndrome; similarly, these COMT gene variants have been found in children without psychiatric disorders and siblings of schizophrenic patients. In the latter two, it may represent a vulnerability to preventable major mental illness.

GENETIC ANALYSES OF TAXONS: UTILIZATION VALIDITY

In general, genetics has contributed little to utilization validity, although it remains an important standard and guide for current research. However, in numerous areas of research, this possibility may soon materialize. For example, pharmacogenetics is beginning to identify genetic variations in medication responses (e.g., Baumann et al. 2004), which may help clinicians to select the appropriate medication for a particular patient. Although the genetic basis of enzymatic differences is not a direct taxon of diagnosis, it may be a useful adjunctive piece of information to be "coded" in DSM as a specifier for the major disorder because it may help direct treatment planning.

Genetic Strategies for Delineating Relational Disorders

CAN RELATIONSHIPS BE PHENOTYPES?

As we have shown, genetic analyses are useful in clarifying individual disorders with at least two starting points. First, they can analyze the similarity (concordance) of taxon assignment in genetically related individuals. The phenotype here is defined by the consensus process and empirical research supporting the DSM taxonomy. Genetic analysis can also point to revising taxons—as in the case of common genetic origins for GAD and major depressive disorder—or it can help to define simpler dimensions of behavior that are more closely tied to well-delineated genetic or neurobiological systems. Some additional complexities exist for relational disorders. Although DSM-IV includes several categories of relational problems that may be considered relational taxons (e.g., the V code of "parent-child relational problem"), they are not currently defined with much precision. This is because of a lack of an authoritative consensus process within the DSM consortium for relational problems, even though we have many excellent clinical studies of dimensions of caregiver-child and adult-partner relationships.

Another possible impediment to genetic research on relationship disorders is that the use of a relationship as a phenotype is novel, particularly in human, clinical genetic research. It is perhaps easier to accept that an individual's *perceptions* of relationships are genetically influenced; negative perceptions of this kind are an integral part of personality disorders. In fact, many twin and sibling studies confirmed that one's perceptions of relationships with a parent or with one's family show notable genetic influence (e.g., Plomin et al. 1988; Rowe 1983). Not surprisingly, these genetic influences on perceived relationships reflect genetic influences on personality. For example, an adult's remembered warmth in relationship to parents during childhood and adolescence can be attributed in part to genetic influences on the adult's current personality traits of optimism, low aggression, and good humor (Lichtenstein et al. 2003).

It is more difficult to conceive that genetic factors would influence the observed behavior of an individual in a particular relationship (e.g., variation in marital conflict). Many interpersonal theories regard the patterns and dynamics of relationships as prepotent, muting the contributions of individual heritable factors to relationship patterns (e.g., Gottman 1994). Even those who might grant the possibility that heritable factors might have some influence on how a target individual behaves with a specific other would be surprised to see that the genotype of the target individual could have profound and systematic effects on how the other responds to the target. Indeed, data are accumulating that genetic factors do influence marital relationships; genetic influences on the risk for divorce are substantial, as suggested by greater concordance for divorce among MZ than among DZ twins (McGue and Lykken 1992). Reiss and colleagues' "Twin Moms" study has shown genetic influences on marital satisfaction as reported by both the wife's (whose own genes may influence her perception) and the husband's reports of marital satisfaction. These data indicate that genetically influenced personality traits may result in a person being a more or less satisfactory spouse, yet they also imply that the genetic traits in one spouse set up a predictable relationship pattern that affects the nongenetically related spouse's satisfaction with the relationship

(Spotts et al. 2004a, 2004b). However, given that the proposition that both care-giver-child and adult-partner relationships are legitimate phenotypes remains controversial, the tools of quantitative and molecular genetics can be deployed to clarify, elaborate, and validate dimensions relevant to a taxonomy of relationships for DSM-V.

CLASSIFICATORY VALIDITY OF RELATIONAL TAXONS

We use as an example parent-child conflict, which currently would be coded in DSM-IV as the V code parent-child relational problem. Beach et al. (Chapter 1, this volume) reviewed good clinical evidence for the importance of this dimension for individual child and adolescent development and for the suffering of both parents and children who show very high levels of conflict. The Nonshared Environment in Adolescent Development (NEAD) study (T.G. O'Connor et al. 1995; Reiss et al. 2000), a comprehensive genetic analysis of this relational problem, used a unique design that included twins, full and half siblings, and genetically unrelated siblings in stepfamilies. The NEAD study found that heritabilities were greater than 50% for parent-child conflict, as measured by a combination of child report, parent report, and direct, in-home observation earlier in adolescence (mean age of child = 12.8 years) and again 3 years later. Therefore, the heritable characteristics of the child evoked parental conflict. Not only was parent-child conflict seen as a discrete aspect of parent-adolescent relationships, but also the genetic analyses could discern the boundaries or *discriminability* of this dimension of parent-child relationship pattern from others. As might be expected, parent-child conflict was inversely correlated with parent-child warmth and positively correlated with each parent's unsuccessful attempts to control his or her child. However, for both mothers and fathers, the genetic influences on conflict were quite distinct from those on warmth and attempted control. This finding is analogous to the distinctive genetic influences on panic and GAD reported by Kendler and colleagues (1995; see subsection, "Genetic Analysis of Taxons: Classificatory Validity" earlier in chapter). These findings suggest that distinctive heritable characteristics of children that evoke conflict and inadequate control from both mothers and fathers delineate parent-child conflict from other qualities of the parent-child relationship.

Reiss and colleagues (2000) also found almost complete overlap in the genetic influences on mother-child conflict as on father-child conflict, suggesting that the same heritable feature in children activates conflict with both parents. The story was entirely different for warmth: although increased parent-child conflict was associated with decreased warmth, little or no overlap in genetic influences on paternal and on maternal warmth was seen. Furthermore, distinctive heritable characteristics in the adolescent evoked warmth in fathers and in mothers.

Taken together, these findings already suggest that descriptors can be more specific in parent-child relational problem. Parent-child conflict can be treated as a unitary and distinct dimension of parent-child relationships shaped substantially by evocative influences of the child. This inference was reinforced by the Twin Moms study: mothers' genes had no measurable influence on observed conflict with their adolescents or conflict as reported by their children when measures identical to those used in the NEAD study were used (Neiderhiser et al. 2004). Thus, parent-child conflict emerges as a dimension of parent-child relationships whose strongest determinants are genetic or neurobiological processes in the child.

Are There Similar Outcomes for Parent-Child Conflict?

Genetic analysis also can be applied to follow-up data on relational problems. Three genetically informed studies have followed up children and adolescents over time. Reiss et al. (2000) showed that, similar to depression in adults (see "Genetic Analysis of Taxons: Classificatory Validity" earlier in this chapter), genetic factors in the child explain almost all of the stability of parent-child conflict across time, reinforcing the view that stable genetic or neurobiological processes in the child are central to parent-child conflict in adolescence. Importantly, the results are just the reverse for parental warmth and unsuccessful control of their children. Continuity across time is influenced primarily by environmental factors common to both siblings—most likely, dynamics of the entire family system. This view is supported by the fact that the substantial correlation between the mother's and the father's warmth is also accounted for by shared environment (and not influenced by heritable characteristics of the child). The same is true for the relations between parental warmth and sibling warmth. Combining a common-fate analysis of three dimensions of parent-adolescent relationships, along with additional genetically informed data about the relationships of subsystems in the family, provides additional evidence for the distinct genetic underpinnings of conflict in sharp contrast to other features of family life.

Are There Similar Precursors for Parent-Child Relationships High in Conflict?

Three different genetically informed studies converge to identify a common origin for parent-child negativity and conflict; these studies delineate particular heritable traits that precede and probably evoke severe parental responses. Adoption designs provide the most critical information. Investigators observe the relation between behavioral characteristics of birth parents and parental responses of adoptive parents to the child adopted at birth. When investigators control for intrauterine exposure to parental substance use and maternal stress, this design provides the most stringent tests for the role of evocative processes in genetic influences on parenting. These designs also provide clues as to what heritable properties in children evoked the parental responses.

Two adoption studies showed a substantial correlation between antisocial and impulsive behavior in birth parents and harsh, negative parental behavior toward adoptive children. Moreover, these studies identified heritable aggressive and anti-social behavior in the child as the evocative agent (Ge et al. 1996; T.G. O'Connor et al. 1998). These findings were recently confirmed in a large twin study that also identified antisocial and defiant behavior as likely to be evocative of harsh parenting (Jaffee et al. 2004).

Are There Similar Patterns in the Family History of Those in a Relational Taxon?

Studies of human families suggest that parent-child conflict, as well other adverse parenting practices, has family history. Parents who treat their children with hostility and aggression were themselves treated in similar fashion when they were children. Recent findings have documented this continuity with direct observations of grandparent-parent interactions with follow-up a generation later to observe parent-child relational patterns (Conger et al. 2003). Because the human genetic studies discussed earlier have suggested that the offspring's genes influence the harshness of the parent's behavior toward him or her, one might expect that intergenerational transmission of harsh parenting would be partially accounted for by genetic transmission. However, this hypothesis has been tested only in animal models and only with parental behaviors of nurturance, not harshness. We refer to the work by Francis et al. (1999) illuminating the etiological inputs to maternal caregiving behavior in two genetically different strains of rats, one with high nurturing maternal behaviors and the other with reliably lower levels of these behaviors. These investigators used a cross-fostering paradigm, whereby offspring from "high-nurturant" mothers were cross-fostered with "low-nurturant" mothers, and vice versa. Francis et al. reported that the offspring's subsequent nurturing behavior toward his or her own offspring (i.e., third generation) was primarily a result of nongenomic behavioral experiences early in life. In other words, clearly, a "familial" transmission of a relationship pattern (i.e., patterns of high or low nurturing maternal behavior) occurred, and that pattern was transmitted by primarily nongenetic avenues. Studies in humans may allow discrimination between genetically influenced parenting practices (e.g., harshness and poor monitoring) and nongenetically influenced parenting practices (e.g., warmth and nurturance).

PATHOGENIC VALIDITY OF RELATIONAL DIMENSIONS

Thus far, genetic research has yielded little in the way of pathogenic markers that correspond to discrete individual diagnoses or taxons. Some (Charney et al. 2002) have used this fact to suggest that the current taxons are not accurately reflecting the underlying pathogenic mechanisms and may need to be reconsidered from a perspective of pathogenic etiologies. Use of genetics to understand relational patterns is at an early stage in development but may offer paradigms that will be more useful in understanding the genetic bases of behavioral variations. Genetic analyses play a central role in this research in two ways. First, they clarify the role of specific relational processes in *mediating* genetic influences on the development of psychopathology. That is, heritable traits in children, adolescents, and adults evoke responses from the environment that make them vulnerable to psychopathology. As a consequence, these relational factors are integral to the evolution of psychopathology, and as DSM moves toward a pathogenesis-based taxonomy, these relational processes may become central ways of characterizing illness. Second, relational processes also *moderate* genetic influences: under favorable environmental circumstances, genetic risks for major mental disorders may never be expressed. These relational processes should take center stage as DSM evolves in taxonomy relevant not only for treatment of established disorders but also for identification of treatable prodromal conditions, as well as for reduction of well-specified relational risk factors in individuals who show no clear signs of illness yet.

Relationships as Mediators of Genetic Expression

The evidence for specific relationships within the family mediating a genetic vulnerability toward pathology is strongest for adolescent antisocial behavior and derives from two twin studies and two adoption studies. The NEAD study examined cross-lagged correlations comparing parent-child negativity in earlier adolescence with the development of significant antisocial behavior 3 years later, as well as the correlation of earlier antisocial behavior with parent-child negativity in later adolescence. The NEAD study found that the former relation exceeded substantially the latter one and that the cross-lagged correlations were attributable primarily to genetic influence common to *earlier* conflict and *later* antisocial behavior. This outcome suggests that heritable characteristics of the child—perhaps aggressive or oppositional behavior, as suggested earlier—evoked parent-child conflict, which, over time, amplified the child's behavior difficulties into notable antisocial behavior (Reiss et al. 2000). The Minnesota Twin Family Study found similar results in a younger sample, although genetic factors played a less important role, and environmental factors were more important in the cross-lagged analyses (Burt et al. 2003).

The NEAD and Minnesota findings are buttressed by data from two adoption studies already cited (Ge et al. 1996; T. G. O'Connor et al. 1998). Although these studies used different statistical techniques, both studies suggested reciprocal influences of genetically influenced evocative effects of the child on harsh parenting and a reciprocal effect of that harsh parenting on subsequent externalizing behavior in children and adolescents. Child-evoked parent-child conflict may mediate some forms of a disorder but not others. In the domain of substance abuse, this possibility is suggested by Cadoret et al.'s (1996) findings on two pathways that link parental and child disorder: in one pathway, the genetic influences are mediated by childhood aggression, but in the other they are not. To return to relational mediation of genetic influences, if this occurs in only some forms of a disorder, then relational factors are a crucial specifier of the disorder and help to define a more homogeneous subtype. If the relational mediator is essential for all or most cases, it must be included in the description of the disorder.

Relational Factors That Moderate Genetic Expression

Ample evidence now indicates that adverse family relationships moderate the expression of genetic influence both in conduct disorders and in depression. Among the strongest findings are from adoption and twin investigations of the interaction of the entire genotype with adverse family relationships. For example, Cadoret et al. (1996) studied adopted women with and without birth parents with alcoholism. These women had highly variable adoptive experiences—from those whose adoptive parents had severe psychopathology, marital difficulties, and legal problems to those who had none of these problems. Women developed depression only when the biological risk factors combined with an adverse rearing environment (Cadoret et al. 1996). Cadoret and colleagues showed the same type of interaction in the genesis of aggressivity and conduct disorders in both boys and girls: these disorders appeared only in the joint presence of an adverse adoptive rearing environment (assessed as in the depression study) and biological risk indexed by severe antisocial personality disorder or alcoholism in the birth parents. These studies provide some epidemiological clues as to which interpersonal familial patterns may be protective of an at-risk genetic vulnerability and which may amplify the at-risk genetic profile into disorder status. The more specific relational patterns may be noted as relational risk clusters for the development of a specific disorder, when both relational and biological risk factors may be necessary for disorder.

Two recent studies permit a clearer view of critical features of adverse relationship patterns. Button and colleagues (2005) studied gene–environment interaction in the development of conduct problems in children. Genetic influence was estimated directly from comparisons between MZ and DZ twins, and a continuous measure of family problem-solving skills, communication, and support was tested for its interaction with these genetic estimates. They found substantial interaction between genetic and family process variables in the prediction of severe conduct problems in both boys and girls (Button et al. 2005). Even more specific are recent reports by Tienari and colleagues (2004) on gene–environment interaction in schizophrenia with an adoption design. Genetic risk was defined by maternal schizophrenia. Children adopted from these mothers developed schizophrenia or schizophrenia spectrum disorders only if the rearing environment showed high levels of conflict, restricted affect, and poor definition of individual responsibilities and parental leadership (Tienari et al. 2004).

GENETIC ANALYSES AND UTILIZATION VALIDITY

As we have noted, the current DSM system is useless for prevention. However, data we have presented suggest the utility of genetic analyses of relational processes. Recall the data on how family conflict and restriction of affect enhance risk for schizophrenia, but only in genetically vulnerable individuals. Indeed, these specific types of relational patterns may be modifiers of equally specific neurobiological mechanisms, and the interaction between the two may determine whether the individual develops schizophrenia. For example, as we have noted, an allele of the COMT gene is associated with reduced executive functioning. Recently, a locus on chromosome 15 has been associated with a similar psychological deficit: impaired sensory gating, or the inability to resist distracting stimuli. A distinctive neurobiological mechanism is almost certainly involved because this defect is associated with a specific electroencephalogram abnormality: diminished inhibition of the P50 evoked response (Freedman et al. 2003). In DSM-V, the description of schizophrenia might include a section on risk clusters that suggest high vulnerability to the disorder and the need for prevention services. According to current evidence, the cluster would include restricted affect, conflict and poor intergenerational boundaries in the family, *and* deficits in executive functioning and sensory gating.

Conclusion

We have discussed two ways in which genetic analyses can help to establish the role of relationship patterns in a psychiatric taxonomy: 1) relationship dimensions as mediators, which would lead to relationship variables as specifiers of or in the description of disorders, and 2) relationship patterns as moderators, which may lead to description of relational risk clusters for development of disorders.

We described in detail the relational pattern of adolescent-parent conflict, which seems to be driven primarily by the heritable traits of the adolescent, yet needs parental willingness to be involved with reactions of hostility and poor control of child's behavior. This pattern had clear precursors, as well as consistent course over time without treatment. It could be seen as a disorder in its own right, because of the mental anguish and poor outcomes associated with it, or it could be seen as a relationship that mediates the genetic vulnerability for conduct disorder and augments the likelihood that conduct disorder will develop. In DSM-V, parent-child conflict may become a key item in the definition of conduct disorder, to note more clearly the critical role of this pattern in the development of the disorder and the need for a treatment plan to intervene with the pattern.

Genetic analyses also can help in elaborating how relational patterns may be pathogenically involved in the moderation of individual disorders, thus noting the utility for the proper measurement and assessment of relational patterns as specifiers of individual taxons (e.g., a family interactional pattern of diffuse responsibilities and high conflict as being a specifier in the individual diagnosis of schizophrenia). Schizophrenic illness may occur without this risk cluster, and noting it may help to differentiate among the many pathways to the final outcome of schizophrenia, as well as indicate therapeutic approaches that are necessary for that particular individual. Encouraging relationship assessments may stimulate new models of thinking about these conditions that may prove helpful in advancing our ability to provide both more specific prevention and intervention.

References

Akil M, Kolachana BS, Rothmond DA: Catechol-O-methyltransferase genotype and dopamine regulation in the human brain. J Neurosci 23:2008–2013, 2003

Alpert JE, Uebelacker LA, McLean NE, et al: Social phobia, avoidant personality disorder and atypical depression: co-occurrence and clinical implications. Psychol Med 27:627–633, 1997

American Psychiatric Association: Diagnostic and Statistical Manual of Mental Disorders, 3rd Edition. Washington, DC, American Psychiatric Association, 1980

American Psychiatric Association: Diagnostic and Statistical Manual of Mental Disorders, 3rd Edition, Revised. Washington, DC, American Psychiatric Association, 1987

American Psychiatric Association: Diagnostic and Statistical Manual of Mental Disorders, 4th Edition. Washington, DC, American Psychiatric Association, 1994

American Psychiatric Association: Diagnostic and Statistical Manual of Mental Disorders, 4th Edition, Text Revision. Washington, DC, American Psychiatric Association, 2000

Baumann P, Hiemke C, Ulrich S, et al: The AGNP-TDM expert group consensus guidelines: therapeutic drug monitoring in psychiatry. Pharmacopsychiatry 37:243–265, 2004

Benazzi F: The symptoms of atypical depression. Can J Psychiatry 48:350–351, 2003

Blais MA, Hilsenroth MJ, Fowler J: Diagnostic efficiency and hierarchical functioning of the DSM-IV borderline personality disorder criteria. J Nerv Ment Dis 187:167–173, 1999

Burt SA, Krueger RF, McGue M, et al: Parent-child conflict and the comorbidity among childhood externalizing disorders. Arch Gen Psychiatry 60:505–513, 2003

Button TM, Scourfield J, Martin N, et al: Family dysfunction interacts with genes in the causation of antisocial symptoms. Behav Genet 35:115–120, 2005

Cadoret RJ, Winokur G, Langbehn D, et al: Depression spectrum disease, I: the role of gene-environment interaction. Am J Psychiatry 153:892–899, 1996

Charney DS, Barlow DH, Botteron K, et al: Neuroscience research agenda to guide development of a pathophysiologically based classification system, in A Research Agenda for DSM-V. Edited by Kupfer DJ, First MB, Regier DA. Washington, DC, American Psychiatric Association, 2002, pp 31–83

Conger RD, Neppl T, Kim KJ, et al: Angry and aggressive behavior across three generations: a prospective, longitudinal study of parents and children. J Abnorm Child Psychol 31:143–160, 2003

Coryell W, Winokur G, Shea T, et al: The long-term stability of depressive subtypes. Am J Psychiatry 151:199–204, 1994

First MB, Pincus HA, Levine JB, et al: Clinical utility as a criterion for revising psychiatric diagnoses. Am J Psychiatry 161:946–954, 2004

Francis D, Diorio J, Liu D, et al: Nongenomic transmission across generations of maternal behavior and stress response in the rat. Science 286:1155–1158, 1999

Freedman R, Olincy A, Ross RG, et al: The genetics of sensory gating deficits in schizophrenia. Curr Psychiatry Rep 5:155–161, 2003

Ge X, Conger RD, Cadoret RJ, et al: The developmental interface between nature and nurture: a mutual influence model of child antisocial behavior and parent behaviors. Dev Psychol 32:574–589, 1996

Goldberg TE, Egan MF, Gscheidle T, et al: Executive subprocesses in working memory: relationship to catechol-O-methyltransferase Val158Met genotype and schizophrenia. Arch Gen Psychiatry 60:889–896, 2003

Gottman JM: What Predicts Divorce? Hillsdale, NJ, Lawrence Erlbaum Associates, 1994

Hettema JM, Prescott CA, Kendler KS: Genetic and environmental sources of covariation between generalized anxiety disorder and neuroticism. Am J Psychiatry 161:1581–1587, 2004

Hilsenroth MJ, Baity MR, Mooney MA, et al: DSM-IV major depressive episode criteria: an evaluation of reliability and validity across three different rating methods. International Journal of Psychiatry in Clinical Practice 8:3–10, 2004

Jaffee SR, Caspi A, Moffitt TE, et al: The limits of child effects: evidence for genetically mediated child effects on corporal punishment but not on physical maltreatment. Dev Psychol 40:1047–1058, 2004

Kahn DA, Carpenter D, Docherty JP, et al: Treatment of bipolar disorder. J Clin Psychiatry 57 (suppl 12A):3–89, 1996

Keller MB, Klein DN, Hirschfeld RMA, et al: Results of the DSM-IV mood disorders field trial. Am J Psychiatry 152:843–849, 1995

Kendler KS, Neale MC, Kessler RC, et al: A longitudinal twin study of personality and major depression in women. Arch Gen Psychiatry 50:853–862, 1993a

Kendler KS, Neale MC, Kessler RC, et al: A longitudinal twin study of 1-year prevalence of major depression in women. Arch Gen Psychiatry 50:843–852, 1993b

Kendler KS, Walters EE, Neale MC, et al: The structure of the genetic and environmental risk factors for six major psychiatric disorders in women: phobia, generalized anxiety disorder, panic disorder, bulimia, major depression, and alcoholism. Arch Gen Psychiatry 52:374–383, 1995

Kendler KS, Eaves LJ, Walters EE, et al: The identification and validation of distinct depressive syndromes in a population-based sample of female twins. Arch Gen Psychiatry 53:391–399, 1996

Lichtenstein P, Ganiban J, Neiderhiser JM, et al: Remembered parental bonding in adult twins: genetic and environmental influences. Behav Genet 33:397–408, 2003

McGue M, Lykken DT: Genetic influence on risk of divorce. Psychol Sci 3:368–373, 1992

Neiderhiser JM, Reiss D, Pedersen NL, et al: Genetic and environmental influences on mothering of adolescents: a comparison of two samples. Dev Psychol 40:335–351, 2004

O'Connor BP, Dyce JA: A test of models of personality disorder configuration. J Abnorm Psychol 107:3–16, 1998

O'Connor TG, Hetherington EM, Reiss D, et al: A twin-sibling study of observed parent-adolescent interactions. Child Dev 66:812–829, 1995

O'Connor TG, Deater-Deckard K, Fulker D, et al: Genotype-environment correlations in late childhood and early adolescence: antisocial behavioral problems and coercive parenting. Dev Psychol 34:970–981, 1998

Ono H, Shirakawa O, Nushida H, et al: Association between catechol-O-methyltransferase functional polymorphism and male suicide completers. Neuropsychopharmacology 29:1374–1377, 2004

Parker G, Roy K, Mitchell P, et al: Atypical depression: a reappraisal. Am J Psychiatry 159: 1480–1481, 2002

Plomin R, McClearn GE, Pedersen NL, et al: Genetic influence on childhood family environment perceived retrospectively from the last half of the life span. Dev Psychol 24: 738–745, 1988

Reiss D, Neiderhiser J, Hetherington EM, et al: The Relationship Code: Deciphering Genetic and Social Patterns in Adolescent Development. Cambridge, MA, Harvard University Press, 2000

Robins E, Guze SB: Establishment of diagnostic validity in psychiatric illness: its application to schizophrenia. Am J Psychiatry 126:983–986, 1970

Rosa A, Peralta V, Cuesta MJ, et al: New evidence of association between COMT gene and prefrontal neurocognitive function in healthy individuals from sibling pairs discordant for psychosis. Am J Psychiatry 161:1110–1112, 2004

Rowe D: A biometrical analysis of perceptions of family environment: a study of twin and singleton sibling kinships. Child Dev 54:416–423, 1983

Spotts EL, Neiderhiser JM, Ganiban J, et al: Accounting for depressive symptoms in women: a twin study of associations with interpersonal relationships. J Affect Disord 82:101–111, 2004a

Spotts EL, Neiderhiser JM, Towers H, et al: Genetic and environmental influences on marital relationships. J Fam Psychol 18:107–119, 2004b

Strobel A, Lesch KP, Jatzke S, et al: Further evidence for a modulation of novelty seeking by DRD4 exon III, 5-HTTLPR, and COMT val/met variants. Mol Psychiatry 8:371–372, 2003

Tienari P, Wynne LC, Sorri A, et al: Genotype-environment interaction in schizophrenia spectrum disorder. Br J Psychiatry 184:216–222, 2004

Todd RD, Joyner C, Heath AC, et al: Reliability and stability of a semistructured DSM-IV interview designed for family studies. J Am Acad Child Adolesc Psychiatry 42:1460–1468, 2003

Young MA, Keller MB, Lavori PW, et al: Lack of stability of the RDC endogenous subtype in consecutive episodes of major depression. J Affect Disord 12:139–143, 1987

Zanarini MC, Skodol AE, Bender D, et al: The Collaborative Longitudinal Personality Disorders Study: reliability of Axis I and II diagnoses. J Personal Disord 14:291–299, 2000

PART II

ASSESSMENT

CHAPTER 7

CHILDHOOD MALTREATMENT AND ADULT PSYCHOPATHOLOGY

Some Measurement Options

George W. Brown, Ph.D.

Childhood maltreatment can take several forms, including physical or sexual abuse, neglect, and emotional abuse (Garbarino et al. 1986). All can have highly adverse effects on adjustment during childhood and adulthood. Such maltreatment relates to childhood behavior problems, internalizing and externalizing psychopathology (e.g., Cicchetti and Carlson 1989), a variety of adult psychiatric disorders (e.g., Brown 2002a; Craig et al. 1993), and other outcomes such as frequency of medical consultations (Kapur et al. 2004). In this chapter, I comment on some of the measurement options that emerge in the light of the wide-ranging research literature.

Setting the Scene

Two articles based on the New Zealand Dunedin birth cohort illustrate some of the key issues I discuss in this chapter. The first article reported abysmal agreement between adolescent retrospective reports of family life and measures collected dur-

---

This chapter is based on a paper prepared for a Fetzer Institute meeting in Washington, DC, March 24–25, 2005.

ing childhood and concluded by emphasizing the superiority of measures of parental behavior carried out during childhood compared with retrospective reports by older children (Henry et al. 1994). The second article reported that observational measures of parent-child interaction involving rejection and hostile behavior were unrelated to later depression in early adulthood. However, retrospective questioning of adults about unwanted sexual contact before age 11 years did relate to such depression in early adulthood (Jaffe et al. 2002). The authors did not comment, however, how this finding apparently contradicts their earlier conclusion about the shortcomings of retrospective measures (see also Caspi et al. 2005).

In response to such results I will ask in what follows whether retrospective reports are necessarily so inaccurate. How far the disagreement related to how the retrospective material was collected? Why only sexual abuse was considered? And why the observations made in childhood failed to relate to adult depression when there is good reason to expect an association?

Research on Developmental Psychopathology

There has in fact been an overwhelming emphasis in the literature on the study of sexual or physical abuse despite evidence that emotional abuse and neglect may well be the key factors of etiological importance (e.g., Dong et al. 2003; Garbarino and Collins 1999). As a result, a good deal of recent research has overlooked many individuals who have been maltreated and also has failed to document other forms of maltreatment often occurring to children with sexual and physical abuse (Brown 2002a; Fergusson and Mullen 1999).

Often, studies concerned with the long-term effects of family life do not attempt to establish the presence of maltreatment but instead use likely markers of abuse and neglect such as parental discord. These risk indicators are usually based on a simple count of family characteristics, such as discord, poverty, social class, and maternal depression (e.g., Rutter and Quinton 1984), and this has consistently shown associations with child and adolescent outcomes (e.g., Sanson et al. 1991; Williams et al. 1990). However, these associations have not led to convincing causal models of the processes likely to be involved. For this it is essential to deal with the components individually and also acquire detailed information about how parental behavior relates to particular children (Caspi et al. 2004). Without this it has not been possible to explore the implications of the fact that siblings often have different experiences of parental care (J. Dunn and Plomin 1991).

Such failure to identify early maltreatment clearly relates to the practical and legal difficulties of collecting such information during childhood (e.g., Weiss et al. 1992). It also explains why much of the research that has been done has been based on children who have been legally or clinically defined as maltreated. This large body of research has produced many important findings, but it also has had significant limitations. Particularly notable is that children themselves are likely to be highly selected; for example, in the United States, parents often have been involved in substance abuse (M.G. Dunn et al. 2002). There also has been a failure to identify children in comparison series who have experienced maltreatment.

Cut-Points or Correlations?

The use of agency records has understandably accompanied a categorical approach to the measurement of childhood maltreatment. Population studies of maltreatment also have used a similar cut-point approach, usually in the form of a simple dichotomy. By contrast, developmental research and behavioral genetics have been primarily concerned with documenting the full range of parental behavior in ordinary families and typically have used dimensional measures of parental behavior. Nonetheless, it is easy to see what is common in the two approaches—the negative end of the dimension of warmth will probably contribute to a measure of "neglect," and the negative end of the dimension of acceptance will probably contribute to a measure of "emotional abuse," and so on. However, the use of dimensional measures may not disclose very much if the psychosocial origins of psychopathology relate to such extremes (Rutter 1987). Correlations can be expected to be low (Meyer et al. 2000), and Scarr (1992, p. 15) has provocatively concluded, "Ordinary differences between families have little effect on children's development, unless the family is outside the normal developmental range." But, to anticipate my conclusion, the point at issue is not the use of dimensional measures but the danger of using *only* such measures and the variance-based statistics associated with them.

It is now clear that dichotomous measures of maltreatment show substantial associations with adult outcomes. The London (England) Child Experiences of Care and Abuse (CECA) instrument, which uses investigator-based ratings, covers all aspects of childhood maltreatment (Bifulco et al. 1994). The semistructured interview encourages detailed accounts of actual incidents. In a sample of 400 London women, we found that 1 in 5 had experienced significant childhood neglect or abuse according to a simple yes-or-no index (Brown and Moran 1994). This maltreatment was associated with a doubling of the risk for onset of an adult depressive episode. Particularly notable was a fourfold risk that an episode would take a *chronic* course lasting at least 1 year. A second population inquiry involving pairs of adult sisters confirmed these findings (G.W. Brown, T.K. Craig, T.O. Harris, et al.: "A Life-Course Perspective on Chronic Depression, 1: The Role of Parental Maltreatment," manuscript submitted for publication, August 2005). We used an index of maltreatment based on five categories of increasing severity of parental behavior. This showed only a modest increase in risk *within* the three categories used to define maltreatment and none in relation to its two nonmaltreatment categories. To be able to justify the use of such a simple index, we began by using five categories and in doing so accepted the possible importance of dealing with a continuum. As I see it, a decision in this matter should have little to do with whether a case can be made for the presence of a dimension but rather what relates to the outcome of interest: this may be a dichotomy, a trichotomy, or some version of a dimensional measure.

The matter has a further complication. Conclusions about what kind of measure to use may differ for different outcomes. For example, in our current research, our conclusions about the measurement of conduct problems were similar to those for maltreatment. A simple dichotomy was adequate to represent such problems and represented a key mediating factor linking parental maltreatment and adult chronic depression (G.W. Brown, T.K. Craig, T.O. Harris, et al.: "A Life-Course Perspective on Chronic Depression, 3: The Role of Family Wide and Child-Specific Characteristics," manuscript submitted for publication, August 2005). However, another study, which used social achievement as an outcome rather than adult depression, found an index with multiple categories to be relevant (Fergusson and Horwood 1995). There is no reason to doubt the legitimacy of conceiving conduct problems in dimensional terms, but there is equally no point in doing so if a simpler measure is adequate. Indeed, to do so can lead to confusion, including a failure to recognize interactive effects (Brown et al. 1991; Pickles and Angold 2003). Probably for this reason, person-environment interaction has proved to be puzzlingly elusive in developmental and behavioral genetic research (Plomin et al. 1988). As Rutter and Pickles (1991) pointed out, such statistical interactions often apply to small subsections of a population, and it is unwise to restrict attention to effects that hold for the bulk of subjects falling within the "normal" range of a continuous measure. They concluded that in tackling this issue, "the conceptual and statistical tool kit of the epidemiologist can prove more incisive than that of the psychometrician" (Rutter and Pickles 1991, pp. 106–107). Here I suspect the key tool remains that of *cross-tabulation* carried out in an exploratory, but theoretical, mode if this term is used lightly to represent a series of analyses guided by ideas about possible mechanisms. My general conclusion is similar to a few that follow: there is much to be said in our current state of knowledge for use of more than one approach in the same inquiry.

Childhood Maltreatment or Maltreatments?

A related issue is the extent to which different aspects of parental maltreatment can usefully be seen as working together. One way to proceed is to ask how far its components show similar associations with the outcome of interest. My sense of research findings so far has been that overall *severity* of experience has emerged as the key basis for the division between maltreated and nonmaltreated. This is illustrated by the latest research with the CECA instrument. Just three aspects of parental behavior have emerged as of importance for women: a mother's lack of affection, mother's rejection, and father's physical abuse (G.W. Brown, T.K. Craig, T.O. Harris, et al.: "A Life-Course Perspective on Chronic Depression, 1: The Role of Parental Maltreatment," manuscript submitted for publication, August 2005). Such findings illustrate not only the usefulness of an index based on a simple dichotomy but also the possible presence of a core experience common to all aspects of maltreatment, with parental rejection appearing to be a likely candidate (G. W. Brown, T. K. Craig, T. O. Harris, et al.: "A Life-Course Perspective on Chronic Depression, 1: The Role of Parental Maltreatment," manuscript submitted for publication, August 2005).

There are two caveats. The presence of such a core experience is consistent with long-term effects occurring via *different* psychosocial mechanisms. For adult depression, evidence indicates at least two mechanisms. One involves *self concepts* partly influenced by evolutionary evolved systems such as attachment (Bowlby 1969) or submissive responses (Gilbert 2002) that eventually influence a child's ideas about self in a way that can persist into adulthood. Here we have emphasized the importance of feelings of shame and inferiority. A second involves deficits in *self-regulation* that relate to later aggression and hypervigilance and for some a chaotic adult lifestyle (Glaser 2000). A second caveat is that some evidence already shows that sexual abuse may at times have effects that are distinct (Hill et al. 2001; Mullen et al. 1996). Also, some aspects of maltreatment of infants and young children may relate to different outcomes (e.g., Manley et al. 1994). Therefore, one must proceed with both possibilities in mind. And here a relevant feature of the London instrument is its flexibility. The components of the current index of maltreatment can be disaggregated, and the researcher also may take account of other parental behavior such as "role reversal" and "lax supervision," which are not included in the index. My earlier recommendation for the use of more than one approach to measurement is considerably eased by this kind of flexibility.

Retrospective Measurement

A prospective birth cohort design is the approach of choice for tackling many etiological issues in psychiatry, and such birth cohort studies already have contributed significantly to our knowledge (Colman and Jones 2004). However, as discussed earlier, childhood maltreatment has presented particularly difficult problems for this approach, and the strengths of retrospective questioning once children have reached adulthood have been increasingly recognized (e.g., Dadds and Salmon 2003). An obvious bonus is that research questions can be tackled without having to wait until children reach adulthood. (In our latest research, it would have been necessary to wait decades after initial data collection until the children reached at least their mid-30s.) Indeed, one of the problems of large-scale longitudinal research has been that enthusiasm for the methodological payoff of contemporary observation usually has been associated with a failure to invest in the time-consuming business of developing effective ways of collecting data retrospectively in order to establish what has occurred between research contacts in longitudinal studies that can span several years.

Error, of course, is to be expected in retrospective measurement of psychosocial variables. The relevant question is whether this is sufficient to rule out effective research. There is now some reason to believe that intensive interviews and investigator-based ratings are accurate enough for research to proceed. Our own semistructured method of gathering such material can be seen as broadening a purely cognitive approach by the use of autobiographical memory and the emotions such questioning can evoke (e.g., Conway 2001). A recent account of life-course research has gone so far as to argue that only memories that are linked to self through their emotional and motivational significance are truly autobiographical (Bluck and Habermas 2000). By contrast, in the validity study of the Dunedin group, mentioned earlier, only standard questions of the kind "When you were between 7 and 15, how much conflict was there in your family?" were used. This method has proved inadequate for collecting material about adult life events, and it is unlikely to do better when extended into childhood (Brown 1989). An alternative is to use questions, such as "Was the conflict between your parents, or did it involve the children too?"; "Which children?"; "Around what age?"; "How often: more or less than once a week?"; and "Did anyone get physically hurt?" Such questions are used in an attempt to fill out a coherent account. When asking about adult life events via the Life Event and Difficulty Schedule (LEDS), this kind of detailed questioning has aimed to create a coherent "story" and has provided surprisingly stable reports over a period as long as 10 years (Neilson et al. 1989). Evidence also suggests that it can be extended to deal with later childhood and adolescence. As part of a prospective design, Maughan and colleagues (1995) administered such intensive interviews to children in their late 20s and concluded that error came largely from those with adverse childhood experience who *failed* to report such experience as an adult. Retrospective accounts about aversive parental behavior itself appeared to be generally accurate. This also appears to be the conclusion to be drawn about reporting of childhood trauma (McNally 2003).

In the most recent study that used the CECA instrument, different interviewers asked pairs of sisters about their own and the others' experience. Agreement was reasonably high, and the investigators concluded that the material was accurate enough for research to proceed (Bifulco et al. 1997). The association between parental maltreatment and adult chronic depression, although somewhat reduced, also remained substantial when only the account of a paired sister about the subject was used (G. W. Brown, T. K. Craig, T. O. Harris, et al.: "A Life-Course Perspective on Chronic Depression, 2: The Role of Differing Sibling Experience of Parental Maltreatment," manuscript submitted for publication, August 2005).

A Return to the Two Opening Examples

Given that a prima facie case can be made for taking retrospective measurement seriously, there remains the question of why, as noted earlier, observations taken during childhood itself do not necessarily predict adult depression. Several studies hinted that this may relate to shortcomings in measurement. For example, a prospective inquiry of maltreatment (defined by the use of public service records) and outcome in adolescence found that experience in childhood was not predictive of outcome in adolescence (Thornberry et al. 2001). Another prospective study, which used various measures of child-mother relationship before age 6 years, failed to predict adolescent depression in girls (Duggal et al. 2001). One explanation for such negative findings is that *persistence* of maltreatment is critical and that a cross-sectional measure will not necessarily reflect this with sufficient accuracy. Another prospective study, taking account of parental behavior at ages 6, 14, and 16 years, found that the *number* of maladaptive parental behaviors was highly related to psychiatric disorder in late adolescence and early adulthood (Johnson et al. 2001). This study also reported that persistent parental maladaptive behavior was related to a higher risk for psychiatric disorder, although no details were given (Johnson et al. 2001, p. 457). Another study saw families when the children were 5 years old and saw the children again at age 30. Multiple social disadvantages, family instability, and poor parenting were highly related to adult depression (Sadowski et al. 1999). One possibility for this positive result is that these general measures concerning deprivation were related to the likelihood of *subsequent* adversity during childhood.

However, numerous studies of the efficacy of observations of parent-child interaction in shorter-term predictions have been done. Yet the case for the importance of persistence of maltreatment is perhaps strong enough to raise questions about the status of such cross-sectional measures when used for longer-term predictions. For example, expressed emotion measures have proved highly effective in the short-term prediction of the course of several disorders, but these measures may not be as effective in the longer term. The original study that used the return of florid symptomatology in discharged patients with schizophrenia as a criterion of outcome repeated the expressed emotional ratings nearly a year later and found a good deal of change, with a tendency for relatives to make fewer critical comments (Brown et al. 1972). Relatives of patients showing improvement were less likely to have a high expressed emotional rating repeated. Bidirectional effects are therefore indicated, and adverse family behavior is often reversible. For the families of patients with schizophrenia, this may well involve as many as a third of families with high expressed emotion over a period of 1 year (Brown et al. 1972; see also Scazufca and Kuipers 1998).

Although such reversibility may help to explain the modest long-term prediction of cross-sectional measures, it remains relevant to ask about the success of retrospective measures. Paradoxically, one reason may stem from a shortcoming in reporting. My sense of our fairly detailed descriptive data on sister pairs is that in most instances, parental maltreatment had been persistent and had often begun at an early age. If this reasoning is correct, then we may have sometimes missed shorter periods of neglect and abuse. Perhaps a period of marked lack of maternal affection during a period of depression after the children's father had left home, but sandwiched between sustained periods of closeness and warmth, would be less likely to be reported. If so, our informants would be inadvertently correcting a shortcoming in measurement of the child-parent relationship and in doing so enabling it to focus on more persistent maltreatment.

Absolute or Relative Measures?

Another significant issue concerns how parental behavior is to be measured, leaving aside the matter of retrospective reporting. Behavioral genetics has concluded that parents often treat siblings differently, even when they are close in age, and investigators generally agree that "environmental factors important to development are those that two children in a family experience differently" (J. Dunn and Plomin 1991, p. 272). Our recent study of sister pairs found such findings to be equally relevant for the extremes of parental behavior characterized by maltreatment (G.W. Brown, T.K. Craig, T.O. Harris, et al.: "A Life-Course Perspective on Chronic Depression, 2: The Role of Differing Sibling Experience of Parental Maltreatment," manuscript submitted for publication, August 2005).

Although genetic research has carried out direct observation of parents and children usually over a fairly short time (Reiss et al. 1995, 2000), much research has taken an alternative approach that uses perceptions of *differences* in parental treatment. J. Dunn and Plomin (1991) argued that it may be more important that a child is criticized more than his or her siblings than that the overall level of criticism in the home is high. In this context, Rutter (1999, p. 142) has gone so far as to assert that "the concept of some relationship feature such as warmth or criticism or shared parent-child activities being 'high' or 'low' cannot be considered as having any absolute metric." Such assumptions have been built into existing measures by asking questions in comparative terms, such as "Does your mother show more attention to your sister?" (Daniels and Plomin 1985). In other words, measurement has been *relative*, with a focus on who has received more (or less) of a particular parental behavior rather than how much (Jenkins et al. 2003). However, the measures of the London studies that used CECA are, by contrast, *absolute*, with weight placed on the severity of parental behavior toward a particular child irrespective of that directed to other children of the family.

Leaving aside my sense that the case for a relative perspective has been overstated, my understanding of what is at stake is that if extreme parental behavior is of importance, then the approach will be inadequate for tackling issues concerning maltreatment. For example, closely similar experience of negative behavior is not uncommon in dysfunctional families. But a relative approach would probably at times show that nothing untoward had occurred (because neither child reports a difference in treatment) or that only one of the pair had been involved (because only one reports a difference). The reverse problem would hold at the other end of the continuum covering largely satisfactory family settings. However, I do not want to suggest that a relative perspective is irrelevant. It would, for example, be surprising if such perceptions did not play some role in the reports of behavior used to define maltreatment in the alternative absolute approach.

Fortunately, I do not think that settling the matter is at present of primary importance. It would probably be a mistake to try to rule out completely elements of a relative stance in reporting. What is important is to ensure that ratings of severity of maltreatment have some anchoring in detailed descriptions of parental behavior and that instances of maltreatment are not missed. Once this is in place, there is no reason that ratings from a relative perspective cannot also be obtained. Again, the inclusion of elements of more than one approach may be useful.

Context and Meaning

The importance of taking account of context in the kind of research I have been discussing is the subject of a series of recommendations of the MacArthur Network on Psychopathology and Development (Boyce et al. 1998). They refer to the use of context in research in London to assess the likely meaning of an event for a child (Brown and Harris 1978). A married woman, who already had a lover and had discussed with him leaving her husband, would in this approach be assessed as unlikely to have experienced severe threat when her husband unexpectedly left her. In reaching this kind of decision, the investigator takes account of context by reference to apparent plans and commitments held by a subject relevant to the event. However, this is not the route we have followed with childhood maltreatment, in which we have assessed the likely severity of the threat *only* on the basis of accounts of parental behavior.

I think this can be explained by an assumption on our part that context is less relevant for a child because his or her fundamental needs, particularly for security and recognition, will differ little across settings. A child's high level of commitment in the relationship with his or her mother has therefore been assumed by default. In other words, if context is to be taken into account, it is probably best assessed via its effect on the mother. How, for example, have poverty, lone motherhood, and an unrewarding core sexual relationship influenced her relationship with the child in question?

However, context should not be ignored altogether. Two issues stand out. The first concerns the growing body of research dealing with childhood traumatic events such as those surrounding sexual abuse (Fergusson and Mullen 1999). Measurement has largely proceeded on the assumption that agreement on a respondent's part to questions such as "Has anyone touched your private parts?" is sufficient to establish its relevance. However, exactly what such an answer reflects is not explored. For example, a father touched his fully clothed 13-year-old daughter between her legs while she was bent over a sink washing her hair. On further questioning, the daughter explained that at the time, she thought that her father might have mistook her for her mother. My point is not that this incident would be necessarily wrongly classified as abuse but simply that research workers rarely (and readers never) get the chance to consider such accounts.

There are, of course, economic reasons why research on abuse usually lacks a descriptive underpinning. Gelles (1990) has described how in his influential work on family violence, it was decided to use a much larger sample after the first interview-based survey. Because of the expense, a further decision was made to rely on telephone contacts and to halve the length of the interview. Such practices risk cutting research off from the real world; ironically, such diminished instruments are just as commonly used in small-scale inquiries, even though it is not necessary in financial terms.

An equally difficult issue regarding context relates to the implications of population differences in rates of adverse parental behavior (Brown 2002a). As many as 42% of a sample of middle-class professionals in India admitted to abusive violence involving use of objects or acts of kicking, biting, or punching with fists. However, the investigators noted that the use of objects such as a stick, ruler, or hairbrush may be perceived as normal violence in India (Segal 1995). How to deal with this kind of possibility has received little systematic attention. In this instance, for example, adverse long-term effects may well turn on how far rejection is conveyed and the more general closeness of the relationship. (The London instrument does not assume that physical abuse necessarily involves rejection; for this, rejecting comments also would need to be present.)

However, it is reassuring (and perhaps puzzling to many) that the contextual ratings of adult life events developed on the basis of criteria developed in London have proved to be remarkably relevant for quite different cultures. Perhaps most surprising is that the basic event-depression link has been confirmed for women in a black township in Harare, Zimbabwe, with use of the contextual criteria for rating threat developed for the London LEDS (Broadhead and Abas 1998; Brown 2002b). The study did make elaborate efforts to take account of cultural differences: for example, the high value placed on having a male child and the rejection of a wife then could follow failure in this regard. But the required changes proved to be minor and made practically no difference to the findings. While recognizing the relevance of considering context in some of the issues surrounding the measurement of maltreatment, and even trauma, in childhood, my sense is that where long-term effects are concerned, we are often dealing with evolutionarily derived needs that are not easily nullified by cultural influences. The most effective way forward would again appear to be the use of elements of both approaches—an absolute one buttressed when necessary with contextual and self-report measures.

Whatever decision is made, it is important to recognize that with most standardized instruments, there is no way an interesting finding can be explored because it is nothing more at hand than agreement to the several alternatives presented. Implicit in my account of investigator-based instruments has been the need to recognize the importance of collecting descriptive material. Another discussion of measurement put the matter succinctly and more generally: "Virtually all research should be exploratory. Even a study designed to test quantitatively a prespecified hypothesis ought to collect much side information, to enrich thinking about within-cell variation in process and results" (Cronbach 1991, p. 96).

Questionnaire or Interview?

The question of context raises the difficult issue of the use of questionnaires to collect material about childhood maltreatment. There is no straightforward answer, but a choice between a questionnaire and an interview-based instrument should ideally be made on scientific rather than economic grounds. Questionnaires can provide excellent screening instruments, but when they are used more broadly, careful consideration of possible shortcomings is warranted. One of the most frequently used, the 25-item Parental Bonding Instrument, asks adults standard questions about perceptions of poor care (Parker et al. 1979; Plantes et al. 1988). It commonly uses the two dimensions of "care" and "overprotection." It has produced substantial correlations with conditions such as neurotic depression. Studies have shown that associations are restricted to a small group with "low care" and "high protection," termed *affectionless control*. Typically, about one-third of the depressed and only 2% of the comparison series belong to this high-risk group (Parker et al. 1979; Plantes et al. 1988). However, the infrequency in the general population contrasts with that found by interview-based instruments such as the CECA instrument, which suggests rates of approximately 20% as having experienced significant neglect or abuse (Brown 2002a). More comprehensive coverage by the questionnaire is clearly needed. (Another version has been produced that includes parental abuse, but as yet no data are available on its use in the general population; Parker et al. 1997.) We also must determine the reason that in many studies, "low care" without "high protection" has not proved to be predictive.

I refer to this instrument simply to illustrate the kind of consideration that should be taken into account when considering the use of a questionnaire. I believe that questionnaires will likely remain significantly flawed without studies that enable findings to be contrasted with detailed descriptive contextual material and the stimulus this would provide for their further development. If questionnaires are used, the best way forward might be to have a backup interview-based instrument in at least a subsample of the research population.

Conclusion

Several measures of child-parent interaction have produced replicable findings. My impression from reviewing the field of development and psychopathology is that we know very little about the relation of such measures to one another. Research dealing with expressed emotion continues to add to the surprising range of childhood and adolescent conditions that appear to be implicated. Its core measure of critical comments (and the associated one of hostility), however, has never been related to the important studies concerning harsh punishment and conduct disorder or to child maltreatment itself. The likely overlap of the two is obvious because rejection may be the central experience of importance in childhood maltreatment, and ratings of critical comments and hostility are core components of the expressed emotion measures. The need to do more about this failure to relate such core measures to each other is also illustrated by work on insecure childhood attachment. Some studies have now shown this factor to be unrelated to later externalizing problems (Greenberg et al. 1993). By contrast, studies that examine insecure attachment occurring in families with one or more of the risk factors used in cumulative indices (e.g., family discord, parental psychopathology, overcrowding) that are markers for likely maltreatment have shown insecure attachment to be predictive of externalizing problems (Greenberg et al. 1993), and there must be the possibility that persistent maltreatment is implicated. Also, parental rejection, when present, is a particularly toxic component of any family situation and may lead to insecure attachment.

A particularly intriguing consequence of comparing such measures could be the development of more effective measures of childhood maltreatment carried out in childhood itself. But my aim in such a short account is no more than to suggest the need to establish what effective measures have in common, how much they play an etiological role in the longer term, and how much this occurs outside the setting of extreme parental behavior represented by maltreatment. Answers will need to take account of the measurement options I have touched on, but I trust I have conveyed that this kind of integration is possible.

References

Bifulco A, Brown GW, Harris TO: Childhood Experiences of Care and Abuse (CECA): a retrospective interview measure. J Child Psychol Psychiatry 35:1419–1435, 1994

Bifulco A, Brown GW, Lillie A, et al: Memories of childhood neglect and abuse: corroboration in a series of sisters. J Child Psychol Psychiatry 38:365–374, 1997

Bluck S, Habermas Y: The life story schema. Motivation and Emotion 24:121–147, 2000

Bowlby J: Attachment. London, England, Hogarth Press, 1969

Boyce WT, Frank E, Jensen PS, et al: Social context in developmental psychopathology: recommendations for future research from the MacArthur Network on Psychopathology and Development. Dev Psychopathol 10:143–164, 1998

Broadhead J, Abas M: Life events, difficulties and depression among women in an urban setting in Zimbabwe. Psychol Med 28:29–38, 1998

Brown GW: Life events and measurement, in Life Events and Illness. Edited by Brown GW, Harris TO. New York, Guilford, 1989, pp 3–45

Brown GW: Measurement and the epidemiology of childhood trauma. Semin Clin Neuropsychiatry 7:66–79, 2002a

Brown GW: Social roles, context and evolution in the origins of depression. J Health Soc Behav 43:255–276, 2002b

Brown GW, Harris TO: Social Origins of Depression. London, England, Tavistock, 1978

Brown GW, Moran P: Clinical and psychosocial origins of chronic depressive episodes, 1: a community survey. Br J Psychiatry 165:447–456, 1994

Brown GW, Birley JLT, Wing JK: The influence of family life on the course of schizophrenic illness: a replication. Br J Psychiatry 121:241–258, 1972

Brown G, Harris TO, Lemyre L: 'Now you see it, now you don't'—some considerations on multiple regression, in Problems and Methods in Longitudinal Research: Stability and Change. Edited by Magnusson D, Bergman LR, Rudinger G, et al. Cambridge, England, Cambridge University Press, 1991, pp 67–94

Caspi A, Moffitt TE, Morgan J, et al: Maternal expressed emotion predicts children's antisocial behavior problems; using monozygotic-twin differences to identify environmental effects on behavioral development. Dev Psychol 40:149–161, 2004

Caspi A, McClay J, Moffitt TE, et al: Role of genotype in the cycle of violence in maltreated children. Science 297:851–854, 2005

Cicchetti C, Carlson V: Child Maltreatment: Theory and Research on the Causes and Consequences of Child-Abuse and Neglect. Cambridge, England, Cambridge University Press, 1989

Colman I, Jones PB: Birth cohort studies in psychiatry: beginning at the beginning. Psychol Med 34:1375–1383, 2004

Conway M: Phenomenological records and the self-memory system, in Time and Memory: Issues in Philosophy and Psychology. Edited by Hoerl C, McCormack T. Oxford, England, Clarendon Press, 2001, pp 235–255

Craig TK, Boardman AP, Mills K: The south London somatisation study, 1: Longitudinal Course and the Influence of Early Life Experiences. Br J Psychiatry 163:579–588, 1993

Cronbach LJ: Emerging views on methodology, in Conceptualization and Measurement of Organism-Environment Interaction. Edited by Wachs TD, Plomin R. Washington, DC, American Psychological Association, 1991, pp 87–104

Dadds MR, Salmon K: Punishment insensitivity and parenting: temperament and learning as interacting risks for antisocial behavior. Clin Child Fam Rev 6:69–86, 2003

Daniels D, Plomin R: Differential experience of siblings in the same family. Dev Psychol 21:747–760, 1985

Dong M, Anda RF, Dube SR, et al: The relationship of exposure to childhood sexual abuse to other forms of abuse, neglect, and household dysfunction during childhood. Child Abuse Negl 27:625–639, 2003

Duggal S, Carlson EA, Sroufe LA, et al: Depressive symptomatology in childhood and adolescence. Dev Psychopathol 13:143–164, 2001

Dunn J, Plomin R: Why are siblings so different? The significance of differences in sibling experiences within the family. Fam Process 30:271–283, 1991

Dunn MG, Tarter RE, Mezzich AC, et al: Origins and consequences of child neglect in substance abuse families. Clin Psychol Rev 22:1063–1090, 2002

Fergusson DM, Horwood J: Predictive validity of categorically and dimensionally scored measures of disruptive child behaviors. J Am Acad Child Adolesc Psychiatry 34:477–485, 1995

Fergusson DM, Mullen PE: Childhood Sexual Abuse: An Evidence Based Perspective. Thousand Oaks, CA, Sage, 1999

Garbarino J, Collins CC: Child neglect: the family with a hole in the middle, in Neglected Children: Research, Practice, and Policy. Edited by Dubowitz H. Thousand Oaks, CA, Sage, 1999, pp 1–23

Garbarino J, Guttman E, Seeley JW: The Psychologically Battered Child: Strategies for Identification, Assessment and Intervention. San Francisco, CA, Jossey-Bass, 1986

Gelles RJ: Methodological issues in the study of family violence, in Depression and Aggression in Family Interaction. Edited by Patterson GW. Hillsdale, NJ, Erlbaum, 1990, pp 49–73

Gilbert P: Evolutionary approaches to psychopathology and cognitive therapy. Journal of Cognitive Psychotherapy 16:263–294, 2002

Glaser D: Child abuse and neglect and the brain—a review. J Child Psychol Psychiatry 41:97–116, 2000

Greenberg MT, Speltz ML DeKlyen M: The role of attachment in the early development of disruptive problems. Dev Psychopathol 5:191–213, 1993

Henry B, Moffitt TE, Caspi A, et al: On the "remembrance of things past": a longitudinal evaluation of the retrospective method. Psychol Assess 6:92–101, 1994

Hill J, Pickles A, Burnside E, et al: Child sexual abuse, poor parental care and adult depression: evidence for different mechanisms. Br J Psychiatry 179:104–109, 2001

Jaffe SR, Moffitt TE, Caspi A, et al: Differences in early childhood risk factors for juvenile-onset and adult-onset depression. Arch Gen Psychiatry 59:215–224, 2002

Jenkins JM, Rasbash J, O'Connor TG: The role of the shared family context in differential parenting. Dev Psychol 39:99–113, 2003

Johnson JG, Cohen P, Kasen S, et al: Association of maladaptive parental behavior with psychiatric disorder among parents and their offspring. Arch Gen Psychiatry 58:453–460, 2001

Kapur N, Hunt G, MacFarlane J, et al: Childhood experience and health care use in adulthood: nested case-control study. Br J Psychiatry 185:134–139, 2004

Manley JT, Cicchetti D, Barnett D: The impact of subtype, frequency, chronicity, and severity of child maltreatment on social competence and behavior problems. Dev Psychopathol 6:121–143, 1994

Maughan B, Pickles A, Quinton D: Parental hostility, child behavior and adult social functioning, in Coercion and Punishment in Long-Term Perspectives. Edited by McCord J. New York, Cambridge University Press, 1995, pp 34–58

McNally RJ: Remembering Trauma. Cambridge, MA, Harvard University Press, 2003

Meyer JM, Rutter M, Silberg JL, et al: Familial aggregation for conduct disorder symptomatology: the role of genes, marital discord and family adaptability. Psychol Med 30:759–774, 2000

Mullen PE, Martin JL, Anderson JC, et al: The long-term impact of the physical, emotional, and sexual abuse of children: a community study. Child Abuse Negl 20:7–21, 1996

Neilson E, Brown GW, Marmot M: Myocardial infarction, in Life Events and Illness. Edited by Brown GW, Harris TO. London and New York, Guilford, 1989, pp 313–342

Parker G, Tupling H, Brown LB: A parental bonding instrument. Br J Med Psychol 52:1–10, 1979

Parker G, Roussos J, Hadzi-Pavlovic D: The development of a refined measure of dysfunctional parenting and assessment of its relevance in patients with affective disorders. Psychol Med 27:1193–1203, 1997

Pickles A, Angold A: Natural categories or fundamental dimensions: on carving nature at the joints and the rearticulation of psychopathology. Dev Psychopathol 15:529–551, 2003

Plantes MM, Prusoff BA, Brennan J, et al: Parental representations of depressed outpatients in the US. J Affect Disord 15:149–155, 1988

Plomin R, DeFreis JC, Fulker DW: Nature and Nurture During Infancy and Early Childhood. Cambridge, England, Cambridge University Press, 1988

Reiss D, Hetherington EM, Plomin R, et al: Genetic questions for environmental studies: differential parenting and psychopathology in adolescence. Arch Gen Psychiatry 52:925–936, 1995

Reiss D, Neiderhiser JM, Hethrington EM, et al: The Relationship Code: Deciphering Genetic and Social Influences on Adolescent Development. Cambridge, MA, Harvard University Press, 2000

Rutter M: Continuities and discontinuities from infancy, in Handbook of Infant Development, 2nd Edition. Edited by Osofsky J. New York, Wiley, 1987, pp 1256–1296

Rutter M: Social context: meanings, measures and mechanisms. European Review 7:139–149, 1999

Rutter M, Pickles A: Person-environment interactions: concepts, mechanisms, and implications for data analysis, in Conceptualization and Measurement of Organism-Environment Interaction. Edited by Wachs TD, Plomin R. Washington, DC, American Psychological Association, 1991, pp 105–141

Rutter M, Quinton D: Long-term follow-up of women institutionalized in childhood: factors promoting good functioning in adult life. British Journal of Developmental Psychology 2:191–204, 1984

Sadowski H, Ugarte B, Kolvin I, et al: Early disadvantages and major depression in adulthood. Br J Psychiatry 174:112–120, 1999

Sanson A, Oberklaid F, Pedlow R, et al: Risk indicators: assessment of infancy predictors of pre-school behavioral maladjustment. J Child Psychol Psychiatry 32:609–626, 1991

Scarr S: Developmental theories for the 1990s: development and individual differences. Child Dev 63:1–19, 1992

Scazufca M, Kuipers E: Stability of expressed emotion in relatives of those with schizophrenia and its relationship with burden of care and perception of patients' social functioning. Psychol Med 28:453–461, 1998

Segal U: Child abuse by the middle class: a study of professionals in India. Child Abuse Negl 19:217–231, 1995

Thornberry TP, Ireland TO, Smith CA: The importance of timing: the varying impact of childhood and adolescent maltreatment on multiple problem outcomes. Dev Psychopathol 13:957–979, 2001

Weiss B, Dodge KA, Bates JE, et al: Some consequences of early harsh discipline: child aggression and maladaptive social information processing style. Child Dev 63:1321–1335, 1992

Williams S, Anderson J, McGee R, et al: Risk factors for behavioral and emotional disorder in preadolescent children. J Am Acad Child Adolesc Psychiatry 29:413–419, 1990

CHAPTER 8

TAXOMETRICS AND RELATIONAL PROCESSES

Relevance and Challenges for
the Next Nosology of Mental Disorders

Theodore P. Beauchaine, Ph.D.
Steven R. H. Beach, Ph.D.

Relationship researchers often have a somewhat different view of the underlying nature of relationship problems than do clinicians working with disturbed couples and families. On the one hand, relationship researchers often view relational processes as continuously distributed variables, best described by a range of finely graded values. On the other hand, clinicians often view relationships in categorical terms, described at base by a fundamental distinction between pathological versus nonpathological functioning and, for those within the pathological group, a secondary characterization in terms of severity. Finding a way to examine these conflicting views about the best way to characterize the structure of relationship problems has the potential to help bridge the gap between science and practice. In addition, a concern with the fundamental structure of diagnostic entities unites rather than divides discussions about relational processes and other syndromes represented in the DSM.

Questions concerning the reliability, validity, and proper level of analysis for assessing mental disorders are not new to psychiatry and remain among the most

Preparation of this chapter was supported in part by Grant R01 MH63699 to Theodore Beauchaine from the National Institute of Mental Health and support provided to Steven Beach from the Fetzer Institute.

important considerations facing us as we deliberate over the next revision of our nosological system, DSM-V. The necessity of obtaining replicable diagnoses across raters and sites has long been recognized and is in large part responsible for the revolution in psychiatric assessment that began with publication of the DSM-III in 1980 (American Psychiatric Association 1980). Both DSM-I (American Psychiatric Association 1952) and DSM-II (American Psychiatric Association 1968) contained criterion sets for psychiatric disorders that were compiled largely on the basis of expert opinion. Consequently, diagnostic classes were theoretically rather than empirically based and suffered from poor reliability (e.g., Malik and Beutler 2002). Since then, reliability has improved considerably following the formation of empirically informed criterion sets and the application of structured clinical interviews in which all raters assess equivalent diagnostic criteria.

Although there is widespread agreement that diagnostic reliability is now adequate to excellent for many psychiatric disorders, questions of construct validity remain (Beauchaine and Marsh 2006; Kendell 1989). In this context, *validity* refers to the extent to which a symptom criterion set identifies a nonarbitrary class of individuals who suffer from a single condition that confers increased risk of morbidity, mortality, and/or interpersonal distress. A valid diagnostic criterion set should therefore specify a distinct pathological trajectory that follows an insidious course and shares common biological and/or environmental substrates. Construct validity must be evaluated whenever the latent cause of a putative trait or disorder cannot be observed directly (Cronbach and Meehl 1955). This is nearly always the case in psychiatry, where the construct validation process is formidable because all of our criterion sets are composed entirely of manifest behaviors, few if any of which are specific to a single latent psychopathological trait. Because we lack pathognomic signs, the validity of a diagnostic class must be established through a series of deliberate and systematic steps. This need for a deliberate and systematic construct validation process is equally applicable to relational disorders and will therefore pose a challenge for any diagnostic class with a strong relational component.

The Feighner Criteria

At present, the gold standard for establishing the validity of a psychiatric syndrome is the five-step process referred to as the *Feighner criteria* (Feighner et al. 1972; Robins and Guze 1970). An extension of Cronbach and Meehl's (1955) construct validation procedure, this process includes clinical description, laboratory studies, delimitation from other disorders, follow-up studies, and family studies. Diagnostic validity is established when a clinical syndrome is characterized by 1) a cluster of covarying symptoms and etiologic precursors, 2) reliable physiological, biological, and/or psychological markers, 3) readily definable exclusionary criteria, 4) a predictable course, and 5) increased rates of the same disorder among first-degree relatives. This system was adopted by the American Psychiatric Association, beginning with DSM-III, and has strongly influenced all subsequent versions of the DSM (see Cloninger 1989). Unfortunately, the criteria tend to reduce interest in relationship categories under the presumption that such categories would not have heritable bases, an assumption that is now proving false (see Reiss and Wamboldt, Chapter 6, this volume).

When the Feighner criteria are met, much greater confidence in the construct validity of a diagnostic class is warranted because more is known about the etiologic substrates of psychopathology (see Beauchaine and Beauchaine 2002; Beauchaine and Marsh 2006, for extended discussions). This in turn leads to more effective treatments because etiologic mechanisms can be targeted directly. In psychiatry, such mechanisms have usually been presumed to be pathophysiological in nature, following a strict disease model of psychopathology. As a result, environmental risk factors have generally not been considered as putative etiologic agents. Thus, despite widespread recognition that environmental influences and epigenetic effects can hasten the age at onset for complex genetic disorders and are sometimes *required* for phenotypic expression of genetic risk, the environmental context in which psychopathology develops has been largely ignored in the construct validation process.

Relational Processes as Etiologic Mechanisms for Psychopathology

As outlined in other chapters in this volume (see Beach et al., Chapter 1; Benjamin et al., Chapter 10, this volume) and and elsewhere (Beauchaine et al., in press; Reid et al. 2002; Wamboldt and Wamboldt 2000), it is becoming increasingly apparent that relationship processes— particularly coercive, emotionally labile interaction patterns and traumatic experiences within the familial environment— can exert long-term functional effects on developing serotonergic, noradrenergic, and dopaminergic systems that govern aspects of mood, impulse control, and emotion regulation (see Bremner and Vermetten 2001; Pine et al. 1996; Pollak 2003; Schwarz and Perry 1994). Given that mood disturbance, impulsiveness, and/or emotional lability are present in most psychiatric disorders (see Beauchaine 2001), the exclusion of relational processes from our criterion sets as potential etiologic substrates of psychopathology may represent a major oversight for many diagnostic classes. Our intent here is not to review this literature in detail; interested readers are referred to other sources for this information (e.g., Beach et al., Chapter 1, this volume; Beauchaine et al., in press; Reid et al. 2002; Wamboldt and Wamboldt 2000). Rather, our intentions are to 1) reinforce the point made by other authors that relational processes should be considered as etiologic mechanisms for some psychiatric disorders, 2) emphasize the fact that relational processes may be either taxonic or continuous and that this distinction is important, and 3) illustrate how relational processes might be included in the construct validation process using taxometric methods, a set of techniques aimed at identifying discrete psychopathological traits.

Taxometrics and Construct Validation

One of the strongest pieces of evidence for the construct validity of a psychiatric disorder is provided when members of the diagnostic group constitute a discrete latent class of individuals who differ in kind from nonmembers (Meehl 1995). A discrete latent class is suggested when multiple indicators of a psychiatric syndrome cluster together tightly enough to differentiate those affected by the disorder from those who are unaffected. Such patterns suggest differences in kind rather than degree and allow for diagnostic cutoffs that are nonarbitrary. Moreover, when evidence for a discrete psychopathological trait is obtained from multiple levels of analysis, including psychological, biological, and etiologic, the first three of the Feighner criteria are met (Beauchaine and Beauchaine 2002). In the sections that follow, we briefly describe taxometric methods aimed at identifying discrete psychopathological traits and offer recommendations for including relational process variables in future taxometrics studies (see also Heyman and Slep, Chapter 9, this volume).

OVERVIEW OF TAXOMETRICS

The term *taxometrics* is typically applied to a set of 13 interrelated algorithms that were developed by P.E. Meehl and colleagues with the aim of distinguishing between discrete and dimensional latent structure (e.g., Meehl 1999; Meehl and Yonce 1994, 1996). These algorithms search for disjunctions in the distributional properties of two or more markers, or indicators of an observed trait. For example, the maximum slope (MAXSLOPE) procedure searches for a disjunction in the slope of a smoothed regression function run through the bivariate distribution of two variables. This procedure is illustrated in Figure 8–1, where two hypothetical bivariate distributions are depicted, one in which two discrete groups are present and the other in which a purely dimensional relation exists between two variables. In the taxonic case, a disjunction is observed in the slope of the regression line (dy/dx), which is maximized at the point along x that best differentiates between groups. In contrast, the nontaxonic case yields no disjunction in the regression function. Other taxometric methods search for disjunctions in the covariance structure among indicators. It should be noted that MAXSLOPE is neither the most sensitive nor the most frequently used taxometric procedure, but it is intuitively appealing. Interested readers are referred to Waller and Meehl (1998) for a thorough discussion of more commonly used taxometric algorithms (see also Chapter 9, Heyman and Slep, this volume).

Although alternative methods of classifying exist, taxometrics offers a significant advantage over other approaches, including cluster analysis, latent class anal-

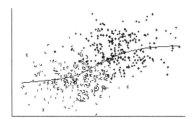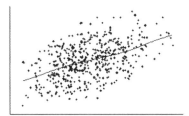

FIGURE 8–1.   Illustration of the MAXSLOPE procedure.

Note.   MAXSLOPE is for two discrete latent classes of equal size ($n=250$; *left panel*) and a single group of continuously distributed scores ($n=500$; *right panel*). In both cases, the correlation between x and y is .50. Note the disjunction observed in the slope of the regression line (dy/dx) in the discrete latent class case. This slope is maximized at the point along x that best differentiates between groups.

Source.   Adapted from Beauchaine and Marsh 2006.

ysis, and mixture modeling techniques. Each of these methods will partition most data sets into two or more subgroups, whether or not those subgroups are actually discrete (Beauchaine and Waters 2003; Beauchaine and Marsh 2006). In contrast, extensive Monte Carlo studies have demonstrated that the maximum covariance (MAXCOV) procedure in particular is quite unlikely to produce false positives under a wide range of operating conditions (Beauchaine and Beauchaine 2002; Haslam and Cleland 1996). Thus, provided that due caution is taken in the selection of candidate indicators, a topic that we consider in detail below, taxometric methods are much less likely to identify arbitrary diagnostic cut-offs. Moreover, taxometric methods have already been used to identify discrete latent structure in a number of disorders and conditions for which compromised interpersonal functioning is a central feature, including antisocial behavior (Ayers et al. 1999; Skilling et al. 2001), avoidant personality disorder (A. Fossati, T. P. Beauchaine, F. Grazioli F, et al.: "Confirmatory Factor Analyses of DSM-IV Cluster C Personality Disorder Criteria," manuscript submitted for publication, 2006), narcissistic personality disorder (Fossati et al. 2005), melancholic depression (e.g., Ambrosini et al. 2002; Beach and Amir 2003), and marital discord (Beach et al. 2005). These studies suggest promise for the inclusion of relational process variables in taxometrics research examining the latent structure of psychopathology. It is important, however, to review a number of considerations that must be addressed in performing rigorous taxometric research. Some of these considerations are especially relevant for relational process variables, as indicated in the following sections.

CHOOSING VALID INDICATORS

The term *validity* has several definitions in the behavioral sciences. In the context of taxometrics, validity refers to the efficiency with which a variable distinguishes between members of a taxon group (those with a discrete disorder) and its complement class (those without the disorder) (see Cole 2004; Meehl 1995). Selection of valid indicators may be the single most important consideration in planning a taxometric analysis because large effect sizes are required for taxonic searches to uncover discrete latent structure among variables. In general, effect sizes separating taxon and complement means should exceed 1.2 standard deviations for all indicators (Meehl 1995), which is about twice the effect size typically observed in psychological research (Cohen 1988). Selecting valid indicators is further complicated by the bootstrapping nature of taxometrics. When performing a taxonic search, we do not know in advance whether separate groups exist in a distribution of scores. Only after the analysis is performed and a positive result is obtained are we in a position to accurately estimate distributional properties, including means and standard deviations, for the taxon and complement class (Waters and Beauchaine 2003). This means that potential indicators should be selected on the basis of strong theoretical considerations and that great care should be taken to ensure that each is measured with precision, or minimal error, so as to maximize effect sizes (Beauchaine and Waters 2003; Lenzenweger 2004; Meehl 1999).

Because measurement precision is so important, certain types of variables are better candidates for taxometric analyses than others. Rating scales, which are commonly used in psychopathology research and which predominate in relationship research, have a number of shortcomings that compromise their efficiency in taxometric and other statistical analyses. As much as 50% of the variance in such measures is attributable to rater biases (Hoyt and Kerns 1999), which necessarily reduces precision. Furthermore, halo effects, which frequently characterize rating scale data, may induce spurious taxonic structure. Using an experimental method in which the cognitive sets of raters were manipulated as dimensional versus categorical, we recently demonstrated that pseudotaxonic structure can be readily imparted in rating scale data (Beauchaine and Waters 2003). Because no single indicator can drive a taxonic outcome, this does not mean that rating scales should be excluded entirely from taxometric analyses. It does suggest, however, that other types of measures should be included. Or, if other types of measures are not included, it should be noted that the construct may be method dependent. Evidence suggests that expert ratings of symptoms may be especially prone to pseudotaxonic biases. Humans are prone toward categorical thinking, gain more confidence in making categorical decisions with increasing expertise, and become more divergent in their beliefs about such decisions over time (Dawes et al. 1989; Simon et al. 2001). Furthermore, experts in psychopathology, similar to clinical experts in the relationship area, are likely to endorse categorical models of at least some disorders. As a consequence, taxometric analyses of scale scores rendered by expert diagnosticians may identify spurious taxonic structure, suggesting caution in the use of diagnostic rating scales as the basis for taxonic conjectures. As we have noted elsewhere, self- and informant-report measures may also be subject to pseudotaxonic biases (Beauchaine and Waters 2003). For these reasons, a pool of candidate indicators should contain at least some objective measures. This requirement has clear implications for relational process variables, which are often measured with Likert scales. For the purposes of taxometrics research, assessments of relational processes should include additional measures such as physiological reactivity, objective behavioral frequency counts, and blindly coded patterns of behavioral and emotional reactivity.

Another consideration of some importance in the study of relational processes is the distinction between "control and influence parameters" and "order parameters" (Nowak and Vallacher 1998). *Control and influence parameters* are variables that influence the stability of an individual's behavior or the degree to which one partner's behavior influences the other. These variables may be very important in forecasting progression from relatively positive relationships to later distress but are not necessarily useful indicators of the actual change in state. In contrast, *order parameters* provide an index of the shift from one "state" to another. In the search for relationship variables that can serve as useful indicators for taxometric purposes, we should seek "order parameters," that is, those variables indicating that a qualitative change in "state" has occurred. For example, a behavioral response tendency, such as withdrawal, that forecasts development of future relationship problems but may not be an indicator of current relationship problems is probably less useful as an indicator of a marital taxon than is evidence of a shift in attributional style for partner behavior.

WINNOWING A SET OF CANDIDATE INDICATORS

Regardless of how carefully one chooses among candidate indicators, some of those indicators are more precise than others and are therefore more efficient at discriminating taxon group members from nonmembers. Because any underlying taxon will go undetected when invalid indicators are used, systematic screening of each candidate variable is required to ensure that failure to find a taxon is not a false negative outcome. Accordingly, we have advocated a two-step process initially proposed by Meehl (1995, 2001) and also used by Waller et al. (1996). This process includes preliminary screening of all candidate variables with the *mean above minus below a cut* (MAMBAC) algorithm, which searches for discrete latent structure among variable pairs. If these preliminary MAMBAC analyses suggest taxonic structure among a subset of indicators, only that subset is subjected to further analyses with taxometric methods such as MAXCOV, the most commonly used and extensively studied taxometric method (Haslam and Kim 2002). This two-stage

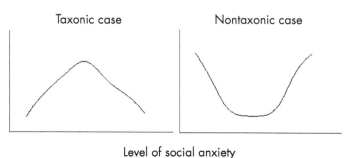

FIGURE 8–2.   Illustrative graphs for the MAMBAC procedure.

Note.   Prototypical *mean above minus below a cut* (MAMBAC) graphs for taxonic (*left panel*) and dimensional (*right panel*) data.

Source.   Adapted from Beauchaine and Waters 2003.

procedure filters the initial set of candidate indicators into a smaller number, providing a more efficient way to differentiate between groups.

Our recommendation is to plot all pairwise combinations of MAMBAC functions in a rectangular matrix (see Beauchaine and Marsh 2006; Beauchaine and Waters 2003). This matrix can then be scanned for indications of taxonic structure. If nearly all of the MAMBAC functions are dish-shaped, which is characteristic of dimensional data (see Figure 8–2), then no further analyses are indicated. If a taxon is present, the most likely scenario is that some MAMBAC plots will be hill-shaped, suggesting latent taxonic structure, whereas others will be dish-shaped. The advantage of plotting all pairwise MAMBAC functions is that specific variables that do not mark the latent taxon can be identified rather easily, because most of the MAMBAC plots in rows and columns representing such variables will be dish-shaped. These variables can be eliminated from the indictor pool. Next, remaining indicators are subjected to further analyses with MAXCOV. Results obtained from MAMBAC and MAXCOV are used as *consistency tests* for judging the plausibility of a taxonic interpretation.

PERFORMING CONSISTENCY TESTS

In performing a taxometric analysis, it is essential that consistent results be obtained both within and across methods for a taxonic interpretation to be supported. For example, if the winnowing procedure described in the previous subsection yields seven indicators of taxon group membership, examining the stability of taxon base rate estimates across the full set of MAMBAC analyses provides the first consistency test. Seven indicators yield $2\binom{7}{2}$, or 42 combinations of variables for

MAMBAC analysis. If a latent taxon is present, these indicators should produce consistent estimates of the taxon base rate across variable pairings. If most baserate estimates fall within a small range, then the taxonic hypothesis is conditionally supported, and the indicators are subjected to MAXCOV (or another taxometric algorithm; see Beauchaine and Marsh 2006). With 7 indicators, there are

$$i \times \frac{(i-1)!}{(i-3)!2!} \text{, or}$$

105 trivariate combinations of variables available for MAXCOV analysis, each of which produces estimates of the base rate and the taxon and complement class means, among other latent parameters. Only when most of these parameter estimates converge on single values is the taxonic hypothesis supported.

It is also important to include a sufficient number of valid indicators for a taxometric analysis to be adequately powered. Monte Carlo studies from our laboratory suggest that power to detect a latent taxon, if present, rises somewhat steeply between 3 and 7 indicators, after which it continues to rise more gradually (Beauchaine and Beauchaine 2002). This suggests that at least six or seven indicators should be included in a taxometric analysis in order to maximize power. Given the discussion above regarding the winnowing of an indicator pool, researchers planning a taxometric study should probably start with about a dozen potential indicators, with the understanding that some will be rejected in the screening process. Fortunately, semiredundant indicators (i.e., alternative measures of the latent construct being assessed) are permissible in taxometric studies. A possible exception to the rule of six or seven indicators occurs in the context of simulations, where fewer variables may be permissible under certain circumstances.

AVOIDING OVERINTERPRETATION OF NULL FINDINGS

Over the past decade or so, several researchers have offered warnings about the potential for committing Type I errors, or identifying spurious latent classes, in taxometrics research (e.g., Beauchaine and Waters 2003; Miller 1996; Ruscio and Ruscio 2002, 2004a, 2004b; Widiger 2001). Few, however, have considered the possibility of committing Type II errors, or concluding that constructs are dimensionally distributed when they are in fact taxonic. We consider this lack of attention to Type II errors to be a serious omission from the discourse on taxometric methods and propose that such errors may in fact be more likely than Type I errors. It has become common practice for researchers to interpret negative findings from taxometric analyses as evidence of dimensional latent structure. However, because taxometric procedures are structure-seeking, the functional null hypothesis is that the analyzed trait or disorder is distributed continuously, and the alternative hypothesis is that it is distributed discretely. Taxometric methods do not identify continua; they identify taxa. This issue maps directly onto both null hypothesis significance testing and signal detection theory. When there is an inadequate effect size separating the null or noise distribution (complement class) from the alternative or signal distribution (taxon), the taxon will go undetected, as Monte Carlo studies in our lab and others indicate quite clearly (Beauchaine and Beauchaine 2002; Meehl and Yonce 1996). Furthermore, in the two-group case using null hypothesis significance testing, the null hypothesis is that both sets of scores derive from one distribution. The alternative hypothesis is that they derive from two discrete distributions. This is fully analogous to the latent multivariate case addressed by taxometrics. Concluding that a negative result from a taxometric procedure suggests a continuous distribution is therefore tantamount to proving the null and should be avoided. If, for example, a latent taxon group and complement class are separated by 0.80 standard deviation units on all indicators, a *large* effect size in psychological research (Cohen 1988), the taxon will not be detected. Yet it would be erroneous to conclude that the latent distribution was continuous. This is particularly important when we consider that, as discussed earlier, the data sources commonly used in taxometrics research are imprecise. Many taxometrics studies are therefore underpowered because of both low measurement precision and the large effect sizes required for a taxon to be detected. It is always possible that more precise measures could yield a latent taxon in future investigations.

Interpreting null outcomes as evidence of continua is particularly problematic when insufficient attention is paid to indicator validity. For example, in their otherwise impressive exploration of the latent structure of attachment, Fraley and Spieker (2003) used all potential indicators with a correlation coefficient of .20 or higher with a given attachment security subtype, assuming implicitly that all such indicators were equally valid markers of the putative latent taxon. For the avoidant subtype, 12 indicators met this criterion and were then subjected to all possible combinations of MAXCOV analyses (*n*=660). Fraley and Spieker concluded, on the basis of null findings, that avoidant attachment is distributed dimensionally. Although this conclusion may be correct, the taxonic hypothesis was not put to a strong test because it is a priori unlikely that all 12 indicators could mark a taxon group of avoidant children with sufficient precision for MAXCOV to detect a discrete latent distribution. For these reasons, we recommend that researchers exercise caution in interpreting null findings, especially when indicators of low to moderate measurement precision are used.

Implications of Taxometrics for Comorbidity Research

Several authors have recently expressed enthusiasm for the potential role that taxometric methods might play in elucidating sources of comorbidity (Meehl 2001; Ruscio and Ruscio 2004a; Waldman and Lilienfeld 2001). For example, suppose one subscribes to the theory that two traits shown to be taxonic in previous research, schizotypy and dissociative experiences, are actually identifying the same latent class using different sets of indicators. In other words, dissociative experiences are simply a marker of schizotypy. Given population prevalence rates of around 5% for each taxon, and given conceptual overlap in criteria, such an argument might be advanced. This hypothesis suggests that the apparent comorbidity is *artifactual*, with the two constructs identifying the same group (Klein and Riso 1993). In such a case, independent error-free taxometric analyses of each trait would yield perfect agreement in a 2×2 contingency table, classifying 5% of individuals into both the schizotypy and dissociative experiences taxa, and classifying 95% of individuals into the complement classes (see Ruscio and Ruscio 2004a). In contrast, suppose another theorist believes that the constructs are independent, in which case the number of individuals assigned to both taxon groups should equal the product of the base rates ($.05 \times .05 = .0025$). This also assumes error-free classification.

Unfortunately, error-free classification is not possible, particularly when base rates are low, as is the case in most psychopathology research. As specified by Bayes' theorem, considerable error will be observed in the classification of any low base rate phenomenon (Baldessarini et al. 1983), regardless of the approach to classification that is used. Monte Carlo simulations of the MAXCOV procedure indicate that under the low base rate conditions typically facing psychopathology researchers, the algorithm is effective at detecting latent taxon *groups*, but yields significant false positive rates when classifying *individuals* into groups (Beauchaine and Beauchaine 2002). With a base rate of 5%, 5 indicators, a sample size of 300, an effect size of 1.25 and within-group correlations of .30, MAXCOV correctly classifies roughly 65% of individuals, with a false positive rate of 30% and a false negative rate of 10%. This means that even if schizotypy and dissociative experiences are independent, MAXCOV analyses with different sets of indicators will place about 10% ($.30 \times .30 = .09$) of individuals into the same taxon. This is roughly double the 5% base rate observed in both populations, which would lead to the incorrect conclusion that the two disorders are etiologically related (see Ruscio and Ruscio 2004a). This example dampens our enthusiasm for the utility of taxometrics for clarifying questions of comorbidity.

Conclusions and Implications for Relational Processes Research

ARE THERE RELATIONAL TAXA?

There is currently no clear and convincing evidence of relational taxa that rises to the standards set forth in this chapter for the domains of greatest interest to clinicians (e.g., parenting, marriage). However, suggestive data are available (Beach et al. 2005), and these data encourage further examination of marital and parenting domains for relational taxa. In addition, complex, nonrecursive systems, such as those that may characterize dyads within families, often show discontinuities and dichotomous outcomes (Gottman et al. 2002; Nowak and Vallacher 1998), suggesting that some relational outcomes could be taxonic. At the same time, there is evidence of genetic influences on some relational processes (e.g., Reiss and Wamboldt, Chapter 6, this volume), further suggesting the potential for the emergence of relational taxa. Moreover, if some relationship events produce long-term, discontinuous changes in central nervous system functioning (e.g., Lim and Young, Chapter 2; Totah and Plotsky, Chapter 3, this volume) or emotion regulation (Beauchaine et al., in press), this might also give rise to relational taxa.

DOES IT MATTER WHETHER THERE ARE RELATIONAL TAXA?

Relational taxa would imply a point of rarity in the distribution of scores for relational problems, thereby constraining theoretical models of the development and maintenance of such problems. In particular, relational taxa would either imply discontinuously distributed individual characteristics that are capable of producing discontinuities in relationship functioning or require systemic models of interaction that produce dichotomously distributed relationship outcomes. As such, the results of taxometric investigations are of considerable importance for theorizing about the development and amelioration of relationship problems and have considerable potential to advance basic theory. In addition, relational taxa have the potential to help refine the search for category indicators, thereby improving clinical understanding of relationship problems. Similarly, relational taxa would provide considerable impetus for the construction of relational diagnoses (Heyman and Slep, Chapter 9, this volume). Clinically, relational taxa would suggest a point at which positive change in the absence of outside help might be more difficult and less likely. As such, cut-points derived from taxometric analyses may be of considerable value in informing clinical decision making regarding the need for services or the likely level of intensity of services that would be required to address a particular relationship problem.

ARE THERE IMPLICATIONS FOR THE REVISION OF THE DSM?

Given the importance of dyadic interaction patterns and their potential to exert a profound influence on the expression of genes and the developmental psychopathology, a DSM revision that ignores such processes would seem incomplete at best. Because dimensional results may be viewed as the "null" hypothesis in taxometric research, it would seem prudent to allow for the possibility that some relational processes of interest in DSM-V might be best considered dimensional, especially in the absence of strong evidence to the contrary. However, it would also seem prudent to allow for the possibility that some relational processes will prove to be well characterized as categories. The results of taxometric investigations can provide a basis for deciding between these competing characterizations and may therefore prove useful in the DSM-V revision process.

References

Ambrosini PJ, Bennett DS, Cleland CM, et al: Taxonicity of adolescent melancholia: a categorical or dimensional construct? J Psychiatr Res 36:247–256, 2002

American Psychiatric Association: Diagnostic and Statistical Manual of Mental Disorders. Washington, DC, American Psychiatric Association, 1952

American Psychiatric Association: Diagnostic and Statistical Manual of Mental Disorders, 2nd Edition. Washington, DC, American Psychiatric Association, 1968

American Psychiatric Association: Diagnostic and Statistical Manual of Mental Disorders, 3rd Edition. Washington, DC, American Psychiatric Association, 1980

Ayers W, Haslam N, Bernstein D, et al: Categorical vs dimensional models of personality disorder in substance abusers: a taxometric analysis. Poster presented at the 152nd annual meeting of the American Psychiatric Association, Washington, DC, May 15–20, 1999

Baldessarini RJ, Finklestein S, Arana GW: The predictive power of diagnostic tests and the effect of prevalence of illness. Arch Gen Psychiatry 40:569–573, 1983

Beach SRH, Amir N: Is depression taxonic, dimensional, or both? J Abnorm Psychol 112: 228–236, 2003

Beach SRH, Fincham FD, Amir N, et al: The taxometrics of marriage: is marital discord categorical? J Fam Psychol 19:276–285, 2005

Beauchaine TP: Vagal tone, development, and Gray's motivational theory: toward an integrated model of autonomic nervous system functioning in psychopathology. Dev Psychopathol 13:183–214, 2001

Beauchaine TP, Beauchaine RJ III: A comparison of maximum covariance and κ–means cluster analysis in classifying cases into known taxon groups. Psychol Methods 7:245–261, 2002

Beauchaine TP, Gatzke-Kopp L, Mead HK: Polyvagal theory and developmental psychopathology: emotion dysregulation and conduct problems from preschool to adolescence. Biol Psychol (in press)

Beauchaine TP, Marsh P: Taxometric methods: enhancing early detection and prevention of psychopathology by identifying latent vulnerability traits, in Developmental Psychopathology, 2nd Edition. Edited by Cicchetti D, Cohen D. Hoboken, NJ, Wiley, 2006, pp 931–967

Beauchaine TP, Waters E: Pseudotaxonicity in MAMBAC and MAXCOV analyses of rating scale data: turning continua into classes by manipulating observer's expectations. Psychol Methods 8:3–15, 2003

Bremner JD, Vermetten E: Stress and development: behavioral and biological consequences. Dev Psychopathol 13:473–489, 2001

Cloninger CR: Establishment of diagnostic validity in psychiatric illness: Robins and Guze's method revisited, in The Validity of Psychiatric Diagnosis. Edited by Robins LN, Barrett JE. New York, Raven, 1989, pp 9–18

Cohen J: Statistical Power Analysis for the Behavioral Sciences, 2nd Edition. New York, Academic Press, 1988

Cole DA: Taxometrics in psychopathology research: an introduction to some of the procedures and related methodological issues. J Abnorm Psychol 113:3–9, 2004

Cronbach LJ, Meehl PE: Construct validity in psychological tests. Psychol Bull 52:281–302, 1955

Dawes RM, Faust D, Meehl PE: Clinical versus actuarial judgment. Science 243:1668–1674, 1989

Feighner JP, Robins E, Guze SB, et al: Diagnostic criteria for use in psychiatric research. Arch Gen Psychiatry 26:57–63, 1972

Fossati A, Beauchaine TP, Grazioli F, et al: A latent structure analysis of DSM-IV narcissistic personality disorder criteria. Compr Psychiatry 46:361–367, 2005

Fraley RC, Spieker SJ: Are infant attachment patterns continuously or categorically distributed? A taxometric analysis of Strange Situation behavior. Dev Psychol 39:387–404, 2003

Gottman JM, Swanson C, Swanson K: A general systems theory of marriage: nonlinear difference equation modeling of marital interaction. Pers Soc Psychol Rev 6:326–340, 2002

Haslam N, Cleland C: Robustness of taxometric analysis with skewed indicators, II: a Monte Carlo study of the MAXCOV procedure. Psychol Rep 79:1035–1039, 1996

Haslam N, Kim HC: Categories and continua: a review of taxometric research. Genet Soc Gen Psychol Monogr 128:271–320, 2002

Hoyt WT, Kerns MD: Magnitude and moderators of bias in observer ratings: meta-analysis. Psychol Methods 4:403–424, 1999

Kendell RE: Clinical validity. Psychol Med 19:45–55, 1989

Klein DN, Riso LP: Psychiatric disorders: problems of boundaries and comorbidity, in Basic Issues in Psychopathology. Edited by Costello CG. New York, Guilford, 1993, pp 19–66

Lenzenweger M: Consideration of the challenges, complications, and pitfalls of taxometric analysis. J Abnorm Psychol 113:10–23, 2004

Malik ML, Beutler LE: The emergence of dissatisfaction with the DSM, in Rethinking the DSM. Edited by Beutler LE, Malik ML. Washington, DC, American Psychological Association, 2002, pp 3–15

Meehl PE: Bootstraps taxometrics: solving the classification problem in psychopathology. Am Psychol 50:266–275, 1995

Meehl PE: Clarifications about taxometric method. Appl Prev Psychol 8:165–174, 1999

Meehl PE: Comorbidity and taxometrics. Clin Psychol Sci Prac 8:507–519, 2001

Meehl PE, Yonce LJ: Taxometric analysis, I: detecting taxonicity with two quantitative indicators using means above and below a sliding cut (MAMBAC procedure). Psychol Rep 74:1059–1274, 1994

Meehl PE, Yonce LJ: Taxometric analyses, II: detecting taxonicity using covariance of two quantitative indicators in successive intervals of a third indicator. Psychol Rep 78:1091–1227, 1996

Miller MB: Limitations of Meehl's MAXCOV-HITMAX procedure. Am Psychol 51:554–556, 1996

Nowak A, Vallacher RA: Dynamical Social Psychology. New York, Guilford, 1998

Pine DS, Wasserman G, Coplan J, et al: Platelet serotonin 2A (5-HT$_{2A}$) receptor characteristics and parenting factors for boys at risk for delinquency: a preliminary report. Am J Psychiatry 153:538–544, 1996

Pollak SD: Experience-dependent affective learning and risk for psychopathology in children. Ann NY Acad Sci 1008:102–111, 2003

Reid JB, Patterson GR, Snyder J: Antisocial Behavior in Children and Adolescents: A Developmental Analysis and Model for Intervention. Washington, DC, American Psychological Association, 2002

Robins E, Guze SB: Establishment of diagnostic validity in psychiatric illness: its application to schizophrenia. Am J Psychiatry 126:983–987, 1970

Ruscio A, Ruscio J: The latent structure of analogue depression: should the Beck Depression Inventory be used to classify groups? Psychol Assess 14:135–145, 2002

Ruscio J, Ruscio AM: Clarifying boundary issues in psychopathology: the role of taxometrics in a comprehensive program of structural research. J Abnorm Psychol 113:24–38, 2004a

Ruscio J, Ruscio AM: A conceptual and methodological checklist for conducting a taxometric investigation. Behav Ther 35:403–447, 2004b

Schwarz ED, Perry BD: The post-traumatic response in children and adolescents. Psychiatr Clin North Am 17:311–326, 1994

Simon D, Pham LB, Le QA, et al: The emergence of coherence over the course of decision making. J Exp Psychol Learn Mem Cog, 27:1250–1260, 2001

Skilling TA, Quinsey VL, Craig WM: Evidence of a taxon underlying serious antisocial behavior in boys. Criminal Justice and Behavior 28:450–470, 2001

Waldman ID, Lilienfeld SO: Applications of taxometric methods to problems of comorbidity: perspectives and challenges. Clinical Psychology: Science and Practice 8:520–527, 2001

Waller NG, Meehl PE: Multivariate Taxometric Procedures: Distinguishing Types From Continua. Newbury Park, CA, Sage, 1998

Waller NG, Putnam FW, Carlson EB: Types of dissociation and dissociative types: a taxometric analysis of dissociative experiences. Psychol Methods 1:300–321, 1996

Wamboldt MZ, Wamboldt FS: Role of the family in the onset and outcome of childhood disorders: selected research findings. J Am Acad Child Adolesc Psychiatry 39:1212–1219, 2000

Waters E, Beauchaine TP: Are there really patterns of attachment? Comment on Fraley and Spieker (2003). Dev Psychol 39:417–422, 2003

Widiger TA: What can be learned from taxometric analyses? Clinical Psychology: Science and Practice 8:528–533, 2001

CHAPTER 9

RELATIONAL DIAGNOSES

From Reliable, Rationally Derived Criteria to Testable Taxonic Hypotheses

Richard E. Heyman, Ph.D.
Amy M. Smith Slep, Ph.D.

> The ability to engage in harmonious social relationships, handle conflict and aggression, and receive and offer nurturance are central to mental health, and aberrations in these behaviors and processes are fundamental in the development, definition, and course of psychopathologies.
>
> *Setting Priorities for Basic Brain & Behavioral Science Research at NIMH*
> (National Advisory Mental Health Council 2004)

In setting priorities for research at the National Institute of Mental Health (NIMH), a workgroup of the National Advisory Mental Health Council recently affirmed the *fundamental* role that aberrant social relationships play in the outcomes that are the hallmark of the NIMH's mission (i.e., the development, definition, and course of psychopathologies). One of the behaviors and processes listed

Preparation of this chapter was supported by the U.S. Air Force/U.S. Department of Agriculture (Contracts CR19245B-545771 and CR 19245–545810), National Institute of Mental Health (Grant R01-MH06704301), National Institute of Child Health and Human Development (Grant R01 HD046901–01), and a Raymond and Rosalee Weiss Think Tank Award.

by the workgroup—"conflict and aggression"—is ubiquitous in American families, with 48% of families with young children reporting physical aggression between the partners in the last year (Slep and O'Leary 2005). If partner emotional maltreatment—for example, severe psychological aggression on the Revised Conflict Tactics Scale (CTS2; Straus et al. 1996)—is included, the rate rises to 63%.[1]

Partner physical assault victims, compared with nonvictims, are at elevated risk for 1) symptoms at or near diagnostic thresholds for major depressive disorder (MDD) (e.g., Magdol et al. 1998), posttraumatic stress disorder (PTSD) (e.g., Jones et al. 2001), generalized anxiety disorder (GAD) (Magdol et al. 1998), alcohol abuse (Magdol et al. 1998), and alcohol dependence (Danielson et al. 1998); and 2) a vast array of acute and chronic health problems (Coker et al. 2002; Gelles and Straus 1990).

However, prevalences such as 63% rightly prompt skeptics to ask what is the proportion of victims who are actually at high risk for serious sequelae. Thus, the very ubiquity of emotional and physical partner assault generates disparate perceptions of partner assault, either as a serious threat to public health (and thus worthy of research funding prioritization and inclusion in the *Diagnostic and Statistical Manual of Mental Disorders* [DSM; American Psychiatric Association 2000]) or as a variably serious "problem of living" (and thus worthy of the NIMH's and the DSM's inattention).

Similar quandaries affect not only other forms of family maltreatment (e.g., child abuse and neglect) but also all relational problems discussed in this volume. Researchers' current inability to distinguish relational problems that are "pernicious public health threats" from unpleasant behaviors that are "problems of living" makes it highly likely that relational problem research and clinical intervention will be increasingly marginalized, especially considering the striking progress in other areas of mental health research and intervention (e.g., neuroimaging, molecular neurobiology, gene-environment interactions, psychopharmacology).

Given space constraints, in this chapter we use partner abuse as an exemplar of how researchers interested in relational disorders can attempt to resolve this quandary. We review 1) fundamental weaknesses in the operationalization of partner abuse that substantially frustrate its ability to inform translational research on psy-

---

[1]The prevalences from this representative study of couples with children between 3 and 7 years of age are substantially higher than those in most prior prevalence studies, likely because 1) parents of young children are at higher risk because they are younger than the general adult population (although most are not in the highest-risk group [people younger than 25 years]); 2) the CTS2 (which has questions ordered randomly) was used instead of the original CTS (which has questions ordered by increasing severity), which was used in all prior prevalence studies; and 3) data were collected anonymously and in writing rather than by interview.

chopathology; 2) a rational approach to creating and testing a diagnostic criteria; and 3) theoretical and empirical work implying that truly abusive relationships are a distinct subgroup (i.e., are "taxonic" and thus appropriate for diagnostic classification). We then propose and discuss the implications for research investigating whether "problems of living" and "public health threats" represent distinct subgroups.

For clarity, we define our terms of interest. *Partner assault*—comprising physical assault, sexual assault, and emotional assault—involves an attack of one intimate partner by another, excluding behaviors enacted to protect oneself from imminent physical harm. *Partner abuse,* in our usage, is a hypothesized construct that constitutes a serious threat to victims' physical and/or emotional health.

Defining Partner Abuse

For nearly three decades, there has been debate about what constitutes partner abuse, in large part because of the existence of two distinct subfields (e.g., Straus 1990). One subfield studies individuals or couples from the general population, while the other studies women in shelters and men in court-mandated treatment programs. Each subfield uses a sole criterion for identifying partner abuse: the former usually classifies on the basis of a report of a single act of physical assault in the last year, whereas the latter classifies on the basis of a woman presenting at a shelter or a man being mandated into treatment.

Defining physical abuse as a "single act of physical assault in the last year" is of questionable validity for two reasons. First, despite near universal belief that partner abuse is almost exclusively a male-perpetrated phenomenon, women are equally or more likely to commit physical partner assault than men in all age groups (Archer 2000). The high prevalence of female-to-male assaults cannot be due to self-defense, as women attribute their actions to self-defense less than a quarter of the time (Cascardi and Vivian 1995). Second, again running counter to expert beliefs about partner abuse, assaults typically are not severe (e.g., Caetano et al. 2000), are infrequent (Straus and Gelles 1990), and often desist spontaneously (e.g., Quigley and Leonard 1996). Furthermore, victims typically are uninjured (e.g., Stets and Straus 1990) and report minimal psychological impact (Ehrensaft and Vivian 1996). On the other hand, defining physical abuse by victims' shelter presentation or perpetrators' arrest is of questionable validity, because many truly abusive relationships never come to be known by shelters or the courts (Gelles 2000).

Because most prevention, intervention, and public policy efforts are targeted at assaults that either directly harm victims or prevent victims from living freely without fear of harm, several recent conceptualizations have gone beyond using only assault or shelter/arrest to define partner maltreatment. Research definitions by the Centers for Disease Control and Prevention (Saltzman et al. 1999) and a growing number of researchers (e.g., Coker et al. 2002; Graham-Kevan and Archer 2003; Heyman 2001; Johnson and Leone 2005; Smith et al. 2002) have made clearer distinctions between impactful assaults (i.e., those that cause or have a high potential to cause, injury, harm, or death) and non-impactful assaults. In the next section we describe our program of research that extends this area by creating and testing reliable diagnostic criteria.

A Rational Approach to Developing Diagnostic Criteria

A rational approach to developing a diagnostic system— exemplified by the neo-Kraepelinian, committee-derived DSM-II (American Psychiatric Association 1968) and DSM–III (American Psychiatric Association 1980)— describes potentially clinically significant syndromes with an initial goal of classifying disorders reliably and an eventual goal of testing the validity of reliable diagnoses. Initial diagnostic criteria are based more on consensus among experts' rationally derived clinical judgments than on data, because reliable criteria necessarily must precede validity investigations.

We recently described a four-stage approach that we used to create reliable family maltreatment diagnoses (Heyman and Slep, in press). First, we conducted content validity studies (e.g., Haynes et al. 1995) of a widely used set of maltreatment criteria, using both experts and clinicians in the field. Second, we adopted a conceptual framework requiring physical and emotional abuse and neglect to comprise both a qualifying act and a significant impact (e.g., injury, fear, or psychological sequelae) or high potential for significant impact (e.g., shooting a gun at a spouse but not hitting him or her).[2] This framework parallels that used in DSM, which requires that mental disorders be associated with distress, disability, or increased potential for death or disability. Third, we developed and fine-tuned our maltreatment operationalizations through a thorough examination of legal, research, and clinical definitions and operationalizations of each form and facet of maltreatment. Fourth, we field-tested the initial definitions ($N=650$ cases) and continued to fine-tune them during the trial. We then tested the final maltreatment definitions' reliability in a second field test ($N=556$ cases).

The final field trial procedures, like those used to assess reliability of the DSM, required raters to vote on each criterion separately. Local community boards (comprising mostly individuals with no mental health background) and master reviewers achieved an agreement level across all eight forms of partner/child abuse and neglect of 92% ($\kappa=.84$, $N=556$), a substantial improvement over the estimated 50% agreement obtained in prior years using the previous definitions. Agreement

---

[2]Because of a presumed significant impact of partner sexual abuse and parent-child sexual abuse, the sexual abuse conceptual framework required only a qualifying act.

for partner physical, emotional, and sexual abuse was 91% ($\kappa = 0.82$, $n = 233$), 89% ($\kappa = 0.76$, $n = 79$), and 88% ($\kappa = 0.75$, $n = 8$), respectively.

When well operationalized, relational disorders can be reliably diagnosed, even by those who are not mental health professionals. Initial, reliable definitions can be rationally derived to balance the need for high sensitivity and specificity in identifying *abuse,* unlike single-criterion approaches such as "single act of physical assault" (high sensitivity, low specificity) and shelter/arrest (low sensitivity, high specificity).

Moving Beyond a Rationally Derived Definition of Partner Abuse

Creating and establishing the diagnostic reliability of family maltreatment diagnoses brings these problems in line with the rest of those in the DSM, for better and worse. Former NIMH chief Steven Hyman (2003, p. xii) recently summarized nearly universally recognized sentiments about incompletely and variably validated rationally derived diagnostic criteria: "If a relative strength of DSM is its focus on reliability, a fundamental weakness lies in problems related to validity. Not only persisting but looming larger is the question of whether DSM-IV-TR truly carves nature at the joints—that is, whether the entities described in the manual are truly 'natural kinds' and not arbitrary chimeras." One could add partner abuse (and child abuse and neglect) to the list of reliable rationally derived diagnoses in search of proof that they are "natural" kinds and, if they are, that the current criteria optimally distinguish them.

Over the past decade, partner assault researchers have been increasingly swayed by "natural kind" hypotheses. For example, Johnson (1995) has asserted that partner assault comprises two "largely nonoverlapping populations, experiencing different forms of violence" (p. 289). As labeled by Johnson and Leone (2005), the maltreatment uncovered in general population surveys and relationship clinics is "situational couple violence," a typically less severe form of assault committed by individuals (both men and women) who are not qualitatively distinct from nonassaultive individuals (Waltz et al. 2000); the maltreatment found in shelters and court-mandated treatment settings is "intimate terrorism," a typically severe form of assault marked by power and control committed by individuals (predominantly men) who are qualitatively distinct from the rest of the population.

Thus, a theoretical supposition exists that partner physical abuse is qualitatively distinct from more ubiquitous low-level assault. The supposition can be extended to make hypotheses that a partner-abusive subgroup (the taxon group, PA+) differs from the rest of the population (the complement group, PA−, comprising both assaultive [but not abusive] and nonassaultive individuals) on risk factors (e.g., Axis II psychopathology) and severity of victim impact (e.g., depression, poor health outcomes). Such supposition has not been put to direct empirical test via taxometric analyses (see Beauchaine and Beach, Chapter 8, this volume). However, a variety of a priori and descriptive (e.g., cluster analysis) typological studies lend credence to the supposition, and we now turn our attention to them.

Typological Studies: Initial Discrimination of Abusive and Nonabusive Groups

Research teams attempting to isolate PA+-like groups—some working with victims (Ehrensaft et al. 2004; Smith et al. 2002) and some working with perpetrators (Holtzworth-Munroe et al. 2000; Langhinrichsen-Rohling et al. 2000 [studies 1 and 2]; Waltz et al. 2000[3])—have all obtained PA+ prevalence estimates of approximately 10% of the general population, despite using radically different operationalizations and methods. This noteworthy convergence suggests these different approaches may be isolating a true latent class—one that is identified regardless of which specific indicators are used and which sample is studied. Of interest, this prevalence is high enough to be important from a public health perspective and yet strikingly lower than the prevalence estimates of all couples reporting any physically or emotionally assaultive behavior.

DIFFERENTIAL OUTCOMES

One measure of the validity of investigators' initial PA+ criteria is whether PA+ victims report significantly worse physical and mental health outcomes than victims in the complement group. Johnson and Leone (2005) found support for their PA+ operationalization: PA+ victims, compared with other victims, were 2.5 times more likely to sustain injuries, missed more work due to the last assault, reported significantly elevated symptoms of depression and PTSD, and used painkillers more often (even after age, education, income, and race were controlled for).

DIFFERENTIAL COURSES

As Pagelow (1981, p. 45) noted, "One of the few things about which almost all researchers agree is that batterings escalate in frequency and intensity over time." Thus, the field hypothesizes that PA+ is characterized by persistence and often escalation.

---

[3]These studies did not include a nonassaultive group. If one assumes the same nonassaultive prevalence as in the Ehrensaft et al. (2004) study (79.1%), one can extrapolate the population prevalence of the PA+ group.

None of the five longitudinal studies of partner assault (Aldorondo 1996; Lawrence and Bradbury 2001; Feld and Straus 1990; O'Leary et al. 1989; Quigley and Leonard 1996) attempted to isolate a PA+-like class. If, however, one uses severity as a crude stand-in for PA+, the results are as hypothesized: 10%–17% of severely physically assaultive men (i.e., putative PA+) desist over a several year period, compared with 35%–66% of non–severely assaultive men (i.e., putative PA–).

IMPLICATIONS

Johnson (1995) first hypothesized the existence of a qualitatively distinct PA+ subgroup. Although this proposition has not been directly tested, several lines of research now point to the soundness of this assertion. Research using multiple indicators to discriminate a PA+ group has consistently identified a base rate of 10%. When this PA+ group is isolated, both perpetrators and victims conform more tightly with hypotheses regarding PA+ (e.g., physical and mental health impacts, persistence).

Thus, a direct empirical test of the existence of a partner abuse subgroup, and of the appropriateness of thereby categorically diagnosing partner abuse, is warranted because 1) the partner-abuse field has, since its inception, implied that abuse is distinguishable from lower-level assault, 2) theory supports the postulated qualitative distinction, 3) multiple studies have converged on a prevalence of the hypothesized partner abuse subgroup, and 4) hypothesized differential outcomes and courses for the partner abuse subgroup have been preliminarily supported.

SUMMARY

Fundamental questions such as "What is partner abuse?" and "Is partner abuse distinct from the continuum of hostile things partners do to each other?" have haunted the partner-abuse area since its inception. Distinguishing whether a construct is dimensional or forms "natural kinds" is important because it "may enhance its theoretical conceptualization, shed light on its etiological origin, facilitate its accurate classification and diagnosis, promote its valid and powerful measurement, specify the most appropriate research designs for its investigation, and help inform its management in clinical and public health settings" (Ruscio and Ruscio 2004, pp. 406–407).

Identification and validation of a PA+ subgroup would allow for much more precise research on the link between psychopathology (e.g., antisocial personality disorder, borderline personality disorder) and partner abuse perpetration and the link between PA+ victimization and specific psychopathological outcomes (e.g., major depressive disorder, PTSD). There is likely no question more fundamental to the partner maltreatment field than "What is partner abuse?"; similar definitional questions must be answered for all purported relational disorders to join the mainstream of psychopathology research and treatment.

Testing Whether Partner Abuse Is Truly Distinctive

OVERVIEW OF TAXOMETRICS

Taxometrics are different from all other analytic strategies available for identifying latent subgroups, such as cluster analysis, latent class analysis, latent profile analysis, finite mixture analysis, growth mixture modeling, and latent transition analysis. All of these other techniques identify subgroups regardless of whether the data do, in fact, reflect a single continuous distribution. Taxometric approaches are the only analyses available to truly answer questions regarding whether a distribution contains a combination of subgroups versus a single continuous dimension. Each taxometric analytic technique revolves around the observation that within distributions containing subgroups (e.g., a sample of dogs and cats), indicators of subgroup membership (e.g., weight and affinity for balls as indicators of "dogness") are likely uncorrelated within each subgroup. When observed in a population that contains both subgroups, indicators are correlated because of the mixture of the groups. The correlation observed is greatest in the segment of the distribution in which the subgroups are most highly overlapping. Taxometric analytic techniques partition the data in multiple ways to identify this local peaking of relations, if present. Thus, by carefully choosing putative indicators, assessing them in an appropriate sample, and subjecting the resulting data to a series of taxometric procedures, one can fairly conclusively determine whether the data reflect discrete subgroups or a continuous dimension. (See Beauchaine and Beach, Chapter 8, this volume, for a more complete introduction to taxometrics.)

Because taxometric analyses test whether the data indicate subgroups, rather than identify subgroups as best as possible (the case for the other analytic approaches listed above), the results of well-conceived and well-conducted taxometric analyses can be considered to reveal more conclusively whether a phenomenon is truly dimensional or whether "natural kinds" exist. If subgroups are found, one can determine 1) the validity (effect size) of each proposed indicator, 2) the base rate of the taxon (e.g., PA+), 3) the indicators that most efficiently discriminate group members, 4) optimally sensitive and specific cutpoints for the indicators, and 5) the probability of taxon membership for each individual in the sample. Alternatively, if dimensionality is found, commonplace analyses (e.g., correlations) can determine relations among indicators and between indicators and outcomes. Further, resesarchers can examine mediators and moderators of indicator-outcome relations, confident in the knowledge that the indicators under investigation are best conceived of and studied as continuous variables and do not reflect inappropriately mixed subgroups.

The likely substantive impacts of determining if partner abuse is a qualitatively distinct subgroup are considerable. First, finding the putative taxon subgroup would allow researchers to search for 1) etiological factors of a more validly defined phenomenon (without embedding these factors in the definition of the construct itself) and 2) outcomes (e.g., physical and mental health impacts on victims and children) in both the PA+ and PA– groups. Second, it would allow researchers to test the differential treatment response of individuals in relationships classified as PA+ and PA–. Because the etiological and maintaining factors are likely different between the two groups, treatments would likely need to be different. For example, victims in intact PA+ relationships with major depressive disorder or PTSD might not respond as well to psychopharmacological or standard cognitive-behavioral treatments as would PA– individuals; couples treatment may be an effective intervention for PA–, but not PA+, couples; and so forth. Knowing PA+/PA– status may help in delivering more effective, targeted interventions for some current treatment nonresponders.

PROPOSED TAXOMETRIC MODEL

Our hypothesized taxonic model of partner abuse includes three classes of taxometric indicators: facets of maltreatment (frequency, severity, and chronicity of episodes of physical, emotional, and/or sexual assault; amount of physical and emotional assault within an episode; ratio of male-to-female physical and emotional acts per episode); power and control behaviors; and affect expression/suppression during conflict (expression of belligerence and contempt; suppression of anger expression). Note that, using an approach befitting a relational disorder, we have chosen relational, rather than individual, indicators. Although individual variables may be useful as risk or etiological factors for (e.g., history of conduct problems, borderline personality features) and sequelae of (e.g., injury, depression) the problem of interest, relational disorders occur solely within a relational context and, we believe, can be most cleanly defined via indicators that recognize the relational context.

We first briefly review the literature for why we believe they are possibly valid indicators of partner abuse and then discuss how we suggest the taxon structure itself could be validated.

Proposed Indicators

Facets of maltreatment. PA+ is believed by most researchers and theorists (e.g., Crowell and Burgess 1996; Dutton 1995; Jacobson and Gottman 1998) to involve frequent, chronic acts that represent an actual or perceived threat to the victim's physical or psychological integrity (i.e., severe acts). Over 90% of PA+ individuals are likely to be male (Johnson and Ferraro 2000).

Traditionally, only overall frequency of acts of varying severities was assessed. However, acts of maltreatment (e.g., insulting, pushing, forced sex) are nested within episodes (i.e., the naturally occurring unit, with a discrete beginning and ending, which comprises a series of connected acts in a coherent whole). We suggest that researchers measure multiple facets of maltreatment thought to distinguish the PA+ and PA– subgroups (frequency, severity, and chronicity of episodes; amount of assault within episodes; ratio of male-to-female acts per episode).

Power and control.   Frequent use of power and control tactics is universally believed to discriminate between PA+ and PA– (e.g., Johnson 1995; Yllo and Bograd 1988). For example, Johnson and Leone (2005) report that all seven power/control behaviors studied were high in frequently violent (M = 18 physical assaults per year, putatively PA+) but not in infrequently violent (M = 3 physical assaults per year, putatively PA–) men.

Affect expression during conflict: belligerence and contempt.   The majority of violent incidents occur during escalating, angry conflict (Cascardi and Vivian 1995; Stamp and Sabourin 1995). More than 200 studies have observed and coded couple conflicts in the laboratory (see Heyman 2001), with a handful focusing on partner maltreatment. Waltz et al. (2000), using Holtzworth-Munroe and Stuart's (1994) typology, reported that men in the two battering (putative PA+) groups emitted more contempt than did men in the two nonbattering groups (putative PA–). Gottman et al. (1995), using a typology based on physiological reactivity, found that putative PA+ men emitted more belligerence and contempt than did putative PA– (but still physically assaultive) men. Jacobson et al. (1994) used high-frequency and/or repeated, severe CTS acts to create their putative PA+ group. As with the Gottman et al. (1995) study, men in the putative PA+ group, compared with those in a non–physically assaultive group (putative PA–), displayed more belligerence and contempt during observed couple conflicts.

Affect suppression during conflict: anger.   In a fascinating series of studies (Gross 1998; Gross and Levenson 1993, 1997; Richards and Gross 1999), Gross found that 1) suppression of the display of an emotion was not accompanied by less intense experience of that emotion; 2) suppression of display when the emotion was experienced exacted significant tolls on physiology, and 3) suppression may "boomerang" if ineffective at ending the provocation (e.g., the suppressor's anger may be displayed at a level significantly higher than if suppression were not used). Such a boomerang effect would be consistent with 1) violent men's explanation that when they try to withdraw or use other suppressive strategies, they often cannot take their partners' aversive display any longer and erupt in anger; and 2) victimized women's description of their partners' anger seemingly exploding out of nowhere during a conflict.

Proposed Descriptive Tests for the Hypothesized PA+ Subgroup

If a PA+ taxon is indeed found, then description of both the prevalence and the location and spread (analogous to mean and standard deviation) of the hypothesized indicators would be central to theory generation about, first, the etiology of partner maltreatment and, second, differential treatment approaches for prevention and treatment research. Determining which of the proposed indicators are indeed taxonic and which are dimensional would provide important information about the construct of partner abuse. For example, if the groups differ on all power and control indicators but none of the affect expression/suppression indicators, this would suggest that future theoretical and empirical work on partner abuse omit affect, since it would not appear to be defining of the phenomenon and class. This further isolation of what constitutes PA+ will support a search for markers that are more etiological proximal (see Beauchaine and Marsh, in press), a critical step if we hope to eventually identify biological diatheses of PA+.

In addition to describing PA+ members, compared with PA− members, in terms of putative indicators, we also suggest comparing the groups on the following variables: sociodemographics (i.e., parent age, family size, age of children, income, occupational status, marital status), observational and self-report measures of couple conflict, generalized aggressive behavior across the lifespan, developmental risk factors for partner maltreatment, and relationship satisfaction. All these variables have been used in previous partner maltreatment studies, and all will provide useful clues about differences between PA+ and PA− individuals.

Summary and Implications

Determining if partner abuse is, in fact, qualitatively distinct from the rest of the population as the field speculates, and, if it is, isolating the distinct structure indicators of PA+, would allow for much more powerful basic research (e.g., functional magnetic resonance imaging, behavioral genetics, and developmental psychopathology studies) and for taking a more focused approach to treatment of physically assaultive men. We believe identifying similarities and differences between PA+ and PA− members on putative indicators of and risk factors for PA+ will prove fruitful for theory generation. Researchers will be able to place the taxon firmly within the existing literature. This will allow them to begin to identify 1) which existing theories and research might be most generalizable to the taxon and 2) where gaps exist in the current literature that need to be filled if we want to understand PA+.

PROPOSED VALIDITY TESTS FOR THE HYPOTHESIZED PA+ SUBGROUP

Demonstrating the existence of a PA+ subgroup and specifying its indicators is only a start in validating a partner abuse diagnosis. The existing definitional criteria must be examined in the context of the supported indicators and their optimal cutpoints, and if necessary, modifications must be made. A series of construct, criterion, and predictive validity tests are still necessary. Results supporting the existence of subgroups may confirm that it is appropriate to think of the population as containing qualitatively distinct groups, and therefore to apply categorical diagnoses, but these results themselves do not constitute construct validity (Cronbach and Meehl 1995; Lenzenweger 2004).

If subgroups are found, we suggest testing the PA+ group's validity, both concurrently and longitudinally, in the following ways.

Victim's Mental and Physical Health

We predict differential health statuses for PA+ victims and PA− group members of the same gender on DSM-IV Axis I psychopathology (especially major depressive disorder, PTSD, dysthymia, and GAD) and on physical health (see results of Coker et al. 2000, 2002 for a broad array of physical health sequelae in victims).

Prevalence and Gender

Theorists believe that men constitute the vast preponderance of PA+ group members (see, e.g., Gelles et al. 2005).

Injury

We hypothesize that physical assaults by those in the PA+ group, compared with those in the PA− group of the same gender, will be significantly more likely to result in an injury (e.g., Leone et al. 2004).

Fear

We hypothesize that physical assaults by those in the PA+ group, compared with those in the PA− group of the same gender, will be significantly more likely to result in fear (e.g., Morse 1995) and fear sequelae (perceived loss of power/control over one's own life, sense of entrapment) (Jacobson and Gottman 1998; Smith et al. 2002).

PA+ Stability

We suggest testing the hypothesized stability of the taxometric findings in three ways: 1) stability of the taxonic indicators across time; 2) consistency of the direction of indicators across repeated assessments (i.e., if taxon members are significantly higher on a validated indicator at time 1, are they significantly higher at all other assessments?); and 3) stability of taxon group membership across repeated assessments.

Risk Factors

We also recommend testing the concurrent and predictive validity of the initial taxon classification by relating it to hypothesized risk factors. In the case of partner maltreatment, we would make the following four predictions. PA+ members, compared with PA− individuals of the same gender, will 1) report higher frequency of generalized aggressive behavior; 2) report more developmental risk factors (e.g., interparental violence; school problems; legal trouble); 3) report and be observed engaging in more couples conflict; and 4) report being more unhappy with their relationships.

Implications of a Taxometric Model

If our hypotheses were tested and supported, indicators of PA+ identified, and the PA+ subgroup validated as detailed earlier, this would suggest a radical shift in how partner maltreatment is assessed and how a partner abuse taxon is defined, both in clinical and in research settings. First, it would strongly support, and provide initial validity evidence for, categorically classifying partner abuse. Further, etiological research could focus on identifying endophenotypic markers and specific developmental pathways to PA+, which is only possible when sensitive and specific markers are known. Prevention research could focus on early identification of this specific group of individuals and developing the technology to deflect a likely narrower set of developmental trajectories. Legal and treatment systems responding to partner maltreatment would be able to more accurately discern who would likely benefit from psychoeducational diversion programs (which could then be targeted for their needs and not the needs of PA+ offenders) and who needs more intensive intervention or possible incarceration.

Of course, implications are equally compelling if partner abuse is not found to represent a distinct construct, but rather is found to fall along a continuum of partner behavior. Such a finding would be a monumental shift for the partner maltreatment field, which has always viewed the phenomenon as categorical. It would suggest that not only is there no qualitative distinction between our hypothesized PA+ and PA− groups, but also there is not a qualitative distinction at any point along the distribution of partner assaultive acts. If this were the case, it would argue for all research on partner assault and abuse to recognize its continuous nature and lessen the reliance on contrasted groups designs.

The implications for diagnosis are also dramatic. Rather than seeking optimal diagnostic criteria for capturing the PA+ group, attempts at developing categorical diagnostic criteria should be abandoned in favor of providing rough clinical guidelines based on a continuous distribution. It should be recognized, however, that cutoffs themselves are arbitrary guidelines that might be useful indicators of what segment of the distribution an individual lies within, but that individuals immediately above and below the cutoff are more similar than distinct.

Conclusion

In this chapter we have attempted to demonstrate the contribution to basic and translational research that searching for a distinct partner abuse construct and subgroup specifically, and relational disorder subgroups more generally, could make.

Even if qualitatively subgroups are not found, carrying out well-conceived and well-conducted research necessary to test taxometric hypotheses (Lenzenweger 2004) would undoubtedly benefit both those interested in relational disorders and those interested in the physical and psychiatric disorders that relational disorders affect or are affected by.

References

Aldorondo E: Cessation and persistence of wife assault: a longitudinal analysis. Am J Orthopsychiatry 66:141–151, 1996

American Psychiatric Association: Diagnostic and Statistical Manual of Mental Disorders, 2nd Edition. Washington, DC, American Psychiatric Association, 1968

American Psychiatric Association: Diagnostic and Statistical Manual of Mental Disorders, 3rd Edition. Washington, DC, American Psychiatric Association, 1980

American Psychiatric Association: Diagnostic and Statistical Manual of Mental Disorders, 4th Edition, Text Revision. Washington, DC, American Psychiatric Association, 2000

Archer J: Sex differences in aggression between heterosexual partners: a meta-analytic review. Psychol Bull 126:651–680, 2000

Beauchaine TP, Marsh P: Taxometric methods: enhancing early detection, diagnosis, and prevention of psychopathology by identifying latent vulnerability traits, in Developmental Psychopathology, 2nd Edition. Edited by Cicchetti D, Cohen D. Hoboken, NJ, Wiley, 2006, pp 931–967

Caetano R, Cundradi CB, Clark CL, et al: Intimate partner violence and drinking patterns among white, black, and Hispanic couples in the U.S. J Subst Abuse 11:123–138, 2000

Cascardi M, Vivian D: Context for specific episodes of marital violence: gender and severity of violence differences. J Fam Violence 10:265–293, 1995

Coker AL, Smith PH, Bethea L, et al: Physical health consequences of physical and psychological intimate partner violence. Arch Fam Med 9:451–457, 2000

Coker AL, Davis KE, Arias I: Physical and mental health effects of intimate partner violence for men and women. Am J Prev Med 23:260–268, 2002

Cronbach LJ, Meehl PE: Construct validity in psychological tests. Psychol Bull 52:281–302, 1995

Crowell NA, Burgess AW (eds): Understanding Violence Against Women. Washington, DC, National Academy Press, 1996

Danielson KK, Moffitt TE, Caspi A, et al: Comorbidity between abuse of an adult and DSM-III-R mental disorders: evidence from an epidemiological study. Am J Psychiatry 155:131–133, 1998

Dutton DG: A scale for measuring propensity for abusiveness. J Fam Violence 10:203–221, 1995

Ehrensaft MK, Vivian D: Spouses' reasons for not reporting existing marital aggression as a marital problem. J Fam Psychol 10:443–453, 1996

Ehrensaft MK, Moffitt TE, Caspi A: Clinically abusive relationships in an unselected birth cohort: men's and women's participation and developmental antecedents. J Abnorm Psychol 113:258–271, 2004

Feld SL, Straus MA: Escalation and desistance from wife assault in marriage, in Physical Violence in American Families: Risk Factors and Adaptations to Violence in 8,145 Families. Edited by Straus MA, Gelles RJ. New Brunswick, NJ, Transaction Publishers, 1990, pp 489–526

Gelles RJ: Estimating the incidence and prevalence of violence against women: National Data Systems and Sources. Violence Against Women 6:784–804, 2000

Gelles RJ, Straus MA: The medical and psychological costs of family violence, in Physical Violence in American Families: Risk Factors and Adaptations to Violence in 8,145 Families. Edited by Straus MA, Gelles RJ. New Brunswick, NJ, Transaction Publishers, 1990, pp 425–430

Gelles RJ, Loseke DR, Cavanaugh MM (eds): Current Controversies in Family Violence, 2nd Edition. Newbury Park, CA, Sage, 2005

Gottman JM, Jacobson NS, Rushe RH, et al: The relationship between heart rate reactivity, emotionally aggressive behavior and general violence in batterers. J Fam Psychol 9:227–248, 1995

Graham-Kevan N, Archer J: Physical aggression and control in heterosexual relationships: the effect of sampling. Violence Vict 18:181–196, 2003

Gross JJ: Antecedent- and response-focused emotion regulation: divergent consequences for experience, expression, and physiology. J Pers Soc Psychol 74:224–237, 1998

Gross JJ, Levenson RW: Emotional suppression: physiology, self-report, and expressive behavior. J Pers Soc Psychol 64:970–986, 1993

Gross JJ, Levenson RW: Hiding feelings: the acute effects of inhibiting negative and positive emotion. J Abnorm Psychol 106:95–103, 1997

Haynes SN, Richard DCS, Kubany ES: Content validity in psychological assessment: a functional approach to concepts and methods. Psychol Assess 7:238–247, 1995

Heyman RE: Observation of couple conflicts: clinical assessment, applications, stubborn truths, and shaky foundations. Psychol Assess 13:5–35, 2001

Heyman RE, Slep AMS: Creating and field-testing diagnostic criteria for partner and child maltreatment. J Fam Psychol (in press)

Hyman SE. Foreword, in Advancing DSM: Dilemmas in Psychiatric Diagnosis. Edited by Phillips KA, First MB, Pincus HA. Washington, DC, American Psychiatric Association, 2003, pp xi–xxi

Holtzworth-Munroe A, Meehan JC, Herron K: Testing the Holtzworth-Munroe and Stuart (1994) batterer typology. J Consult Clin Psychol 68:1000–1019, 2000

Holtzworth-Munroe A, Stuart GL: Typologies of male batterers: three subtypes and the differences among them. Psychol Bull 116:476–497, 1994

Jacobson NS, Gottman JM: When Men Batter Women. New York, Simon & Schuster, 1998

Jacobson NS, Gottman JM, Waltz J, et al: Affect, verbal content, and psychophysiology in the arguments of couples with a violent husband. J Consult Clin Psychol 62:982–988, 1994

Johnson MP: Patriarchal terrorism and common couple violence: two forms of violence against women in U.S. families. J Marriage Fam 57:283–294, 1995

Johnson MP, Ferraro KJ: Research on domestic violence in the 1990s: making distinctions. J Marriage Fam 62:948–963, 2000

Johnson MP, Leone JM: The differential effects of intimate terrorism and situational couple violence: findings from the National Violence Against Women Survey. J Fam Issues 26:322–349, 2005

Jones L, Hughes M, Unterstaller U: Post-traumatic stress disorder (PTSD) in victims of domestic violence: a review of the research. Trauma Violence Abuse 2:99–119, 2001

Langhinrichsen-Rohling J, Huss MT, Ramsey S: The clinical utility of batterer typologies. J Fam Violence 15:37–54, 2000

Lawrence E, Bradbury TN: Physical aggression and marital dysfunction: a longitudinal analysis. J Fam Psychol 15:135–154, 2001

Lenzenweger MF: Consideration of the challenges, complications, and pitfalls of taxometric analysis. J Abnorm Psychol 113:10–23, 2004

Leone JM, Johnson MP, Cohan CL, et al: Consequences of male partner violence for low-income minority women. J Marriage Fam 66:472–490, 2004

Magdol L, Moffitt TE, Caspi A, et al: Developmental antecedents of partner abuse: a prospective-longitudinal study. J Abnorm Psychol 107:375–389, 1998

Morse BJ: Beyond the Conflict Tactics Scale: assessing gender differences in partner violence. Violence Vict 10:251–272, 1995

National Advisory Mental Health Council, Workgroup on Basic Science: Setting Priorities for Basic Brain & Behavioral Science Research at NIMH. Report of the National Advisory Mental Health Council's Workgroup on Basic Sciences. Bethesda, MD, National Institute of Mental Health, May 2004. Available at: https://www.nimh.nih.gov/council/bbbsresearch.pdf. Accessed March 6, 2006.

O'Leary KD, Barling J, Arias I, et al: Prevalence and stability of physical aggression between spouses: a longitudinal analysis. J Consult Clin Psychol 57:263–268, 1989

Pagelow MD: Woman-Battering: Victims and Their Experiences. Thousand Oaks, CA, Sage 1981

Quigley BM, Leonard KE: Desistance of husband aggression in the early years of marriage. Violence Vict 11:355–370, 1996

Richards JM, Gross JJ: Composure at any cost? The cognitive consequences of emotion suppression. Pers Soc Psychol Bull 25:1033–1044, 1999

Ruscio J, Ruscio AM: A conceptual and methodological checklist for conducting a taxometric investigation. Behavior Therapy 35:403–447, 2004

Saltzman LE, Fanslow JL, McMahon PM, et al: Intimate partner violence surveillance: uniform definitions and recommended data elements (ver. 1.0). Atlanta, GA, National Center for Injury Prevention and Control, Centers for Disease Control and Prevention, 1999

Smith PH, Thornton GE, DeVellis R, et al: A population-based study of the prevalence and distinctiveness of battering, physical assault, and sexual assault in intimate relationships. Violence Against Women 8:1208–1232, 2002

Stamp GH, Sabourin TC: Accounting for violence: an analysis of male spousal abuse narratives. J Appl Commun Res 23:284–307, 1995

Stets JE, Straus MA: Gender differences in reporting marital violence and its medical and psychological consequences, in Physical Violence in American Families. Edited by Straus MA, Gelles RJ. New Brunswick, NJ, Transaction Publishers, 1990, pp 151–165

Straus MA: The Conflict Tactics Scales and its critics: an evaluation and new data on validity and reliability, Physical Violence in American Families: Risk Factors and Adaptations to Violence in 8,145 Families. Edited by Straus MA, Gelles RJ. New Brunswick, NJ, Transaction Publishers, 1990, pp 3–16

Straus MA, Gelles RJ (eds): Physical Violence in American Families: Risk Factors and Adaptations to Violence in 8,145 Families. New Brunswick, NJ, Transaction Publishers, 1990

Straus MA, Hamby SL, Boney-McCoy S, et al: The Revised Conflict Tactics Scales (CTS2): development and preliminary psychometric data. J Fam Issues 17:283–316, 1996

Waltz JB, Babcock JC, Jacobson NS, et al: Testing a typology of batterers. J Consult Clin Psychol 68:658–669, 2000

Yllo K, Bograd M (eds): Feminist Perspectives on Wife Abuse. Beverly Hills, CA, Sage, 1988

DEFINING RELATIONAL DISORDERS AND IDENTIFYING THEIR CONNECTIONS TO AXES I AND II

Lorna Smith Benjamin, Ph.D.

Marianne Z. Wamboldt, M.D.

Kenneth L. Critchfield, Ph.D.

The Comorbidity Problem: Challenges to Categorical Interpretations of DSM-IV

Many research studies have shown that comorbidity is rampant within both Axis I (e.g., Newman et al. 1998) and Axis II (e.g., Kupfer et al. 2002), as well as between Axis I and Axis II (e.g., Petrocelli et al. 2001). The comorbidity problem is so well recognized that an early and preliminary workgroup for DSM-V suggested that "reification of DSM-IV entities, to the point that they are considered to be equivalent to diseases, is more likely to obscure than to elucidate research findings." The workgroup further noted, "All these limitations in the current diagnostic paradigms suggest that research exclusively focused on refining the DSM-defined syndromes may never be successful in uncovering their underlying etiologies. For that to happen, an as yet unknown paradigm shift may need to occur" (Kupfer et al. 2002, p. xix). No such theoretical paradigm has been established, and any such proposals must be supported by data.

Dimensional Alternatives to DSM

Empirically based diagnostic paradigms based on factor analysis have been proposed as a solution to the comorbidity problem. In the case of Axis II disorders, favored candidates for a revised nomenclature, according to First and colleagues (2002), include Livesley's Dimensional Assessment of Personality Pathology (DAPP; Livesley and Jackson 2002), the Five-Factor Model (e.g., Costa and McCrae 1992), Cloninger's Temperament and Character Inventory (Cloninger et al. 1994), and Clark and Watson's Schedule for Nonadaptive and Adaptive Personality (SNAP; Clark 1993). These methodologies yield a profile that assigns an individual a position on each of the proposed underlying dimensions. Dimensional models might apply to Axis I, too. For example, a dimensional description that accommodates comorbidity between anxiety and depression was offered by Clark and Watson. It has performed well in validation studies (e.g., Clark et al. 1994). Whether applied to Axis I or II, dimensional models solve the comorbidity problem by assessing everyone on each presumed underlying continuous dimension.

Required Features of a Relational Disorder

First and colleagues (2002, pp. 157–159) examined the possibility of creating a new dimension in DSM-V that describes relational disorders. They identified needed features, which included the following:

1. The diagnostic description must be of the relationship, not just of the individual.
2. The relational problems must have distinctive features.
3. The relational problems must cause severe emotional, social, and occupational impairment.
4. The relational problems must have a recognizable clinical course.
5. The relational problems should show recognized patterns of comorbidity.
6. The relational problems are expected to appear in patterns of family aggregation.
7. The relational problems should involve both biological and psychosocial factors.
8. Relational disorders should show response to specific treatments.
9. Relational disorders should be preventable.
10. There would be evidence of repeated instances of having impact on the course of Axis I disorders and on medical conditions.
11. The relational dimensions should clarify the role of parent-child and marital disorders in the expression of biological influence on psychiatric disorders.

Many of these features might be expected of all DSM descriptions, and although few Axis I and no Axis II categories actually meet those standards, the goals are worthy.

Use of Structural Analysis of Social Behavior in Diagnosing Relational Disorders

Structural Analysis of Social Behavior (SASB) is a dimensional model that helps clinicians and researchers clearly and reliably describe social interactions via patient self-ratings or objective observers. Use of SASB can contribute significantly to the challenge of addressing all 11 requirements for defining relational disorders, including a viable approach to comorbidity. Self ratings on SASB Intrex questionnaires can quickly assess key relationships that can be related to Axis I or Axis II diagnoses. Each key relationship (usually one's relationship with a spouse) can be rated on a 36-item questionnaire. If the assessment shows that the relationship is, for example, 2 or more standard deviations from the norm in the direction of pathology, clinicians could be directed to interview the patient to explore that relationship in greater depth. Alternatively, a T score of 70, as is the convention in psychological testing, might serve to identify relationships that require investigation. An optional observational coding method provides assessment by objective observers that is in the same metric as that generated by self-ratings on the questionnaires. Differences in results between self and observer ratings can, among many things, identify treatment targets. For example, Humes and Humphrey (1994) found that parents of drug-abusing adolescent females described themselves as more friendly to their daughters than did objective observers. Validity of the SASB model has been tested in many ways, and support is strong (e.g., Benjamin 1996b, 2000; Benjamin et al. 2006; Constantino 2000; Lorr 1991).

Patient ratings of views of self and others show orderly and significant associations with symptoms from Axis I and Axis II. Groups of subjects whose ratings deviate from the norm in the direction of hostility by 2 or more standard deviations have significantly greater symptomatology than subjects with less extreme scores. It follows that marital or family or individual therapy focused on the problem relationships could lessen severity of the associated Axis I or Axis II pathology. A prototype for this approach is provided by the successful expressed emotion (EE) research that has established the importance of helping families change specific hostile patterns of relationship that are associated with exacerbation of psychiatric disorders such as schizophrenia, bipolar disorder, and eating disorders (e.g., Weissman et al. 2000).

THE SASB MODEL

The SASB model is built on three dimensions. The first dimension, *focus,* comprises three types: transitive interpersonal action directed toward other (prototypically parentlike) (designated 1); intransitive interpersonal action focused on self (prototypically childlike) (designated 2); and introjection, or transitive action directed toward self (designated 3). A study of maternal ratings of siblings of 171 pediatric outpatients suggested that intransitive actions (focus on self) of infants and toddlers past 6 months in age showed good internal consistency.[1] Maternal ratings of transitive actions (focus on other) by children of various ages showed progressively greater internal consistency through the age group 7–9 years, in which adult levels in consistency of focus on mother were demonstrated. In a normal adult relationship, focus is distributed approximately equally between focus on other and on self, and internal consistency for the two domains is comparable in normal populations (Benjamin 2000 [see Tables 10 and 11 of that manual]).

The horizontal and vertical dimensions for each type of focus are presented in Figure 10–1A, along with two versions of the SASB model (quadrant and cluster). The horizontal dimension (Figure 10–1B) runs from Hate on the left to Love on the right. The vertical dimensions for the three types of focus define enmeshment at the lower end of the vertical dimension and differentiation at the upper end. For transitive action directed toward another person, represented in **bold** in Figure 10–1C, the vertical dimension runs from **Control** to **Emancipate**. If the focus is an intransitive state in relation to another person, the vertical dimension runs from Submit to Separate. Enmeshment is defined in terms of **Control** by one person and Submission by the other. Differentiation, the opposite of Enmeshment, is defined in terms of **Emancipation** by one person and Separation by the other. *Italics* represent transitive focus directed back upon the self rather than toward another person. For example, **Control** becomes *Self-Control*.

The quadrant version of the model, shown in Figure 10–1B, depicts (starting at 3 o'clock and moving clockwise) friendly enmeshment and hostile enmeshment; hostile differentiation and friendly differentiation. The octant version, shown in Figure 10–1C, adds names to points midway between each of the axes. For example, **Affirm** represents transitive action directed toward another person that consists of moderate amounts of **Active Love** and moderate amounts of **Emancipate**. Its opposite, **Blame**, appears 180 degrees away and consists of moderate amounts of **Control** plus moderate amounts of **Attack**. So starting at 3 o'clock

---

[1]Measured for each individual by a correlation between a normal curve and the pattern that emerged from 35 progressively lagged autocorrelations of the 36 scores on the SASB Intrex long form for a given domain, such as intransitive focus on self (Benjamin 1974, pp. 400–405). Internal consistency for the medium form is measured by correlating the eight items for version 1 with the eight corresponding items for version 2. The developmental study just described has not been performed with the medium form, nor has it been replicated for the long form. In normal adult populations, internal consistency for all types of focus typically is very high when either the medium or the long form is used.

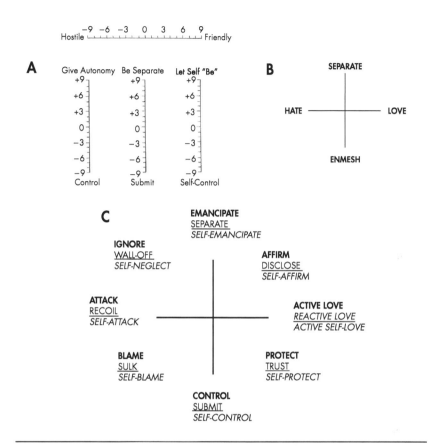

FIGURE 10–1. SASB dimensions applied to quadrant and octant models.

The horizontal and vertical dimensions (**A**) and the quadrant version of the SASB model (**B**) appear on top, while the octant version (**C**) is on bottom. See text for details about how the dimensions can be combined to define the quadrant and the octant models.

Source.   (**A**) Reprinted with permission from Benjamin LS: "Use of the SASB Dimensional Model to Develop Treatment Plans for Personality Disorders, I: Narcissism." *Journal of Personality Disorders* 1:43–70, 1987. Copyright 1987, Guilford Press. Used with permission. (**B**) Reprinted with permission from Benjamin LS: "Structural Analysis of Differentiation Failure." *Psychiatry* 42:1–23, 1979. Copyright 1979, William Alanson White Psychiatric Foundation. (**C**) Reprinted with permission from Benjamin LS: *Interpersonal Diagnosis and Treatment of Personality Disorders,* 2nd Edition. New York, Guilford, 1996. Copyright 1996, Guilford Press.

on the octant model, one can progress stepwise through the transitive group from **Active Love** to **Protect** to **Control** to **Blame** to **Attack** to **Ignore** to **Emancipate** to **Affirm**, back to **Active Love** again. The same orderliness exists for <u>intransitive</u> focus and for *introjected* focus. The full SASB model, not shown in Figure 10–1, subdivides quadrants into eighths, so that there are $9 \times 4 = 36$ points for each type of focus.

Individuals and relationships can be assessed in terms of self-ratings on the SASB Intrex questionnaires. One set is based on the octant model (the medium form, with two items per cluster[2] on Figure 10–1), and the other set is based on the full model (the long form, with four or five points per cluster). Each item was written to correspond to the dimensions it represents. For example, one of the items in the SASB Intrex medium form for the point **Affirm** is "X lets Y speak freely and warmly tries to understand Y even if they disagree." An item representing the opposite point, **Blame,** is "X puts Y down, blames Y, punishes Y." Items on the medium form require a sixth-grade reading level. Raters assign items a score that ranges between 0 (does not apply at all, never) and 100 (applies perfectly, all the time).

A rater assesses four aspects of a relationship. The first two come from rating the other person (he/she or they forms) for each type of interpersonal focus (other and self). This yields 1) he or she focuses on me (transitive action), and 2) he or she reacts to me (intransitive reaction). Then, the relationship is assessed by rating self with the other person (I forms). This yields 3) I focus on him (transitive action) and 4) I react to him (intransitive reactive state). In the standard series of SASB Intrex ratings, it is recommended that the relationship with significant other person (SO) be assessed twice: once when the relationship is at its best, and once when the relationship is at its worst. All data that follow are for ratings of the worst state. Introject ratings assess a different set of eight points, which are rated independently of any particular relationship, also usually in the best and in the worst states.

THE PREDICTIVE PRINCIPLES

Predictive principles are useful in understanding interactions between couples, making links between prior and current relationships, marking interpersonal antecedents to self concept, and much more. The main predictive principles of the SASB model are similarity, opposition, complementarity, introjection, and antithesis. *Similarity* is defined when two people behave in the same way and are coded at the same point on the model. For example, if both the husband and wife try to **Control** the relationship, they are similar. *Opposite* behaviors occur 180 degrees across from each other on the model (e.g., **Blame** and **Affirm**). In Figure 10–1C, *complementarity* is shown by adjacent bolded and underlined points. For example, **Affirm** and <u>Disclose</u> are complementary points. Their respective opposites are the complementary pair: **Blame** and <u>Sulk</u>. *Introjection,* as mentioned before, marks transitive action directed inward. For example, **Control** that is introjected becomes

---

[2]There also is a short form, but that form is not recommended because it offers only one item per model point, and it is not possible to compute internal consistency.

Self-Control. Finally, *antithesis* is demonstrated when one person in a relationship chooses to behave in a noncomplementary manner to another, e.g., responding to **Blame** with <u>Disclose</u>.

There are many methods to test the validity of the predictive principles. Complementarity and introjection are most frequently tested, and evidence for their validity is supportive (e.g., Benjamin 2000; K.L. Critchfield, L.S. Benjamin, "Repetition of Early Interpersonal Experiences in Adult Relationships," manuscript submitted for publication; Gurtman 2000).

ORDERLY CONNECTIONS BETWEEN SASB-BASED MEASURES OF RELATIONSHIP AND SYMPTOMS

In a psychiatric inpatient sample of 151 patients, a general association between internalized representations of relationship at worst and symptoms was established by Canonical correlations between eight SASB clusters for an aspect of relationship and nine Symptom Checklist–90—Revised (SCL-90-R) (Derogatis 1977) symptom scales. For each of the four relationship aspects, the Canonical R was highly significant. The same results were obtained for Canonical R between sets of 8 SASB relational measures and the 11 personality disorder (PD) scales developed by Morey and colleagues (1985) on the basis of Minnesota Multiphasic Personality Inventory–I scores. In sum, both Axis I and Axis II showed significant overall associations between ratings of the relationship with significant other (he/she and I/me) and symptoms from Axis I (SCL-90-R) and Axis II (Morey PD scales).

A graphical representation of the connections between perception of relationship and Axis I symptoms appears in Figure 10–2. The correlations between relationship and symptoms of anger, anxiety, and depression show orderly cosinelike patterns consistent with the underlying theoretical structure shown in Figure 10–1. Single asterisks indicate the correlations between ratings of the relationship and a symptom (anger, anxiety, or depression) that were significant at $P<.05$, while double asterisks indicate significance of $P<.01$ or better. An asterisk appears by H, A, or D, indicating whether the significant correlation involved hostility (H), anxiety (A), or depression (D).

The orderliness in the patterns suggests there is an inherent connection between the perceived relationship described by the SASB model and the symptoms. The similarities among the three curves are accounted for by the well-established comorbidity among these symptoms. The differences are interesting and are discussed at length by Benjamin (L.S. Benjamin, manuscript in preparation). Depression is marked by a *deficit in friendly behaviors,* shown by the marked negative correlations in the friendly section of the model, while anger is marked by an *increase in hostile behaviors,* shown by higher positive correlations in the hostile section of the model. Anxiety appears to fall between anger and depression and is significant only for the point <u>Recoil</u>, which is the theoretical complement of **Attack.**

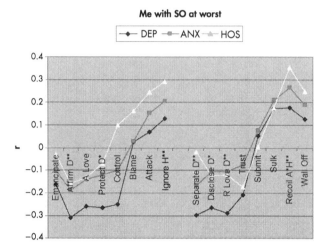

Me with SO at worst

FIGURE 10–2.   Orderly correlations between symptoms and relationship.

One-hundred fifty-one psychiatric inpatients rated symptoms on the SCL-90-R and items assessing "me with my SO [significant other] at worst." Single asterisks mark the correlations between ratings of the relationship and a symptom (anger, anxiety, or depression) that were significant at $P<.05$, while double asterisks indicate significance at least $P<.01$. An asterisk attached to H, A, or D shows that the significant correlation involved hostility, anxiety, or depression, respectively. ANX=anxiety; DEP=depression; HOS=hostility.

Source. Reprinted from Benjamin LS: *Interpersonal Reconstructive Therapy for Anger, Anxiety and Depression.* Washington, DC, American Psychological Association (in press). Used with permission.

Identifying Relationships That May Require Treatment

After a general connection is established between the relationship measures and Axis I and Axis II symptoms, it is appropriate to consider how individual pathological relationships (relational disorders) might be defined. As is the tradition in medicine, the diagnostic task begins with defining "normal."

DEFINING "NORMAL"

Normal relationships have been defined theoretically with the SASB model (Benjamin 2003) and tested empirically (Benjamin 2000). The hypothesis is that normal (and ideal) relationships have a baseline of friendliness, show moderate degrees of enmeshment and moderate degrees of differentiation, and demonstrate a balance of focus between self and others. Nonpatient populations do tend to endorse items in the theoretically normal region of the model, shown in the octant version of Figure 10–1 (C) as the three clusters around the affiliation pole (Benjamin 2000). Pathological relationships and patient populations are more hostile, as shown in the three clusters around the hostility pole in Figure 10–1C. Many published studies have confirmed a robust association between hostility as measured by the SASB Intrex questionnaires and psychopathology.

Patients also are predicted to show extremes of enmeshment or of differentiation. That possibility is not frequently assessed, and when it is, results appear to vary according to context, such as roles, stages of relationship, and cultural values. The association between hostility and pathology is very clear, whereas connections between extreme enmeshment or differentiation and pathology have received limited support and require further study.

ASSESSING RELATIONSHIPS FROM THE PATIENT'S PERSPECTIVE

The four aspects of a relationship can be located in interpersonal space on the basis of a vector that estimates position on the horizontal and the vertical dimensions. The central tendency on the horizontal axis for a given set of eight items is computed by multiplying the value assigned by the rater to items representing each model point times the weights that orient around the horizontal axis, and dividing by 8 (the Affiliation score, or AF), The position on the vertical axis is computed in the same way except that weights orient around the vertical axis (the Autonomy score, or AU).[3]

The top section of Figure 10–3 presents a scatterplot of the (AF, AU) vectors for 191 psychiatric inpatients rating the first aspect, "My SO [significant other] focuses on me at worst."[4] The shaded region includes raters whose vectors fall within 2 standard deviations of the norms. About 25 raters reported having an SO whose hostility was extraordinary ($Z \leq -2$). Seven had partners who were extreme in giving autonomy, and 9 described excessive control.

The lower part of Figure 10–3 shows that more than 20 patients reported that they engaged in much hostile walling off from their partner (AF Z score ≤ -2) compared with the normal standard. Nine showed extreme hostile submission (AU Z ≤ -2), and 6 exhibited extreme autonomy taking (AU Z ≥ 2). Both parts of Figure 10–3 have denser representation in the lower-left-hand quadrant, which suggests that patients had partners who engaged in hostile control of them (top

---

[3]Affiliation weights are greatest for items close to the affiliation pole and progressively decrease as the hostility pole is approached. Autonomy weights are greatest at the differentiation pole and minimal in the enmeshment region.

[4]The SASB Intrex long form is being used.

My SO focuses on me at Worst

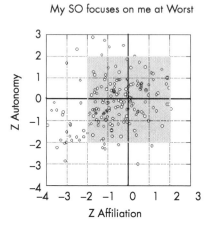

I react to my SO at Worst

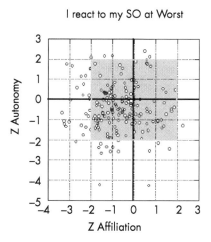

FIGURE 10–3. Identification of individuals with relationship problems–I.

Scatterplot for 191 psychiatric inpatients who rated "My SO [significant other] focuses on me" *(top)* and "I react" *(bottom)*. The horizontal Z scores are the weighted Affiliation scores relative to norms, while the vertical Z scores are the weighted Autonomy scores relative to norms. The shaded box marks individuals within 2 standard deviations of the normal means.

part) and that patients showed more hostile submission (bottom part) to their more controlling partners. The fact that lower-left-hand quadrants were most densely populated for these two sets of ratings (aspects 1 and 4) is consistent with prediction according to the principle of complementarity (hostile control is complemented by resentful submission).

Figure 10–4 shows the scatterplot for the remaining two aspects, "I focus on my SO [significant other] at worst" (aspect 3) and "My SO reacts to me at worst" (aspect 2). Here, the greater clustering of individuals appears in the upper-left-hand quadrant, which suggests there is a trend for patients to dismiss or ignore their partners (top part of Figure 10–3) compared with normal controls. As expected according to complementarity theory, partners tend to match the hostile dismissal by engaging in hostile withdrawal (bottom part of Figure 10–4) from patients.

DIAGNOSING RELATIONAL DISORDERS IN TERMS OF EXTREME Z SCORES

Patients whose Z scores are plotted outside the norms (i.e., Z≥absolute value of 2 in the directions of extreme hostility, enmeshment, or differentiation) in Figures 10–3 or 10–4 would be marked as having relational disorders. Clinicians would be directed to pursue understanding of relationship problems for patients whose view of their relationship falls outside the normal limits for relationships.

Just over 150 psychiatric inpatients were assigned to groups on the basis of their extremity scores shown in Figures 10–3 and 10–4. Repeated measures analysis was performed on the nine SCL-90-R scale scores to assess whether there was a significant between-groups difference (i.e., within normal limits vs. Z less than −2 for the test of AF; within normal limits vs. Z greater than +2 or less than −2 for the test of AU). There also was a test of the groups by SCL-90-R scale score interaction. Either finding would indicate that extremity in relationship score was significantly associated with Axis I symptoms as measured by the SCL-90-R. For the Affiliation dimension, significant group effects were obtained for all four aspects of relationship in the worst state: "my SO focuses on me"; "my SO reacts to me"; "I focus on my SO," and "I react to my SO." Three also showed a significant interaction between group and symptom scales. Figure 10–5 shows the complementary set, each aspect of which showed a significant association between extreme affiliative group membership and psychopathology. Tests of extremity scores on the Autonomy dimension showed no significant differences on the SCL-90-R.

The same exercise was repeated with relationship extremity groups and Axis II symptoms as measured by Morey's definition of 11 DSM-III personality disorders. On the affiliation dimension, significant differences emerged between extreme groups, and in the groups by personality disorder interaction for "I focus on my SO" and "I react to my SO." For the autonomy dimension, the univariate *P* value between groups was <.068 for "I react to my SO at worst."

PROCESSING SASB INTREX RATINGS TO LEARN MORE ABOUT THE INDIVIDUAL

The SASB Intrex provides detailed information about the patterns of relationship with self and others. Raters might be asked, as is recommended in standard uses

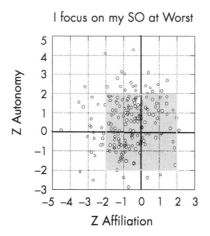

I focus on my SO at Worst

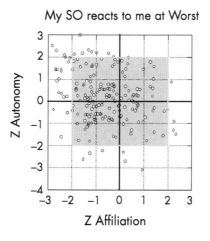

My SO reacts to me at Worst

FIGURE 10–4.   Identification of individuals with relationship problems–II.

Scatterplot for 191 psychiatric inpatients who rated "I focus on my SO [significant other]" *(top)* and "My SO reacts" *(bottom).* Z scores are relative to norms as in Figure 10–3. The shaded box encloses individuals within 2 standard deviations of the normal means.

of SASB Intrex, to rate key figures from the past as well as from the present. Current problems can be linked to past ones by the predictive principles. Software for processing SASB ratings is available through http://www.psych.utah.edu/benjamin/sasb. Output includes the (AF, AU) vectors shown in Figures 10–3 and 10–4, graphical profiles for individuals, one- or two-word statistically based best-fit descriptions of each aspect of each relationship, among other features. Both the graphs

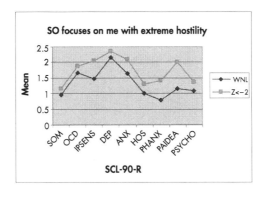

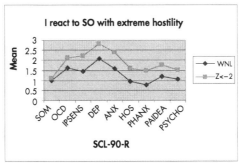

FIGURE 10–5. Relationship problems and psychopathology.

Correlations between Symptom Checklist–90—Revised (SCL-90-R) scores and weighted affiliation scores for 154 psychiatric inpatients who rated "My SO [significant other] focuses on me" *(top)* and "I react" *(bottom)*. The top lines present average symptom scores for the subgroup with extremely hostile relationships, and the bottom lines represent average symptom scores for patients having relationships with affiliation scores greater than −2 standard deviations from the norm. ANX=anxiety; DEP=depression; HOS=hostility; IPSENS= interpersonal sensitivity; OCD=obsessive-compulsive behaviors; PAIDEA=paranoid ideation; PHANX=phobic anxiety; PSYCHO=psychoticism; SOM=somatization; WNL= within normal limits.

and the brief descriptions make it easy to identify predictive principles and copy processes (defined in the next section).

Figure 10–6 gives examples of identification for a patient at the Interpersonal Reconstructive Therapy Clinic at the University of Utah. The patient's pretherapy ratings of his relationship with his father and with his (older male) lover are separated according to transitive focus on other (top) and intransitive focus on self (bottom). The brief descriptions from the summary report are as follows: Patient with his SO at worst: *Rater focuses on the other person: Attacking* (.82); *Rater reacts to the other per-*

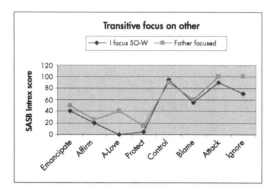

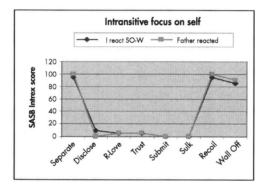

FIGURE 10–6.   Operationalizing the copy process of identification.

The patient whose Structural Analysis of Social Behavior (SASB) data are depicted here focused on *(top)* and reacted to *(bottom)* his male lover almost exactly as his father had focused on and reacted to him when he was a child. SO-W=significant other at worst.

son: Walling Off (0.87).[5] Comparable reports for the patient's father as remembered from childhood were: Attacking (0.82); Walling Off (0.86). Names for the best-fit curves were identical for father and son. That similarity also is reflected in very high correlations between the profiles at the top (*r* for transitive behaviors=0.92) and bottom (*r* for intransitive behaviors=1.00) of Figure 10–6. For both types of interpersonal focus, the patient "becomes" (identifies with) his father in his love relationship.

---

[5]The numbers in parentheses are correlations (best fits) between an actual profile and an 8-point theoretical profile that best matches the observed pattern (e.g., Attacking; Walling Off). A fit between data and theory of 0.71 or more (50% of the variance) is considered adequate to summarize the quality of the relationship aspect.

Hypotheses for How Relational Disorders Connect to Axis I and Axis II Disorders

Benjamin (2003) suggests that problem behaviors (e.g., personality disorder) can be linked to early learning of behavioral patterns by one of three *copy processes,* which frequently conform to the SASB predictive principles of similarity, complementarity, and introjection: 1) be like him or her (identification), illustrated by the man whose data were shown in Figure 10–6; 2) continue to act as if he or she is still there and in control (recapitulation); and 3) treat yourself as you have been treated (introjection). The present data suggest that if there is relational disturbance (measured by the SASB Intrex), there will be corresponding disturbances in Axis I symptoms (as measured by the SCL-90-R) and Axis II disturbances (as measured by Morey et al.'s scales on the MMPI-I). Other measures of Axis I and Axis II symptoms in independent databases show comparable results (Benjamin, manuscript in preparation).

Benjamin (2003) provided a testable theory that could explain how and why Axis I and Axis II covary in this way. The SASB predictive principles and copy process theory can link current relationship patterns to key relationships during development. Through use of the logic of *parallelism theory*—namely, that affect, behavior, and cognition evolved together and move together—it is argued that Axis I (diagnostic categories or dimensions that focus largely on affect and cognition) and Axis II (diagnostic categories or dimension that focus largely on behavior) *should* covary.

If confirmed, copy process theory and parallelism theory would provide draft answers to the 11 challenges for the definition of relational disorders posed by Kupfer et al. (2002). As required, relationship disorder is defined in terms of assessment of a relationship, not of an individual. The recommended procedure involves rating the interpersonal behaviors of a significant other person and of the rater with that person. Also as required, comorbidity is addressed by the proposed definition. If affect, cognition, and behavior are closely linked, comorbidity confirms, rather than contradicts, the associated theory of psychopathology. Another required feature is to develop preventative implications. These would be addressed by copy process theory, because it shows specifically how relationship problems reflect developmental learning. In addition, parallelism plus copy processes (e.g., Figures 10–5 and 10–6) could help account for the "role of parent-child and marital disorders in the expression of biological influence on psychiatric disorders." Hypotheses for each of the other requirements could be offered, but given that not much evidence has yet been developed, these few examples presume only to illustrate the promise of the approach, perhaps justifying further research.

More specific articulation of relational disorders might follow further data gathering on connections between SASB-based dimensional assessments of relationship and psychopathology. Additional tests of the validity of copy process and parallelism theories would help further address the 11 challenges to the definition of relational disorders posed by Kupfer, First, and Regier (2002). Treatment implications also need to be developed, with follow-up on relevant suggestions that appeared in Benjamin (2003). Finally, if this approach were to be pursued, extensive norms in a variety of contexts would be needed. Software and manuals need to be made more user-friendly.

Conclusion: Revisiting the Standards for Defining Relational Disorders

The discussion of SASB-based figures illustrates how relationship disorder can be defined in terms of standard deviations from norms in directions that are significantly associated with examples of Axis I and Axis II symptomatology. Excessive hostility, and perhaps also enmeshment or differentiation, could be targeted by specific treatments. Setting aside considerations of how valid the principles of copy process and parallelism will turn out to be, and whether or not the 11 challenges can be met by applying those principles to definitions of psychopathology, the present data nonetheless provide clear *empirical* support for the need to add a relational dimension to the diagnostic nomenclature. The significance of associations, and the orderliness in Figures 10–2 and 10–5, show that relationship difficulties are directly related to Axis I pathology, as represented by anger, anxiety, and depression, and to Axis II pathology, as represented by personality disorders. Since SASB data on introjection correlate even more powerfully with psychopathology than do the measures of interpersonal patterns with significant others, addition of SASB-based measures of self concept to the definition of "relational disorders" would allow a new relational disorders axis that could account for even more of the variance in psychopathology.

References

Benjamin LS: Structural Analysis of Social Behavior (SASB). Psychol Rev 81:392–425, 1974

Benjamin LS: Structural analysis of differentiation failure. Psychiatry 42:1–23, 1979

Benjamin LS: Use of the SASB dimensional model to develop treatment plans for personality disorders, I: narcissism. J Pers Disord 1:43–70, 1987

Benjamin LS: Interpersonal Diagnosis and Treatment of Personality Disorders, 2nd Edition. New York, Guilford, 1996a

Benjamin LS: Introduction to the special section on Structural Analysis of Social Behavior (SASB). J Consult Clin Psychol 64:1203–1212, 1996b

Benjamin LS: Intrex User's Manual. Salt Lake City, Department of Psychology, University of Utah, 2000

Benjamin LS: Interpersonal Reconstructive Therapy: Promoting Change in Nonresponders. New York, Guilford, 2003

Benjamin LS, Rothweiler JC, Critchfield KL: The use of Structural Analysis of Social Behavior (SASB) as an assessment tool. Ann Rev Clin Psychol 2:83–109, 2006

Benjamin LS: Interpersonal Reconstructive Therapy for Anger, Anxiety and Depression. Washington, DC, American Psychological Association (in press)

Clark LA: Manual for the Schedule for Nonadaptive and Adaptive Personality. Minneapolis, University of Minnesota Press, 1993

Clark LA, Watson D, Mineka S: Temperament, personality and the mood and anxiety disorders. J Abnorm Psychol 103:103–116, 1994

Cloninger CR, Przybeck TR, Svrakic DM, et al: The Temperament and Character Inventory: A Guide to Its Development and Use. St Louis, MO, Center for Psychobiology of Personality, Washington University, 1994

Constantino MJ: Interpersonal process in psychotherapy through the lens of the Structural Analysis of Social Behavior. Applied and Preventive Psychology 9:153–172, 2000

Costa PT, McCrae RR: Revised NEO Personality Inventory (NEO-PI-R) and NEO Five-Factor Inventory (NEO-FFI) Professional Manual. Odessa, FL, Psychological Assessment Resources, 1992

Derogatis LR: SCL-90 Administration, Scoring and Procedures Manuals for the Revised Version. Baltimore, MD, Author, 1977

First MB, Bell CC, Cuthbert B, et al: Personality disorders and relational disorders, in A Research Agenda for DSM-V. Edited by Kupfer DJ, First MB, Regier DA. Washington, DC, American Psychiatric Association, 2002, pp 123–199

Gurtman M: Interpersonal complementarity: integrating interpersonal measurement with interpersonal models. J Couns Psychol 48:97–110, 2000

Humes DL, Humphrey LL: A multimethod analysis of families with a polydrug-dependent or normal adolescent daughter. J Abnorm Psychol 103:676–685, 1994

Kupfer DJ, First MB, Regier DA (eds): A Research Agenda for DSM-V. Washington, DC, American Psychiatric Association, 2002

Livesley WJ, Jackson D: Manual for the Dimensional Assessment of Personality Pathology—Basic Questionnnaire. Port Huron, MI, Sigma Press, 2002

Lorr M: A redefinition of dominance. Pers Individ Dif 12:877–979, 1991

Morey LC, Waugh MH, Blashfield RK: MMPI scales for DSM-III personality disorders: their derivation and correlates. J Pers Assess 49:245–251, 1985

Newman DL, Moffitt TE: Caspi A, et al: Comorbid mental disorders: implications for treatment and sample selection. J Abnorm Psychol 107:305–311, 1998

Petrocelli JV, Glaser BA, Calhoun GB, et al: Personality and affect characteristics of outpatients with depression. J Pers Assess 77:162–175, 2001

Weissman AG, Nuechterlein KH, Goldstein MJ, et al: Controllability perceptions and reactions to schizophrenia: a within-family comparison of relatives with high and low expressed emotion. J Abnorm Psychol 109:167–171, 2000

CHAPTER 11

EXPRESSED EMOTION AND DSM-V

Jill M. Hooley, D.Phil.
David J. Miklowitz, Ph.D.
Steven R. H. Beach, Ph.D.

The construct of expressed emotion (EE) is well established as an important measure of the family environment. Much research has also been conducted on the assessment of this construct, providing a useful background for the discussion of measurement issues related to relational processes in psychopathology. By examining the literature on alternative ways of assessing EE, we can highlight several issues that may be common across efforts to codify relational processes. EE may also be one of the constructs that should be given a higher profile in the *Diagnostic and Statistical Manual* (DSM). A discussion of assessment issues related to EE may therefore be useful in setting the stage for the DSM revision process.

Expressed Emotion and Relapse of Severe Mental Illness

Developed by George Brown and his colleagues (Brown and Rutter 1966; Brown et al. 1972), EE reflects the extent to which the close family members of an identified patient express critical, hostile, or emotionally overinvolved attitudes toward the patient during a private interview with a researcher. The criterion measure of EE is the 1- to 1.5-hour semistructured Camberwell Family Interview, usually administered to the relative when the patient is acutely ill (Vaughn and Leff 1976). The interview examines the development of the patient's episode, the history of the illness, and the emotional impact of the disorder on the family. "High EE" relatives are those who express six or more critical comments (statements of dislike or resentment; e.g., "I dislike his self-serving attitude about things"), make one or more statements of hostility (personalized or generalized criticism or rejection; e.g., "I like nothing about him"), or fulfill criteria for elevated scores (3 or higher) on a 0–5 scale of emotional overinvolvement (e.g., "I worry about her constantly...I get myself sick sometimes").

The importance of expressed emotion for understanding the course of severe mental illness is supported by several decades of research. The research indicates that EE is a highly reliable psychosocial predictor of psychiatric relapse across a number of different disorders. Patients with schizophrenia, mood disorders, or a broad range of other psychiatric conditions who live in family environments that are characterized by critical, hostile, or emotionally overinvolved or intrusive attitudes (i.e., in high EE families) are at significantly elevated risk of early relapse compared with patients who do not live in such family environments (Butzlaff and Hooley 1998; Leff and Vaughn 1985). For example, patients with schizophrenia who live with or are in close association with high-EE relatives are at least twice as likely to relapse in the 9–12 months following a hospitalization than are patients who live with low-EE relatives. A meta-analysis revealed that of the 27 published studies examining EE and relapse in schizophrenia, 23 replicated the longitudinal association between levels of EE and relapse. Across studies, the expected 9- to 12-month relapse rate for patients with schizophrenia was 65% in high-EE families and 35% for patients in low-EE families (Butzlaff and Hooley 1998).

The EE–relapse association also extends to other psychiatric disorders, including mood disorders, eating disorders, anxiety disorders, and substance abuse problems (Butzlaff and Hooley 1998; Chambless et al. 2001; O'Farrell et al. 1998). In fact, the weighted mean effect size for the EE–relapse association across six studies of major mood disorder was slightly higher than the mean effect size for schizophrenia ($r=.39–.45$ vs. $.31$; see Butzlaff and Hooley 1998).

Adding to the construct validity of EE, relatives who are classified as high in EE behave in more negative ways when they interact with patients than do relatives who are classified as low in EE (Hooley 1986; Miklowitz et al. 1984). High levels of EE are also associated with *reciprocal* negativity within the relative-patient relationship (Cook et al. 1991; Hahlweg et al. 1989; Hooley 1990; Simoneau et al. 1998). Patients who interact with high-EE relatives have higher levels of physiological arousal than do patients who interact with low-EE relatives (Tarrier and Turpin 1992). Moreover, interacting with low-EE relatives appears to have a calming effect on patients (Tarrier et al. 1988). For these reasons, EE is appropriately regarded as measuring characteristics of the *patient-relative relationship* that are important for the relapse process.

Understanding the mechanisms through which EE and relapse are associated is now a major topic on the research agenda. Issues here include understanding patterns of brain activation in response to critical remarks (see Hooley et al. 2005), better understanding of the biological cascade initiated by high-EE environments, and the specific interactions between EE and genetic vulnerability. Progress in these areas will no doubt facilitate the continued development of the conceptual basis of EE.

The predictive validity of EE provides one rationale for including EE as a model relational process in DSM-V. EE is also a relational process of considerable interest to clinicians, because family-based interventions that seek to reduce EE have had success in decreasing patients' relapse rates (although it is not clear that reductions in EE are a necessary condition for family interventions to be effective) (Hogarty et al. 1986; Leff et al. 1982; Miklowitz and Tompson 2003). This combination of predictive validity and a conceptual connection to efficacious interventions provides a powerful argument for increased discussion of EE in a revised DSM. Inclusion of EE is likely to help a revised DSM better describe etiology, predict course, guide intervention, and understand the burden of severe mental illness.

However, there are at least two obstacles to the inclusion of EE in the DSM that require attention: one historical and the other practical. We focus the bulk of our attention in this chapter on the practical issue of measuring EE in clinical contexts. However, we begin with a brief consideration of the historical legacy that has slowed progress in the area and that may provide an obstacle to the inclusion of EE or other relational processes in the DSM.

Historical Challenges

Attention to family processes in severe mental illness has a long history, and this history complicates the use of well-validated family measures and the intervention programs that are tied to them. Early attempts to develop models of the influence of relational processes in severe mental illness were overtly parent-blaming. Parents were considered to be responsible for their children's conditions, and it was posited that these conditions had "poor parenting" or "double-bind messages" (Bateson et al. 1956) or "schizophrenogenic" mothering (Fromm-Reichmann 1948) at their root. Although such theoretical notions of etiology have long been discredited, even today any focus on "relational processes," much less "relational disorders," and their role in severe mental illness can provoke negative reactions from family members. For legitimate reasons, these family members view the challenges they face as being similar to the challenges faced by families coping with physically based illnesses, and they are often concerned that efforts to involve the family may end up in efforts to blame the family.

Fortunately, modern approaches to relational and family processes in severe mental illness no longer regard the family as the primary causal agent in the patient's illness. Nor do they view the patient as a "scapegoat" in a dysfunctional family. Now, these approaches are centered on how the family reacts to and organizes around a psychiatrically impaired member and on how these reactions protect against or contribute to the risk of recurrences of illness. Illness is seen as a developmental event or "punctuation point" to which families must respond. Just as physical illnesses require a biopsychosocial model to account for course of illness, and especially the emergence of chronicity (Engel 1977), so too do severe mental illnesses. The biopsychosocial model posits that illness in one family member affects the psychological health and relationships of other members and, in turn, that the reactions of these members affect the functioning of the person with the illness. Working from a biopsychosocial model makes it easier for family members to understand that although they are not responsible for the patient's illness, they can be key players in helping the patient recover and remain well.

Consistent with the modern biopsychosocial and interactional perspective, it is important to note that EE levels typically decline as patients improve. From 25%–50% of relatives of patients with schizophrenia who are rated as high EE during an acute phase of the patient's illness will be reclassified as low EE 1 year later, when patients are in remission (e.g., Brown et al. 1972; Tarrier et al. 1988). However, even as EE levels decline, the most critical relatives initially are still the most critical relatives months later when the patient's illness has remitted (e.g., Hooley et al. 1995). In addition, emotional overinvolvement appears to be even more stable than highly critical or hostile attitudes and declines more slowly over time (Brown et al. 1972; Leff et al. 1990). Taken together, these findings suggest that EE has both traitlike and statelike properties. Consistent with a diathesis-stress perspective, some relatives may be temperamentally predisposed to high-EE attitudes, and the onset of the patient's symptoms may be sufficient to push them across threshold for high EE (Hooley and Gotlib 2000). These observations provide a rationale for discussing relational processes in severe mental illness in a manner that is both empirically grounded and acceptable to families. However, addressing these issues systematically in a clinical context and in guiding work with families requires that we have a practical measurement technology that can be used by clinicians.

Practical Problems in Measuring Expressed Emotion

The criterion measure of EE, the Camberwell Family Interview, is generally viewed as being somewhat long and cumbersome for many clinical settings, particularly those with limited staffing. The average length of the interview is 1.5 hours, and EE can only be assessed reliably by raters who have received rather extensive training (typically 40–80 hours). In addition, training in rating EE is both expensive and difficult to obtain for use in clinical settings. Further, even if one is trained to code the interviews, the CFI takes 2–3 hours to code, which creates an additional potential burden on clinical staff. Moreover, until differential treatment decisions can be tied empirically to the results of EE assessments there may be relatively little clinical incentive to use expensive criterion measures of EE in clinical practice. At present, there may be a perception of too little immediate clinical pay-off to justify such elaborate assessment procedures.

Although the CFI remains the "gold standard" for EE assessment, the need for "practical" assessment alternatives has given rise to several shorter methods for measuring EE. These measures respond to the potential practical need for relatively brief assessments of EE in clinical practice and may serve some clinical needs well. For example, the results of brief measures provide a natural context within which to discuss family involvement in treatment. However, there is a trade-off between brevity and important psychometric properties, in addition to the trade-off between comprehensiveness and cost discussed above. Brief methods for assessing EE often do not provide information that is equivalent to that obtained with the CFI.

To highlight practical issues and to illustrate the potential alternatives to use of the CFI, we describe four different approaches that have been developed for the brief assessment of EE and that have been compared with the CFI and used to predict relapse. A more extended discussion of these instruments is provided by Hooley and Parker (in press).

THE FIVE MINUTE SPEECH SAMPLE

The Five Minute Speech Sample (FMSS; Magana et al. 1986) requires the family member to talk about his or her thoughts and feelings about the patient for 5 uninterrupted minutes. The FMSS is structurally similar to the CFI, in that family members talk about the patient and their relationship. The FMSS is a less costly alternative to the CFI, however, because it requires less time to administer (5 minutes) and score (20 minutes). The speech is recorded and later coded for the overall level of EE (FMSS-EE), criticism (FMSS-CRIT), and emotional overinvolvement (FMSS-EOI). So, the FMSS assesses two important subscales of EE. However, there is no hostility rating on the FMSS. Warmth is also not assessed, although the FMSS does provide a frequency count of the number of positive comments relatives make about the patient that is incorporated into the EOI rating.

These considerations suggest that the FMSS can be directly compared with the CFI on at least some dimensions. Magana and colleagues (1986), in comparing the FMSS and CFI, found that 15 or 23 relatives who were rated as high EE on the CFI were also rated as high EE on the FMSS (sensitivity=65.2%). Of the 17 relatives who were rated as low EE on the CFI, 15 were correctly identified by the FMSS (specificity=88.2%). Virtually identical results were obtained with a Spanish-speaking sample (Magana et al. 1986). Further, even more impressive results for sensitivity (sensitivity=80%; specificity=71%) were reported in a German sample (Leeb et al. 1991). The overall pattern of results suggests that high-EE relatives tend to be under-identified with the FMSS (low sensitivity), but low-EE relatives are well identified (high specificity) with the FMSS. For example, Fujita and colleagues (2002) reported that of 13 high-EE relatives of schizophrenia patients in Japan whose EE level was identified by CFI, only 4 were identified as high EE with the FMSS (sensitivity=.36). In contrast, 37 out of 44 low-EE relatives were correctly identified (specificity=.80) by the FMSS.

The coding instructions for the FMSS specifically instruct raters to be conservative and to stay away from ratings that would lead to a high-EE assessment if they are in doubt. However, sensitivity of the FMSS may increase markedly when relatives who score at the borderline EE level are assigned to the high-EE group (Shimodera et al. 1999, 2002).

Balancing potential enthusiasm for the FMSS is evidence of reduced predictive validity for the FMSS relative to the CFI. Thompson and colleagues (1995) reported that the FMSS did not predict exacerbation of psychotic symptoms in 33 male patients with schizophrenia over a 1-year follow-up. Similar negative findings between FMSS-rated EE and relapse in psychotic patients have been reported elsewhere (Jarbin et al. 2000; Kurihara et al. 2000; Nugter 1997; Tattan and Tarrier 2000; Uehara et al. 1997). In contrast, a significant association between FMSS-EE and relapse in schizophrenia was reported in a large-scale study conducted by Marom and colleagues (2002). Moreover, when relatives who were borderline in their ratings were assigned to the high-EE group, Uehara et al. (1997) did find a significant association between the FMSS and relapse in outpatients with schizophrenia.

One possible explanation for the relatively poor predictive validity of the FMSS is its lower reliability compared with the CFI. A relatively straightforward solution would be aggregation of multiple FMSS samples over time. Aggregation might improve the clinical utility of the FMSS as well as its reliability. Consistent with this hypothesis, Jarbin and colleagues (2000) found that neither FMSS-EE assessed at hospital admission nor FMSS-EE assessed at hospital discharge predicted 1- and 2-year relapse rates in adolescents with psychotic disorders. However, when the results of the two FMSS assessments were combined (and especially if borderline ratings were included as high EE), the aggregated classification of EE did significantly predict patients' 2-year relapse rates. There is also evidence that EE assessed with the FMSS is associated with worse clinical outcomes in mood disorders among children (Asarnow et al. 1993) and depressed outpatients in Japan (Uehara et al. 1996), and in depressive symptoms among patients with bipolar I disorder (Yan et al. 2004).

In summary, the FMSS has advantages and disadvantages as a measure of EE. On the positive side, the measure is shorter than the CFI and takes less time to code, and it does not require extensive training to administer. It is possible to imagine the FMSS being used in standard clinical practice, with FMSS samples being sent to coding laboratories with results returned to clinicians. In this model FMSS samples would be used in clinical practice in a manner similar to other lab tests. The FMSS also has the advantage of being available to assess relationships in which the respondent does not know the patient especially well and would not be able to answer all the questions contained in the CFI (e.g., a treatment team member). The FMSS has demonstrated predictive validity with respect to depression and, to a lesser degree, schizophrenia. However, as an alternative measure of EE, the FMSS has significant shortcomings. Although the FMSS takes less time to administer, this benefit may be offset by the need to have multiple assessments to attain good reliability and predictive validity. The FMSS also tends to under-identify high-EE relatives, and so additional work may be required in developing guidelines to enhance its utility in clinical settings.

LEVEL OF EXPRESSED EMOTION SCALE

The Level of Expressed Emotion (LEE) scale (Cole and Kazarian 1988) is a 60-item, self-report measure that assesses the emotional environment in the patient's most important relationships. The LEE scale comprises four subscales—Intrusiveness, Emotional Response, Attitude Toward Illness, and Tolerance and Expectations—with items based on the EE construct. Items are rated in a true-false format, and the scale generates a score for the level of EE overall as well as four subscale scores. Adding some flexibility, both patient and relative versions of the LEE scale are available. The patient version (LEE-Patient) asks patients to evaluate their relationship with their closest relative (i.e., the relative with whom they live). The relative version (LEE-Relative) requires the close relatives to evaluate their relationship with the patient. Because the LEE scale is a self-report measure, it is easier to administer and requires less time to score than either the CFI or the FMSS.

The initial report on the LEE scale demonstrated the scale's good psychometric properties, including high internal consistency for the total scale and the subscales, as well as high test-retest reliability among patients with schizophrenia (Cole and Kazarian 1988). However, the correlation between the total LEE-Relative score and the number of critical comments relatives made during the CFI was only .38 (Kazarian et al. 1990). In addition, the total LEE-Patient score was only modestly correlated with the number of critical comments relatives made during the CFI (r=.32). So, neither the patient nor the relative forms of the original 60-item LEE scale have demonstrated strong concurrent validity.

Despite its modest association with the CFI, Cole and Kazarian (1993) found that the patient version of the LEE scale was a good predictor of relapse among patients with schizophrenia (relatives' LEE scale scores were not obtained). In addition, when a median split of 9 was used, those who scored high on the LEE scale at the initial assessment were significantly more likely to be rehospitalized 1, 2, and 5 years later (Cole and Kazarian 1993) than were those scoring below the median (see also Donat et al. 1992).

A modified, 33-item version of the LEE scale using 4-point scales rather than true-false items was developed by Gerslma and colleagues (1992), and has an additional subscale to assess perceived criticism. Gerlsma and Hale (1997) reported that, when the modified 33-item LEE was used, the subscales of Emotional Support and Intrusiveness did not significantly predict how well patients fared but that depressed patients who reported higher levels of irritability in their partners fared less well over in the following 6 months. The best predictor of clinical outcome for the new LEE scale was the newly added Perceived Criticism scale. The more the patients rated their partners as being critical, the less change they showed in scores on the Beck Depression Inventory and on the Symptom Checklist–90 over the 6-month follow-up. With regard to concurrent validity, there is also evidence from a sample of patients with schizophrenia that the Perceived Criticism subscale of the LEE scale has a higher correlation with criticism assessed using the CFI ($r=.44$) than either the Total LEE scale ($r=.36$) or the Emotional Support, Intrusiveness, or Irritation subscales (Van Humbeeck et al. 2004).

The LEE scale has also been examined in the context of eating disorders (Moulds et al. 2000), but it did not show consistent evidence of predictive validity. The LEE scale total scores for siblings, mothers, and fathers failed to predict weight gain following treatment.

In sum, correlations between the LEE scale and the CFI, where available, appear to be quite modest, and clinical use of the LEE scale suggests that it is not conceptually parallel to the CFI. Although the 60-item version of the LEE scale appears to have some predictive validity, at least with respect to patients with psychotic disorders, much more research needs to be conducted to establish the validity of this measure for other disorders. Until there is more evidence showing that the revised LEE scale predicts the kinds of negative psychiatric outcomes predicted by the CFI, it cannot be considered to be a viable alternative to the CFI for this purpose. In brief, the LEE scale is promising as a brief descriptive measure, but additional work is required before it can be recommended for use as a clinical tool with predictive validity for particular disorders.

FAMILY ATTITUDE SCALE

The Family Attitude Scale (FAS; Kavanagh et al. 1997) is a 30-item self-report measure of EE. Examples of items are "I wish he were not here," "I lose my temper with him," and "I feel very close to him." The FAS is similar to the LEE scale in that either relatives or patients may complete it. Psychometrically, the FAS appears sound. Kavanagh and colleagues (1997) reported that the FAS had very high internal consistency in a sample of students' parents, as well as with both female and male students. It also has demonstrated good concurrent validity. For instance, fathers' and mothers' FAS scores were associated with expression of anger, trait and state anger, trait and state anxiety, argument frequency, seriousness of worst argument, and duration of argument. Moreover, in a sample of patients with schizophrenia and schizoaffective disorder and their relatives, the FAS showed high internal consistency for mothers, fathers, and other relatives.

Most importantly, the FAS has been shown to have some validity with respect to the CFI. Kavanagh et al. (1997) reported that mothers' and fathers' total FAS scores were correlated with criticism as measured by the CFI ($r=.38$ for fathers and $r=.66$ for mothers). Total FAS scores also correlated with hostility ratings made from the CFI. Although FAS scores were not associated with CFI-assessed emotional overinvolvement, there was an association between the FAS and CFI for warmth. Given the brevity of the measure, this finding must be considered promising. In a subsequent study of schizophrenia patients in Japan, Fujita and colleagues (2002) found that FAS scores were significantly associated with criticism ($r=.47$), hostility ($r=.37$), and warmth ($r=-.39$) as assessed with the CFI. Likewise, Pourmand (2005) reported that FAS scores were higher in high-EE families than in low-EE families. When a cut-off score of 55 on the FAS was used, 65% (22/34) of high-EE cases and 75% (15/20) of low-EE cases were correctly identified. Finally, in a small sample of patients with anorexia nervosa and their siblings, Moulds et al. (2000) also found that siblings' scores on the FAS were correlated ($r=.53$) with patients' scores on the 38-item LEE.

Overall, the early findings with the FAS are encouraging. The measure has overlap with the CFI, although the size of the correlations indicates that only a modest percentage of the variance in CFI scores can be predicted with the FAS. In addition, like the FMSS, the FAS may have low sensitivity. These considerations suggest that the FAS may have some advantages for those seeking a brief measure of EE, but it may not provide a substitute for the CFI when the goal is to maximize the prediction of relapse. For example, in a sample of 62 patients diagnosed with psychosis and comorbid substance abuse, Kavanagh and Pourmand reported baseline family FAS scores were higher in patients who subsequently relapsed. However, the strongest predictor of patient relapse was EE as assessed with the CFI (D.J. Kavanagh, D. Pourmand: "Utility of the FAS in the Prediction of Psychotic Relapse in People With Schizophrenia and Cannabis Misuse," manuscript in preparation, 2005).

PERCEIVED CRITICISM

A particularly simple measure of EE is the Perceived Criticism (PC) measure (Hooley and Teasdale 1989). Hooley and Teasdale (1989) asked patients to rate, using a 10-point Likert-type scale, how critical they thought their relative was of them. Patients were also asked to rate, using the same scale, how critical they thought they were of their relative. A subsequent revision added a question to assess degree of upset ("When [your relative] criticizes you, how upset do you get?" or "When you criticize [your relative], how upset does he or she get?"). In all cases, these items can also be completed by the relatives themselves, providing some flexibility in the way the scale can be used.

Given the brevity of the scale, it is somewhat surprising that it demonstrated concurrent validity in a sample of depressed patients and their spouses. Hooley and Teasdale (1989) found that patients' scores on the perceived criticism scale were correlated ($r=.51$) with spouses' overall EE ratings (high or low) as assessed with the CFI. At the same time, the correlation with spouses' criticism assessed with the CFI was more modest ($r=.27$). Nonetheless, patients' perception of their partner's criticism level (assessed during the index hospitalization) was highly predictive of patient relapse over the course of a 9-month follow-up. Patients who had a relapse in their illness rated their spouses as significantly more critical than patients who did not have a relapse rated their spouses as being. Of interest, none of the patients who gave their spouse a PC score of less than 2 had a relapse in their illness during the follow-up period. In contrast, all of the patients who assigned their spouses a PC rating of 6 or higher had a relapse in their illness.

Depressed patients' PC scores were not related to their Beck Depression Inventory scores or to clinical symptomatology at the time the scale was completed (Hooley and Teasdale 1989; see also Chambless et al. 2001; Riso et al. 1996), suggesting that the predictive power of the PC ratings was not an artifact of symptoms. The PC ratings also showed good test-retest reliability from initial assessment to 3 months later (Hooley and Teasdale 1989), suggesting stability over time.

Of potential relevance to clinical assessment, patients' ratings of PC may provide a more valid assessment of the EE level of the person being rated than do self-report ratings obtained directly. Spouse ratings of how critical they thought they were of the patient were uncorrelated ($r=.00$) with the number of critical comments those spouses actually made during the CFI (Hooley and Teasdale 1989). In a study of patient-therapist relationships in schizophrenia, therapists' self-report ratings of how critical they were with their patients were correlated ($r=.21$) with how critical they were as assessed on the CFI. However, patients' ratings of therapists' criticism were significantly correlated ($r=.45$) with therapists' criticism rated on the CFI (Van Humbeeck et al. 2004).

PC has demonstrated good predictive validity not only for unipolar depression but also for anxiety disorders (Chambless and Steketee 1999), obsessive-compulsive disorder (Renshaw et al. 2001, 2003), and substance abuse problems (Fals-Stewart et al. 2001). For bipolar illness, however, the research findings look a little different. In a study of 360 bipolar patients, Miklowitz et al. (2005) reported that patients' symptomatic outcomes were not predicted by the amount of criticism patients reported receiving from their relatives. Instead, patients who had reported feeling most upset when they were criticized by family members had more severe depressive and manic symptoms at 1-year follow up. So, for bipolar patients it may be patients' responses rather than relatives' behaviors that are more predictive of course of illness. Limiting the practical utilty of simple, single-item measures of PC, however, are various cultural factors. When Okasha et al. (1994) tried to use the PC measure in a sample of unipolar and bipolar depressed patients in Egypt, they noted that the use of a 10-point scale to detect opinions was not familiar in Egyptian culture. They also noted that some patients did not want to evaluate their caregivers with "mere numbers," and some expressed concern about the "real motive or meaning" behind the question. The researchers tried to simplify the scale by reducing it to three categories of criticism (low, moderate, or high). However, no association between this modified scale and relapse was found. These difficulties may suggest limitations to rating scales in general in some cultural contexts.

In summary, PC ratings are not a substitute for the CFI. However, they can be obtained from patients extremely quickly. Like the FMSS and the FAS, PC ratings may be useful as a means of quickly assessing relapse-proneness in settings in which more comprehensive assessments cannot be undertaken. PC ratings appear to be relatively independent of current levels of psychopathology and tend to be rather stable across time. They also correlate reasonably well with EE as assessed by the CFI, although correlations with the criticism subscale of the CFI can sometimes be much more modest. Despite these features, patients' PC ratings have been shown to predict poor clinical outcomes in depressed patients, patients with anxiety disorders, and patients with substance abuse problems. Unfortunately, there are no data concerning the predictive validity of PC for patients with schizophrenia. Moreover, for patients with bipolar disorder, how upset patients report being when they are exposed to criticism may have more predictive validity than the PC ratings themselves. Taken together, these considerations suggest that perceived criticism ratings may have a place among brief alternative measures of EE but that the CFI remains secure as the criterion measure of EE.

CONCLUSIONS REGARDING PRACTICAL MEASUREMENT OF EE

To make EE more clinically useful and accessible, it may be necessary to further develop the potential of brief alternatives to the CFI. In addition, use of brief alternative measures may accelerate research on various aspects of EE. At the present time, however, the brief alternatives have significant weaknesses relative to the CFI, and the CFI remains the best available measure of EE.

It may be that because it is an interview coded by a trained rater, the CFI provides a better context and method for assessing family processes related to relapse than do any of the brief measures. Moreover, clinical use of the CFI would allow clinicians to interpret their results in light of the large body of EE research that has been conducted over the last five decades. The CFI is also the only form of EE assessment that provides data on all five EE variables (criticism, hostility, emotional overinvolvement, warmth, and positive remarks). Given the growing interest in measuring family warmth as a possible moderating variable (e.g., Lopez et al. 2004), the comprehensive coverage of family emotions provided by the CFI is a potential asset to clinicians.

Another major advantage of the CFI for clinical purposes is that when it is conducted by a skilled clinical researcher, it can be a remarkably positive experience for the relative being interviewed. During the CFI the relative is given an opportunity to tell his or her story about what it has been like to be with the patient and deal with mental illness in the family. It is not unusual for family members to express gratitude to the interviewer for listening to what they have to say and taking their perspective seriously. As such, administration of the CFI may provide a solid foundation for further work with the family at the same time that it provides assessment information. In both research and clinical settings, the advantages of this kind of positive connection with families cannot be underestimated. The CFI also allows the clinician to obtain a wealth of information about symptom history and family beliefs about the causes of psychiatric illness that may prove clinically useful. Therefore, the CFI may be the assessment method of choice in some clinical settings. In particular, in settings with a treatment team, it may be possible for one member of the treatment team to be trained to administer and score the CFI.

These considerations suggest the CFI may be an appropriate clinical tool in many cases and may provide a useful starting point for assessment guidelines in the DSM. Focused psychometric work may help the FMSS become a valid and useful measure of EE. However, the FMSS is perhaps best suited for use in situations where there is a need to quickly identify high-EE relatives. In this context, relatives could be screened with the FMSS, and the CFI could be used to provide a more thorough assessment of those who are rated as low in EE. Those rated high on the FMSS could be given high priority for attention to family processes.

The FMSS is also a good substitute for the CFI when the latter might not be feasible for other reasons. For example, an informant (e.g., health care worker) may not know the patient well enough to answer all the questions contained in the CFI. However, he or she may be able to talk briefly about his or her relationship with the patient in a manner that would permit an FMSS rating. Likewise, because of its ease of use, in cases in which a clinician is interested in how family attitudes change over time in response to treatment, repeated administrations of the FMSS are probably more feasible than repeated assessments of the CFI. Focused psychometric work with the FMSS may allow determination of adjusted cut-off scores that better capture the discontinuity between high and low EE (see Beauchaine and Beach, Chapter 8, this volume).

One relevant factor with regard to the questionnaire-based assessments is who is available to complete the measure. Of the measures completed by relatives, the FAS shows greatest promise. Although more data are needed, the FAS correlates modestly with EE as measured with the CFI and predicts relapse in patients with schizophrenia. The original 60-item LEE scale also correlates well with the CFI and has predictive validity for psychotic disorders. However, both of these instruments have not been validated for any other diagnoses. So, considerable focused research would be necessary before they could be recommended generally. The revised version of the LEE scale is still in need of further validation and cannot be recommended for clinical use at this time.

Of the measures completed by the patient, the PC rating appears to have a number of advantages. It is not clear if ratings of PC are measuring characteristics of relatives or heightened sensitivities of patients to criticism. However, of all the alternative measures of EE, PC has the advantage of speed and efficiency. It can be added to assessment batteries without any appreciable time burden. It also has some overlap with the EE ratings obtained from the CFI. Most important, however, when completed by patients, the PC has demonstrated predictive validity for mood, anxiety, and substance abuse disorders. Although there are no indications to support its use in schizophrenia (where the LEE scale or the FAS may be preferred on the basis of available data), and with the caveat that PC ratings provide an estimate of only one aspect of EE (criticism), the measure of PC may have some general clinical utility. Perceived criticism ratings are in no way a substitute for the CFI. However, in circumstances that call for a fast estimate of the affective climate in the family, the time-cost of a PC assessment appears to be greatly outweighed by its possible benefits as negative prognostic indicator.

Implications for Revision of the DSM

Measures of EE describe relational processes with considerable importance for severe mental illness. Including information about the relevance of EE for the prediction of the course of mental illness would enhance the DSM as a clinical tool. The ways in which EE could be incorporated into DSM-V could take a number of different forms (see Beach et al., Chapter 1, this volume). However, it is unlikely the format currently used to describe "relational problems" in DSM-IV will be adequate to capture EE or any of the facets of EE.

In particular, research on EE indicates that considerable care needs to be taken with regard to assessment, because decisions about assessment method and the content of different measures can have consequences for concurrent and predictive validity. The research on brief methods of assessment suggests that even rigorous attempts at creating brief assessments can produce a substantial decline in predictive validity. Likewise, giving clinicians the "gist" of the construct does not appear sufficient to ensure reliable or valid assessment of EE. For example, although it might be natural to think that clinicians who are familiar with the EE construct and aware of its importance might be able to make EE assessments in the absence of formal training and explicit criteria, empirical research suggests that this is not the case. When psychiatrists who were aware of the construct were asked to rate the EE status of their patient's relatives (for whom formal EE ratings had been obtained using the CFI), they performed no better than chance (King et al. 1994). This research suggests the wisdom of better specification of "relational problems" in DSM-V.

The current data suggest that the CFI may be a better model for comprehensive assessment of family environment than are the available brief alternatives. Each of the brief alternative versions of the CFI that have been developed introduces limitations even as they reduce the time required to conduct the assessment.

However, several of the alternative brief measures have desirable characteristics that may be further enhanced through targeted psychometric research. With more focused research, it should be possible to develop guidance for the practical, clinical assessment of EE and to develop guidelines in time for the revision of the DSM.

Research also needs to continue to bridge measures of EE with changes in neurophysiological processes and to clarify the role of EE as a moderator or mediator of treatment outcome. By gaining a better understanding of the link between EE and the biological cascade that leads to relapse, we will make EE a more clinically useful tool. Likewise, by identifying the facets of EE that serve as moderators and mediators of family treatment effects, we will increase the clinical utility of the CFI as well as brief assessments of EE. Current information suggests that assessment of EE can be clinically useful in many cases. By introducing families to the idea that they can play an important role in the recovery process without being blamed, valid assessment of EE can promote positive family engagement in the treatment process.

References

Asarnow JR, Goldstein MJ, Tompson M, et al: One-year outcomes of depressive disorders in child psychiatric inpatients: evaluation of the prognostic power of a brief measure of expressed emotion. J Child Psychol Psychiatry 34:129–137, 1993

Bateson G, Jackson DD, Haley J, et al: Toward a theory of schizophrenia. Behavioral Science 1:251–264, 1956

Brown GW, Rutter M: The measurement of family activities and relationships: a methodological study. Human Relations 19:241–263, 1966

Brown GW, Birley JLT, Wing JK: Influence of family life on the course of schizophrenic disorders: a replication. Br J Psychiatry 121:241–258, 1972

Butzlaff RL, Hooley JM: Expressed emotion and psychiatric relapse. Arch Gen Psychiatry 55:547–552, 1998

Chambless DL, Steketee G: Expressed emotion and behavior therapy outcome: a prospective study with obsessive-compulsive and agoraphobic outpatients. J Consult Clin Psychol 67:658–665, 1999

Chambless DL, Bryan AD, Aiken LS, et al: Predicting expressed emotion: a study with families of obsessive-compulsive and agoraphobic outpatients. Journal of Family Psychology 15:225–240, 2001

Cole JD, Kazarian SS: The Level of Expressed Emotion scale: a new measure of expressed emotion. J Clin Psychol 44:392–397, 1988

Cole JD, Kazarian SS: Predictive validity of the Level of Expressed Emotion (LEE) scale: readmission follow-up data for 1, 2, and 5-year periods. J Clin Psychol 49:216–218, 1993

Cook WL, Kenny DA, Goldstein MJ: Parental affective style risk and the family system: a social relations model analysis. J Abnorm Psychol 100:492–501, 1991

Donat DC, Geczy B Jr, Helmrich J, et al: Empirically derived personality subtypes of public psychiatric patients: effect on self-reported symptoms, coping inclinations, and evaluation of expressed emotion in caregivers. Journal of Personality Assessment 58:36–50, 1992

Engel GL: The need for a new medical model: a challenge for biomedicine. Science 196:129–136, 1977

Fals-Stewart W, O'Farrell TJ, Hooley JM: Relapse among married or cohabiting substance-abusing patients: the role of perceived criticism. Behavior Therapy 32:787–801, 2001

Fromm-Reichmann F: Notes on the development of treatment of schizophrenics by psychoanalytic psychotherapy. Psychiatry 11:263–273, 1948

Fujita H, Shimodera S, Izumoto Y, et al: Family Attitude Scale: measurement of criticism in the relatives of patients with schizophrenia in Japan. Psychiatry Res 110:273–280, 2002

Gerlsma C, Hale WW 3rd: Predictive power and construct validity of the Level of Expressed Emotion (LEE) scale: depressed outpatients and couples from the general community. Br J Psychiatry 170:520–525, 1997

Gerlsma C, van der Lubbe PM, van Nieuwenhuizen C: Factor analysis of the Level of Expressed Emotion scale, a questionnaire intended to measure "perceived expressed emotion." Br J Psychiatry 160:385–389, 1992

Hahlweg K, Goldstein MJ, Nuechterlein KH, et al: Expressed emotion and patient-relative interaction in families of recent-onset schizophrenics. J Consult Clin Psychol 57:11–18, 1989

Hogarty GE, Anderson CM, Reiss DJ, et al: Family psychoeducation, social skills training, and maintenance chemotherapy in the aftercare treatment of schizophrenia. Arch Gen Psychiatry 43:633–642, 1986

Hooley JM: Expressed emotion and depression: interactions between patients and high-versus low-expressed emotion spouses. J Abnorm Psychol 95:237–246, 1986

Hooley JM: Expressed emotion and depression, in Depression and Families. Edited by Keitner GI. Washington, DC, American Psychiatric Press, 1990, pp 55–83

Hooley JM, Gotlib IH: A diathesis-stress conceptualization of expressed emotion and clinical outcome. Journal of Applied and Preventive Psychology 9:135–151, 2000

Hooley JM, Parker HA: Measuring expressed emotion: an evaluation of the short cuts. J Fam Psychol (in press)

Hooley JM, Teasdale JD: Predictors of relapse in unipolar depressives: expressed emotion, marital distress, and perceived criticism. J Abnorm Psychiatry 98:229–235, 1989

Hooley, JM, Rosen LR, Richters JE: Expressed emotion: toward clarification of a critical construct, in The Behavioral High Risk Paradigm in Psychopathology. Edited by Miller G. New York, Springer-Verlag, 1995, pp 88–120

Hooley JM, Gruber SA, Scott LA, et al: Activation in dorsolateral prefrontal cortex in response to maternal criticism and praise in recovered depressed and healthy control participants. Biol Psychiatry 57:809–812, 2005

Jarbin H, Grawe RW, Hansson K: Expressed emotion and prediction of relapse in adolescents with psychotic disorders. Nord J Psychiatry 54:201–205, 2000

Kavanagh DJ, O'Halloran P, Manicavasagar V, et al: The Family Attitude Scale: reliability and validity of a new scale for measuring the emotional climate of families. Psychiatry Res 70:185–195, 1997

Kazarian SS, Malla AK, Cole JD, et al: Comparisons of two expressed emotion scales with the Camberwell Family Interview. J Clin Psychol 46:306–309, 1990

King S, Lesage AD, Lalonde P: Psychiatrists' ratings of expressed emotion. Can J Psychiatry 39:358–360, 1994

Kurihara T, Kato M, Tsukahara T, et al: The low prevalence of high levels of expressed emotion in Bali. Psychiatry Res 94:229–238, 2000

Leeb B, Hahlweg K, Goldstein MJ, et al: Cross-national reliability, concurrent validity, and stability of a brief method for assessing expressed emotion. Psychiatry Res 39:25–31, 1991

Leff JP, Vaughn CE: Expressed Emotion in Families. New York, Guilford, 1985

Leff J, Kuipers L, Berkowitz R, et al: A controlled trial of social intervention in the families of schizophrenic patients. Br J Psychiatry 141:121–134, 1982

Leff J, Berkowitz R, Shavit N, et al: A trial of family therapy versus a relatives' group for schizophrenia: two-year follow-up. Br J Psychiatry 157:571–577, 1990

Lopez SR, Hipke KN, Polo AJ, et al: Ethnicity, expressed emotion, attributions, and course of schizophrenia: family warmth matters. J Abnorm Psychol 113:428–439, 2004

Magana AB, Goldstein JM, Karno M, et al: A brief method for assessing expressed emotion in relatives of psychiatric patients. Psychiatry Res 17:203–212, 1986

Marom S, Munitz H, Jones PB, et al: Familial expressed emotion: outcome and course of Israeli patients with schizophrenia. Schizophr Bull 28:731–743, 2002

Miklowitz DJ, Tompson MC: Family variables and interventions in schizophrenia, in Textbook of Family and Couples Therapy. Edited by Sholevar GP, Schwoeri LD. Washington, DC, American Psychiatric Publishing, 2003, pp 585–617

Miklowitz DJ, Goldstein MJ, Falloon IR, et al: Interactional correlates of expressed emotion in the families of schizophrenics. Br J Psychiatry 144:482–487, 1984

Miklowitz DJ, Wisniewski SR, Miyahara S, et al: Perceived criticism from family members as a predictor of the 1-year course of bipolar disorder. Psychiatry Res 136:101–111, 2005

Moulds ML, Touyz SW, Schotte D, et al: Perceived expressed emotion in the siblings and parents of hospitalized patients with anorexia nervosa. Int J Eat Disord 27:288–296, 2000

Nugter A: Family factors and interventions in recent onset schizophrenia. Unpublished doctoral dissertation, Universiteit van Amsterdam, Amsterdam, 1997

O'Farrell TJ, Hooley JM, Fals-Stewart W, et al: Expressed emotion and relapse in alcoholic patients. J Consult Clin Psychol 66:744–752, 1998

Okasha A, El Akabawi AS, Snyder KS, et al: Expressed emotion, perceived criticism, and relapse in depression: a replication in an Egyptian sample. Am J Psychiatry 151:1001–1005, 1994

Pourmand D: Expressed emotion as predictor of relapse in patients with comorbid psychosis and substance use disorder. Unpublished doctoral thesis, University of Queensland, Australia, 2005

Renshaw KD, Chambless D, Steketee G: Comorbidity fails to account for the relationship of expressed emotion and perceived criticism to treatment outcome in patients with anxiety disorders. J Behav Ther Exp Psychiatry 32:145–158, 2001

Renshaw KD, Chambless DL, Steketee G: Perceived criticism predicts severity of anxiety symptoms after behavioral treatment in patients with obsessive-compulsive disorder and panic disorder with agoraphobia. J Clin Psychol 59:411–421, 2003

Riso LP, Klein DN, Ouimette PC, et al: Convergent and discriminant validity of perceived criticism from spouses and family members. Behavior Therapy 27:129–137, 1996

Shimodera S, Mino Y, Inoue S, et al: Validity of a five-minute speech sample in measuring expressed emotion in the families of patients with schizophrenia in Japan. Compr Psychiatry 40:372–376, 1999

Shimodera S, Mino Y, Fujita H, et al: Validity of a five-minute speech sample for the measurement of expressed emotion in the families of Japanese patients with mood disorders. Psychiatry Res 112:231–237, 2002

Simoneau TL, Miklowitz DJ, Saleem R: Expressed emotion and interactional patterns in the families of bipolar patients. J Abnorm Psychol 107:497–507, 1998

Tarrier N, Turpin G: Psychosocial factors, arousal, and schizophrenia relapse: the psychophysiological data. Br J Psychiatry 161:3–11, 1992

Tarrier N, Barrowclough C, Porceddu K, et al: The assessment of psychophysiological reactivity to the expressed emotion of the relative of schizophrenic patients. Br J Psychiatry 152:618–624, 1988

Tattan T, Tarrier N: The expressed emotion of case managers of the seriously mentally ill: the influence of expressed emotion on clinical outcome. Psychol Med 30:195–204, 2000

Thompson MC, Goldstein MJ, Lebell LB, et al: Schizophrenic patients' perceptions of their relatives' attitudes. Psychiatry Res 57:155–167, 1995

Uehara T, Yokoyama T, Goto M, et al: Expressed emotion and short-term treatment outcome of outpatients with major depression. Compr Psychiatry 37:299–304, 1996

Uehara T, Yokoyama T, Nakano Y, et al: Characteristics of expressed emotion rated by the Five Minute Speech Sample and relationship with relapse of outpatients with schizophrenia. Clin Psychiatry 39:31–37, 1997

Van Humbeeck G, Van Audenhove C, Declercq A: Mental health, burnout and job satisfaction among professionals in sheltered living in Flanders: a pilot study. Soc Psychiatry Psychiatr Epidemiol 39:569–575, 2004

Vaughn CE, Leff JP: The influence of family and social factors on the course of psychiatric illness: a comparison of schizophrenia and depressed neurotic patients. Br J Psychiatry 129:125–137, 1976

Yan LJ, Hammen C, Cohen AN, et al: Expressed emotion versus relationship quality variables in the prediction of recurrence in bipolar patients. J Affect Disord 83:199–206, 2004

PART III

PREVENTION AND TREATMENT

CHAPTER 12

PREVENTION AS THE PROMOTION OF HEALTHY PARENTING FOLLOWING PARENTAL DIVORCE

Irwin N. Sandler, Ph.D.
Sharlene A. Wolchik, Ph.D.
Emily B. Winslow, Ph.D.
Clorinda Schenck, Ph.D.

The thesis of this chapter is that theoretically guided prevention research provides a powerful model for studying the role of relational processes in the development of mental health problems and disorders. A model of prevention research is presented, and each step in the model is illustrated. We primarily used the program of studies conducted by our team at Arizona State University's Prevention Research Center. We first consider divorce as a risk factor for mental disorder and social adaptation difficulties and identify potentially modifiable causal processes that theoretically account for this increased risk. We then discuss research that indicates that postdivorce parent-child relationships are an underlying process that theoretically has a causal effect on the development of problems following divorce. We then describe a program

Preparation of this chapter was supported by grants from the National Institute of Mental Health (NIMH) (2R01MH049155-06 and 5T32MH018387-15).

to improve postdivorce parenting—the New Beginnings Program (NBP)—and discuss findings from an efficacy trial that reported positive effects to improve postdivorce parenting, reduce the prevalence of diagnosed mental disorder and mental health problems, and improve adaptive outcomes 6 years later, particularly for those who had higher risk for problems when they entered the program. Finally, we describe mediation analyses that showed that program-induced improvements in parenting partially accounted for reductions in problem outcomes 6 years after participation. This program of research illustrates how correlational and experimental intervention studies on relationship processes can inform each other both to advance theory about the etiology of mental disorder and to develop effective approaches to prevent the development of disorder and promote healthy developmental outcomes.

Prevention Research Cycle Model

Over the past decade, a prevention research model has emerged that involves epidemiological studies of risk for disorder, correlational studies of underlying etiological processes, and experimental studies of the effects of changing theoretical risk processes to reduce incidence and prevalence of disorder (Mrazek and Haggerty 1994). This model provides a powerful framework for studying the role of relational processes in the development of mental disorder. In the first phase, epidemiological studies identify risk factors associated with higher prevalence of disorder. Although study of these risk factors identifies populations at increased risk, additional studies are needed to test theories of causal processes that underlie the identified risk, many of which involve critical interpersonal relationships. On the basis of these studies, a "small theory" is developed that identifies potentially malleable causal processes to target in a preventive intervention. An intervention is then designed and pilot tested to change these processes. To maximize the potential that the intervention will eventually be adopted, the match between the intervention and the setting in which it may be applied is studied. Experimental field trials of the intervention are then conducted to assess the intervention's ability to change theoretical processes, its short- and long-term effects on disorder, and the mediators and moderators of program effects. Finally, large-scale studies are conducted on factors that influence implementation and sustainability of the intervention in community service delivery systems. We illustrate the application of this model through a program of research to prevent mental health problems experienced by children following parental divorce and promote healthy developmental outcomes for these children.

Parental Divorce: Increased Risk and Theoretical Etiological Processes

Parental divorce places offspring at risk for a wide range of negative outcomes in childhood, adolescence, and adulthood. In childhood, parental divorce is associated with internalizing and externalizing behavior problems, academic and social problems, and poor physical health (Amato 2001; Amato and Keith 1991; Troxel and Matthews 2004). In adolescence, parental divorce predicts continued academic, mental health, and physical health problems, as well as risk for substance use and teenage childbearing (Hetherington et al. 1992; Hoffmann and Johnson 1998; McLanahan 1999). Adults who experienced parental divorce during childhood have an increased risk for multiple mental disorders, including major depression and dysthymia, anxiety disorders, personality disorders, and alcohol and drug dependence (Kessler et al. 1997). Parental divorce also predicts lower educational attainment; occupational problems; physical health problems, including shortened life span; and poorer relationships with spouses, parents, and peers in adulthood.

Although convincing evidence indicates that parental divorce is associated with a variety of maladaptive outcomes, the effects of divorce per se may not be causal but rather may reflect the effects of underlying processes. Kraemer and colleagues (1997) presented a useful model for elucidating the role a specific risk factor plays in producing a particular outcome. They defined a *risk factor* as a characteristic in a population that predicts the outcome of interest (i.e., the factor precedes the outcome). If an association between a characteristic and an outcome has been established only contemporaneously, the characteristic is considered a *correlate* of the outcome. For many outcomes, including mental health and substance use disorders and adult developmental task difficulties (e.g., occupational, marital), parental divorce precedes the outcome, thereby qualifying it as a risk factor (Chase-Lansdale et al. 1995; Furstenberg and Teitler 1994). For example, in a prospective British birth cohort study, Chase-Lansdale and colleagues (1995) reported a 39% increase in the odds of being above the clinical cut point for mental health problems at age 23 as a function of parental divorce during childhood, after they controlled for predivorce childhood emotional problems, school achievement, and family socioeconomic status.

Kraemer and colleagues (1997) further differentiated the type of risk factor by considering whether the factor could be changed and the effects of risk factor change on the outcome of interest. If manipulation of the risk factor changes the outcome, then the factor is termed a *causal* risk factor; otherwise, it is considered a *marker* risk factor. No evidence shows that changing parental divorce (i.e., preventing the occurrence of divorce between parents who would otherwise divorce) leads to changes in offspring outcomes. Therefore, parental divorce is best understood as a marker for other underlying causal processes that precede, coincide with, or follow the divorce event.

Considerable research has identified multiple factors that may play a causal role in mental health problems for children from divorced families, many of which involve relationship processes, including parenting quality, exposure to interparental conflict, and the numerous stressful events that follow divorce (e.g., multiple transitions in caregivers) (Hetherington et al. 1998). Although some of these pro-

cesses, such as interparental conflict (Block et al. 1986), may precede as well as follow divorce, it is hypothesized that changing them following the divorce will lead
to improvements in subsequent mental health problems. Because of the central
role one critical relationship process, *postdivorce parenting*, has played in our program of research, we focus on studies concerning this process. Postdivorce parenting is delivered by estranged mothers and fathers in different households and is
made more difficult because parents are coping with increased levels of stress and
depression, which disrupt quality parenting (Hetherington and Hagan 1999).

PARENTING BY THE RESIDENTIAL MOTHER

Compelling evidence from correlational studies shows that the custodial mother's
parenting is one of the most central influences on children's postdivorce functioning. Postdivorce mother-child relationship quality and discipline effectiveness are
the two most widely studied dimensions of parenting. High-quality mother-child
relationships involve a variety of behaviors, such as affection, positive verbal and
physical exchanges, valuing of the child's ideas and behaviors, effective listening
skills, responsiveness, and empathy. In addition, in high-quality mother-child relationships, children spend individual time with their mothers on a regular basis,
view their mothers as emotionally available, and turn to their mothers in times of
need. Effective discipline involves clear communication of expectations; developmentally appropriate expectations; adequate monitoring and supervision; selection of developmentally appropriate, meaningful, and nonharsh consequences;
and consistent application of these consequences.

The various changes that occur to mothers during divorce, such as increased
household and work responsibilities, fewer financial resources, and increased psychological distress, take a significant toll on their ability to parent effectively. Declines in mother-child relationship quality include poorer communication,
diminished affection and warmth, and decreased responsiveness (Hetherington et
al. 1998; Simons 1996). Also, after divorce, mothers have less control over their
children's behaviors, are more inconsistent in their discipline, and are less able to
monitor their children's activities (Hetherington et al. 1998). Although these parenting decrements are greatest immediately after the separation, in many families, they
persist for several years after the divorce.

Mother-child relationships characterized by warmth, supportiveness, effective
problem-solving skills, positive communication, and low levels of conflict and negativity are associated with fewer adjustment problems (e.g., Hetherington et al.
1992; Simons 1996). Discipline that is consistent and appropriate is related to better postdivorce adjustment (Wolchik et al. 2000b), and high levels of parental
monitoring and joint decision making are associated with low levels of externalizing, substance use, and academic difficulties (e.g., Buchanan et al. 1996). In addition, mother-child relationships have been shown to moderate the negative effect

of divorce-related stressors on adjustment problems (Hetherington et al. 1998). For example, Wolchik and colleagues (2000b) showed that relations between divorce stressors and internalizing and externalizing problems were strongest for children who reported both low warmth and low consistency of discipline; those who reported high levels of both warmth and consistency of discipline had the fewest internalizing and externalizing problems.

High-quality mother-child relationships may protect children from developing adjustment problems in the aftermath of divorce via several plausible pathways. First, by communicating a sense of warmth, caring, and concern, these relationships may allay fears of abandonment, which are significantly related to children's postdivorce adjustment problems (Kurdek and Berg 1987), and may partially mediate the effects of divorce stressors on adjustment problems (Wolchik et al. 2002b). Second, high-quality mother-child relationships may reduce adjustment problems through their effect on coping. Such relationships may promote a more varied repertoire of coping responses (Power 2004), enhance children's perceptions of their coping efficacy, and help children to interpret stressors in more hopeful ways (Kliewer et al. 1994). Also, high-quality relationships may enhance self-esteem, which buffers the negative effects of divorce-related stressors on adjustment problems (Conley et al. 2001).

Effective discipline may act as a protective resource by affecting children's sense of the predictability of their environments. The consistent occurrence of expected outcomes for misbehavior may promote a sense of control, which could influence adjustment problems through its effect on threat appraisals, coping efficacy, or coping efforts (Skinner and Wellborn 1994). Effective discipline also may reduce coercive interactions between mothers and children, which increases children's use of mothers as resources.

PARENTING BY THE NONRESIDENTIAL FATHER

Evidence also indicates that the nonresidential father-child relationship has a significant effect on children's postdivorce mental health problems, an effect resulting from the quality rather than the quantity (i.e., amount of contact between father and child) of the relationship. Amato (1993) summarized 32 studies on divorced families and found that only about half reported that contact was significantly and positively related to children's well-being. Moving beyond examining the father-child relationship in terms of amount of contact, the recent literature has considered two potential roles of fathers—the role of a social companion or friend to the child and a more traditional parent role that includes activities such as helping with homework or talking about things happening in the child's life. Research has shown that noncustodial fathers' participation in leisure or recreational activities with their children is unrelated to child mental health outcomes, but engagement in more daily activities typical of traditional parent-child relationships is positively related to child well-being (Clarke-Stewart and Hayward 1996; Stewart 2003). Similarly, researchers have shown that authoritative parenting behaviors, such as inductive reasoning, monitoring, and consistent discipline, by the noncustodial father are negatively related to externalizing behaviors in the child (Simons et al. 1994) and that children of noncustodial fathers who are more involved (i.e., celebrating holidays together, attending school- or church-related functions, providing comfort and sympathy, and participating in leisure or educational activities) have higher academic performance and greater popularity with their peers than do their counterparts with less involved fathers (Bronstein et al. 1994).

New Beginnings Program: A Theoretically Based Preventive Intervention

The New Beginnings Program was developed to change processes that, according to theory and correlational research, were hypothesized to affect the development of mental health problems for children following parental divorce. The program had two components—one worked directly with children; the other worked with the residential mother. The small theory of the program articulates both a psychosocial theory (links between the putative mediators and outcomes based on psychosocial research) and a program theory (links between the putative mediators and change strategies based on theories of behavior change) (West and Aiken 1997). Four empirically supported putative mediators were targeted that were believed to be modifiable by working with mothers, each of which involves a critical relationship process: 1) mother-child relationship quality, 2) effective discipline, 3) father-child relationship quality, and 4) interparental conflict. Although mothers were thought to have less control over the latter two processes, changes in the mother's behaviors could lead to changes in the father's behaviors in these two relational processes.

Figure 12–1 illustrates the concept of a theory-guided program by presenting the theory for the residential mother component of the NBP. The intervention column on the left shows the program strategies used to change each selected mediator. Use of these strategies is hypothesized to change the relational process (middle column); changes in each relational process are hypothesized to reduce the development of mental health problems and to improve developmental competencies (right column). Illustratively, the program teaches mothers to increase positive family activities, one-on-one time, and attention to positive behaviors and to use active listening skills to improve the quality of the mother-child relationship. Improvement in mother-child relationship quality is predicted to reduce the development of mental health problems. The program was highly structured, and sessions included short didactic presentation, modeling of specific skills, and practice of these skills in session. Homework was given after each session, in which mothers practiced the relationship skills with their children. Homework was cumulative so that skills taught early in the program (i.e., positive family time) were practiced throughout.

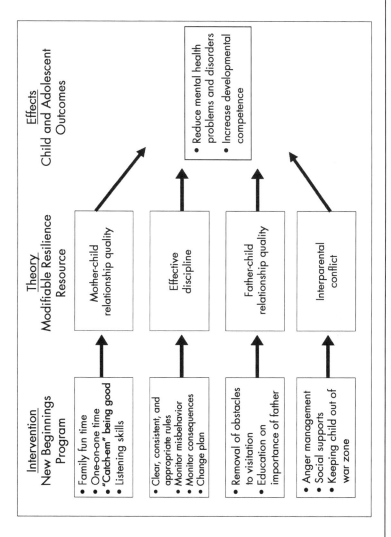

FIGURE 12–1.   The New Beginnings Program: a theory-based intervention to change postdivorce relational processes.

RANDOMIZED EXPERIMENTAL EVALUATION
OF NEW BEGINNINGS PROGRAM

The parenting component was initially evaluated in a small-scale ($N=70$) randomized experimental trial in which the program was compared with a literature control group (Wolchik et al. 1993). Positive program effects occurred on relationship quality, effective discipline, divorce stressors, and children's mental health problems. Program effects on mental health problems were moderated by initial level of problems, such that the program had the greatest benefit for those who had higher levels of problems when they entered the program. Mediational analyses indicated that improvement in parent-child relationship quality partially mediated improvements in children's mental health problems.

A second randomized experimental trial had four objectives: 1) assess whether the positive effects of a slightly modified version of the program for mothers described earlier (Mother Program) could be replicated with a larger sample; 2) test whether a dual-component program involving concurrent, separate groups for mothers and children (Combined Program) produced additive effects; 3) assess whether program effects persisted over time; and 4) examine mediators and moderators of program effects. The trial included 240 children ages 9–12 whose parents had divorced in the prior 2 years. Families were randomly assigned to one of the three conditions.

Groups, which were co-led by two master's level clinicians, met for 11 sessions (1.75 hours each); mothers had two individual sessions (1 hour each) that tailored the program skills to their families. Mothers and children in the literature control group each received three books on children's divorce adjustment and a syllabus. To ensure high fidelity, sessions were delivered with the use of manuals, and extensive training and supervision were provided. Independent ratings of videotapes of all sessions showed exceptional completion of program segments. Attendance, which was high, did not differ significantly across condition.

Five waves of data were collected on one randomly selected child per family—prior to random assignment; immediately after the program; and at 3 months, 6 months, and 6 years following the program. Assessments included multiple measures of each targeted mediator as well as children's mental health problems. Illustratively, measures of parenting included parent and child report of parental acceptance and rejection, family routines and open communication, and behavioral observation ratings of parent-child interactions. Similarly, standardized measures were used to assess child, parent, and teacher report of internalizing and externalizing problems at each wave of data collection, and a structured diagnostic interview of mental disorders was administered at the 6-year follow-up.

Attrition from assessments was low, with 98% of the participants who entered the program being assessed at 3- and 6-month follow-ups and 91% at the 6-year follow-up. Tests of biases in attrition provided little evidence that attrition differed across intervention groups or that attrition biases would threaten the internal or external validity of inferences concerning program effects (Jurs and Glass 1971). All analyses of program effects used an intent-to-treat design, in which all participants who were randomly assigned to conditions were included in the analyses, regardless of their level of attendance in the program.

Effects of NBP in Childhood

Analysis of program effects initially compared the Mother Program and Combined Program with the control condition (Wolchik et al. 2000a). Similar to the initial trial, at immediate posttest, a significant program-by-baseline interaction was seen for externalizing problems—the Mother Program led to the largest improvements for children with higher initial externalizing problems. In addition, main effects of the Mother Program were significant for reducing internalizing problems and improving discipline and observer-rated mother-child relationship quality. The proportion of children scoring in the clinical range on the Child Behavior Checklist (CBCL) internalizing or externalizing subscale was significantly lower in the Mother Program than in the control condition (odds ratio [OR] = 2.79). Significant program-by-baseline interaction effects also were seen on questionnaire measures of parental warmth and attitudes toward the father-child relationship. In both cases, program benefits were strongest for those who entered the program with more negative scores. At 6-month follow-up, significant program-by-baseline interactions occurred for externalizing problems as assessed by mother or child as well as teacher report. For both interactions, those with higher baseline externalizing scores showed greater program benefits. Comparisons of the Mother Program with the Combined Program showed few differences between the conditions on measures of mental health problems, providing little evidence that the child component added to the effects of the parenting component.

Mediational analyses were conducted to test the theoretical proposition that program-induced changes on the targeted mediating variables accounted for improvements in mental health outcomes (Tein et al. 2004). Analyses showed that Mother Program effects on internalizing at posttest were mediated by improvements in mother-child relationship quality; effects on externalizing at posttest and 6-month follow-up were mediated by improvements in relationship quality and effective discipline. Mediation occurred for those with higher baseline problems. These findings provide experimental support for two of the four relational processes that were putative mediators in the small theory of the Mother Program: mother-child relationship quality and effective discipline.

Long-Term Effects of NBP Into Adolescence

The goals of prevention programs are to prevent the development of mental disorder and associated behavior problems and to promote the achievement of developmental competence over time. Thus, assessment of long-term outcomes across developmental periods is critical to evaluating the preventive effect of these interventions. However, the effects of prevention programs are not uniform, and many evaluations are finding that effects are strongest for those who are more at risk when they enter the program (see Brown and Liao 1999; Olds 2002). Short-term evaluation of NBP showed that the program effects were strongest for those with higher levels of problems at baseline. The long-term follow-up determined whether program effects 6 years after participation were moderated by initial level of risk.

Prevention programs are also interested in how the program achieved its effects. The NBP design was based on a theory that changing specific relational processes would lead to reduced problem outcomes, and the short-term evaluations indicated that program effects to improve parental warmth and discipline mediated program effects on mental health problems. The long-term evaluation extended this research by assessing the developmental pathways by which the NBP affects mental health problems from childhood to adolescence over a 6-year period.

Effects of the NBP on Mental Health Problems at 6-Year Follow-Up

A full report of the 6-year effects is presented in Wolchik et al. (2002a). We briefly review the main findings here. Of the families randomly assigned to conditions, 91% completed interviews. No evidence of differential attrition across conditions was found. We compared each program (Mother and Combined Program) to the control condition separately. Analyses provided strong support for preventive effects of the Mother Program and the Combined Program as compared with the control condition. Significant program-by-baseline interactions occurred for 6 of the 15 variables tested (40%): parent or adolescent report of externalizing, symptoms of mental disorder, alcohol use, marijuana use, other drug use, and grade point average (GPA). The pattern of all interactions showed that program benefits were strongest for those with higher initial problems. Analyses also provided strong support for the preventive effects of the Combined Program compared with the control condition. Positive main or interactive effects occurred for 5 of 15 (33%) of the variables tested. The Combined Program differed significantly from the control condition on percentage meeting diagnostic criteria for mental disorder in the past year. Of the adolescents in the control group, 24% met criteria, compared with 11% in the Combined Program (OR=4.50). Significant program-by-baseline interactions occurred for parent or adolescent report of externalizing and symptoms of mental disorder; the benefit of the Combined Program was greater for those with higher baseline problems. Although the Mother Program and the Combined Program each showed benefits as compared with the control condition, post-hoc comparisons of the Mother Program with the Combined Program for the 15 outcome variables showed no significant main or interactive effects. Thus, no evidence indicated that program effects were enhanced by adding a child component to the Mother Program.

Benefits of NBP Participation in the High-Risk Group

To examine whether program effects were moderated by a broader measure of baseline "risk" for later problems, we developed an index of the best baseline predictors of outcomes 6 years later (Dawson-McClure et al. 2004). This risk index, which consisted of the sum of standardized scores on baseline level of child externalizing problems and environmental stress (i.e., interparental conflict, negative life events experienced by the child, maternal distress, reduced contact with father, financial hardship), was highly predictive of internalizing, externalizing, substance use, mental disorder, and competence 6 years later. When the optimal cut point identified through receiver operating characteristic curve analysis was used, the sensitivity and specificity of this index to predict diagnosis of mental disorder in the control group were 0.75 and 0.73, respectively. The odds of having a diagnosis were 8.14 times higher in the group above the cut point compared with the group below the cutpoint.

Because comparisons of the Mother Program and Combined Program found no differences in effects across these two program conditions, we combined the groups that received these two programs and compared them with the control group to provide a parsimonious view of the program effects in adolescence. These analyses used the composite risk variable as the baseline covariate, and the risk-by-program interaction was tested for all outcomes. Significant main or interactive effects occurred for 12 of the 15 (80%) outcomes assessed. Significant main effects occurred for three outcomes: number of sexual partners, GPA, and mental disorder in the past year (OR=2.70). Significant program-by-risk interactions occurred for nine outcomes: parent or adolescent report of externalizing, teacher report of externalizing, parent or adolescent report of internalizing, mental disorder symptoms, alcohol use, marijuana use, other drug use, polydrug use, and competence. For all interactions, program benefits were greater for those with higher baseline risk. Interestingly, inspection of program effect sizes on mental health problems indicated that effects grew over time.

Mediation of NBP Effects on Adolescent Outcomes

As discussed earlier, the theoretical framework for the long-term effects of the NBP posits that program-induced changes in putative mediators lead to reduced mental health problems and mental disorder. Analyses of short-term program effects provided support for both maternal warmth and discipline as mediators of program effects on internalizing and externalizing problems. At the long-term follow-up, program-induced improvements in discipline partially mediated program effects to improve GPA. For the nine outcomes in which the effects of the NBP were moderated by baseline level of risk, a two-group mediational model was used in which the mediators were tested at high and low levels of the baseline risk score (Sandler et al., manuscript in preparation, March 2006). For three of these variables—total psychiatric symptom count, total internalizing problems, and total externalizing problems—significant mediation effects were found to account partially for changes in mental health problems in the high-risk group. In each case, program-induced improvement in maternal warmth at posttest was a significant mediator of program effects to reduce mental health problems 6 years later.

Conclusion

The program of research described in this chapter illustrates a powerful model by which epidemiological studies, theory-testing correlational studies, and experimental intervention trials can be used to study the effects of relational processes on the development of mental disorder. The findings provide strong support that a critical relational process—postdivorce parenting by the residential mother—contributes to the development of mental health problems and disorders following parental divorce. Correlational studies that supported the role of mothers' parenting were complemented by experimental prevention trials that showed that parenting is malleable and that experimentally induced changes in parenting accounted for program effects to reduce mental health problems and disorder over 6 years. Findings that experimentally induced improvements in parenting led to reductions in mental health problems and disorder strengthen the inferences of the causal role of parenting over evidence from passive correlational studies (Rutter et al. 2001).

The research on prevention summarized in this chapter is highly relevant for the maturing empirically based psychiatric nosology and, along with similar evidence from other prevention trials, should be weighted heavily in the formulations of DSM-V. Prevention trials can be considered as carefully controlled experiments that test theories of the pathogenesis of mental disorders. In this program of prevention studies, we found clear evidence that in response to well-defined interventions, specific features of family relationships were altered, and as a consequence, mental disorders in children were prevented. This is the same order of evidence as an experiment that might, preventively, alter the function of the amygdala and thereby prevent anxiety disorders and related psychopathology. Such a preventive experiment would be regarded as strong evidence for the role of the amygdala in the development of anxiety disorders. Indeed, a current workgroup on DSM-V is focusing on "fear circuit disorders" that focus on limbic system research as a way of reconceptualizing psychiatric disorder. From the perspective of objective research, there is no reason that the limbic system should be given more or less causal priority than the family relational systems. While advances in neurobiology are mapping a detailed nexus of brain process implicating the limbic system in psychiatric disorder, as this research makes clear, research on a nexus of systems highly connected to parent-child relationships is also at an advanced state. In this sense, characterization of relationships that are central to the development of psychiatric disorders can be regarded as providing a base of scientific evidence for our developing nosology as rich as that provided by neurobiology.

References

Amato PR: Children's adjustment to divorce: theories, hypotheses, and empirical support. J Marriage Fam 55:23–38, 1993

Amato PR: Children of divorce in the 1990s: an update of the Amato and Keith (1991) meta-analysis. J Fam Psychol 15:355–370, 2001

Amato PR, Keith B: Parental divorce and the well-being of children: a meta-analysis. Psychol Bull 110:26–46, 1991

Block JH, Block J, Gjerde PF: The personality of children prior to divorce: a prospective study. Child Dev 57:827–840, 1986

Bronstein P, Stoll MF, Clauson J, et al: Fathering after separation or divorce: factors prediction children's adjustment. Fam Relat 43:469–479, 1994

Brown CH, Liao J: Principles for designing randomized preventive trials in mental health: an emerging developmental epidemiology paradigm. Am J Community Psychol 27:673–710, 1999

Buchanan C, Maccoby E, Dornbusch S: Adolescents After Divorce. Cambridge, MA, Harvard University Press, 1996

Chase-Lansdale LP, Cherlin AJ, Kiernan KE: The long term effects of parental divorce on the mental health of young adults: a developmental perspective. Child Dev 66:1614–1634, 1995

Clarke-Stewart K, Hayward C: Advantages of father custody and contact for the psychological well-being of school-age children. J Appl Dev Psychol 17:239–270, 1996

Conley C, Hilt I, Metalsky G: The Children's Attributional Style Interview: developmental tests of cognitive diathesis-stress theories of depression. J Abnorm Child Psychol 29:445–463, 2001

Dawson-McClure SR, Sandler I, Wolchik SA, et al: Prediction and reduction of risk for children of divorce: a six-year longitudinal study. J Abnorm Child Psychol 32:175–190, 2004

Furstenberg FF Jr, Teitler JO: Reconsidering the effects of marital disruption: what happens to children of divorce in early adulthood? J Fam Issues 15:173–179, 1994

Hetherington EM, Hagan MS: The adjustment of children with divorced parents: a risk and resiliency perspective. J Child Psychol Psychiatry 40:129–140, 1999

Hetherington EM, Clingempeel WG, Anderson ER, et al: Coping with marital transitions: a family systems perspective. Monogr Soc Res Child Dev 57 (Serial No 227):1–242, 1992

Hetherington EM, Bridges M, Insabella GM: What matters? What does not? Five perspectives on the association between marital transitions and children's adjustment. Am Psychol 53:167–184, 1998

Hoffmann JP, Johnson RA: A national portrait of family structure and adolescent drug use. J Marriage Fam 60:633–645, 1998

Jurs SG, Glass GV: The effect of experimental mortality on the internal and external validity of the randomized comparative experiment. Journal of Experimental Education 48:62–66, 1971

Kessler RC, Davis CG, Kendler KS: Childhood adversity and adult psychiatric disorder in the U.S. National Comorbidity Survey. Psychol Med 27:1101–1119, 1997

Kliewer W, Sandler IN, Wolchik SN: Family socialization of threat appraisal and coping: coaching, modeling, and family context, in Social Networks and Social Support in Childhood and Adolescence: Prevention and Intervention in Childhood and Adolescence. Edited by Hurrelman K, Nestmann F. Oxford, England, Walter De Gruyter, 1994, pp 271–291

Kraemer H, Kazdin A, Offord D, et al: Coming to terms with the terms of risk. Arch Gen Psychiatry 54:337–343, 1997

Kurdek L, Berg B: Children's Beliefs About Parental Divorce Scale: psychometric characteristics and concurrent validity. J Consult Clin Psychol 55:712–718, 1987

McLanahan S: Father absence and the welfare of children, in Coping With Divorce, Single Parenting, and Remarriage. Edited by Hetherington EM. Mahwah, NJ, Lawrence Erlbaum, 1999, pp 117–144

Mrazek PJ, Haggerty RJ: Reducing Risks for Mental Disorders: Frontiers for Prevention Research. Washington, DC, National Academy Press, 1994

Olds DL: Prenatal and infancy home visiting by nurses: from randomized trials to community replication. Prev Sci 3:153–172, 2002

Power T: Stress and coping in childhood: the parent's role. Parenting: Science and Practice 4:271–317, 2004

Rutter M, Pickles A, Murray R, et al: Testing hypotheses on specific environmental causal effects on behavior. Psychol Bull 127:291–324, 2001

Sandler IN, Millsap R, Zhou Q, et al: Mediation of six-year effects of the New Beginnings Program for Children of Divorce. (in preparation)

Simons RL: Understanding Families, Vol 5: Understanding Differences Between Divorced and Intact Families: Stress, Interaction, and Child Outcome. Thousand Oaks, CA, Sage, 1996

Simons RL, Whitbeck LB, Beaman J, et al: The impact of mothers' parenting, involvement by nonresidential fathers, and parental conflict on the adjustment of adolescent children. J Marriage Fam 56:356–374, 1994

Skinner EA, Wellborn JG: Coping during childhood and adolescence: a motivational perspective, in Life Span Development and Behavior, Vol 12. Edited by Featherman DL, Lerner RM, Perlmutter M. Hillsdale, NJ, Erlbaum, 1994, pp 91–133

Stewart SD: Nonresident parenting and adolescent adjustment: the quality of nonresident father-child interaction. J Fam Issues 24:217–244, 2003

Tein J-Y, Sandler IN, MacKinnon DP, et al: How did it work? Who did it work for? Mediation and mediated moderation of a preventive intervention for children of divorce. J Consult Clin Psychol 72:617–624, 2004

Troxel WM, Matthews KA: What are the costs of marital conflict and dissolution to children's physical health? Clin Child Fam Psychol Rev 7:29–57, 2004

West SG, Aiken LS: Towards understanding individual effects in multiple component prevention programs: design and analysis issues, in New Methodological Developments in Prevention Research: Alcohol and Substance Abuse Research. Edited by Bryant KJ, Windle M, West SG. Washington, DC, American Psychological Association, 1997, pp 167–209

Wolchik SA, West SG, Westover S, et al: The Children of Divorce Parenting Intervention: outcome evaluation of an empirically based program. Am J Community Psychol 21:293–331, 1993

Wolchik SA, West SG, Sandler IN, et al: An experimental evaluation of theory-based mother and mother-child programs for children of divorce. J Consult Clin Psychol 68:843–856, 2000a

Wolchik SA, Wilcox KA, Tein J-Y: Maternal acceptance and consistency of discipline as buffers of divorce stressors on children's psychological adjustment problems. J Abnorm Child Psychol 28:87–102, 2000b

Wolchik SA, Sandler IN, Millsap RE, et al: Six-year follow-up of a randomized, controlled trial of preventive interventions for children of divorce. JAMA 288:1874–1881, 2002a

Wolchik SA, Tein J-Y, Sandler IN, et al: Fear of abandonment as a mediator of the relations between divorce stressors and mother-child relationship quality and children's adjustment problems. J Abnorm Child Psychol 30:401–418, 2002b

CHAPTER 13

CULTURAL AND RELATIONAL PROCESSES IN DEPRESSED LATINO ADOLESCENTS

Guillermo Bernal, Ph.D.
Eduardo Cumba-Avilés, Ph.D.
Emily Sáez-Santiago, Ph.D.

Cultural processes frame human relations. The experience of depression and depression as a disorder are bound to have different expressions, and perhaps even differ in essence, given that a particular culture has a unique construction of reality and meaning system and distinct patterns of socialization (Marsella 2003). Culture may be defined as "shared learned meanings and behaviors that are transmitted within social activity contexts for the purpose of promoting individual and societal adjustment, growth, and development" (Marsella 2003, p. 4). Thus, the study of depression demands a study of human relationships embedded in a particular cultural context.

In this chapter, we focus on cultural and relational processes in depressed Latino youth. The Latino culture(s) serves as a case in point, since Latinos are generally described as valuing interdependence over independence, and family and interpersonal needs over individual ones. Other values include *personalismo, familismo,* and spirituality, which allude to the importance of social supports, the use of both nuclear and extended family, and the reliance on spiritual support systems, respectively. These values give meaning to the experience of depression that is, by its very "nature" (or more precisely "culture") relational.

We focus our review on depression in adolescents (specifically Puerto Rican youth), since it is during adolescence that relational processes converge with psychological and biological ones, affecting mood and behavior. First, we examine the epidemiology of depression and discuss family and relational issues associated with youth depression. Subsequently, we review the evidence for the relational hypothesis in psychosocial interventions with this population. We conclude the chapter with recommendations for future work.

Epidemiology of Depression

Research in the last two decades has confirmed the extensive prevalence of adolescent depression. Estimates of the point prevalence of youth depression in population studies have ranged between 0.4% and 8.3% (Birmaher et al. 1996). In the National Comorbidity Survey, lifetime prevalence of major depression in 15- to 18-year-olds was 14%, with an additional 11% of respondents in this age group reporting minor depression (Kessler and Walters 1998). Both prevalence rates are comparable with those found in adult populations, suggesting that depression might be a disorder of childhood or adolescence onset with a chronic or recurrent course (Hammen and Rudolph 2003).

The consequences of depression in youth can be devastating and include a decrease in school performance, withdrawal from social relationships, and increased family conflict and suicide risk. In addition, depression often occurs in conjunction with other psychiatric disorders, particularly conduct and anxiety disorders, further complicating the developmental trajectory of these youth (Birmaher et al. 1996; Hammen and Rudolph 2003). In short, adolescent depression has a deleterious effect on individuals and families.

According to the U.S. Census Bureau's Report for the year 2000, the largest minority group of youth in the United States was Latinos (11.06 million), constituting, as of that year, 16% of the population younger than 18 years (Ramirez and Patricia de la Cruz 2002). No national study addressing the mental health of Latino youth has ever been published. However, smaller studies have revealed that Latino youth tend to have lower self-esteem and self concept and higher levels of depression than do non-Latino youth. A Surgeon General's report (Office of the Surgeon General 2001) concluded that Latino youth are more likely to have difficulties finishing school, manifest more symptoms of depression and anxiety, and contemplate suicide more often than non-Latino youth. In fact, the National Comorbidity Survey (Blazer et al. 1994) and the Hispanic Health and Nutrition Examination Survey (Potter et al. 1995) found higher rates of depression among Latinos. Potter et al. (1995) reported a 6-month prevalence rate of major depression of 7.19% among Puerto Rican children in New York City. Using DSM-IV criteria, a more recent epidemiological study in Puerto Rico revealed a last-year prevalence rate of 4.1% (3.4% when a diagnosis-specific impairment criterion was included) for major depression and dysthymia in children and adolescents (Canino et al. 2004). Although few studies have included sufficient ethnically diverse samples to examine differences in depression rates, a study that examined the rate of major depression in nine ethnic groups found higher rates among those of Mexican descent (Roberts et al. 1997).

Family Relational Issues and Processes Associated With Depression in Adolescents

The development, course, and prognosis of depression in youth have been associated with dysfunctional family interactions. Although the specificity of these findings to depression has been questioned, family interactions of depressed youth are characterized by more conflict, rejection, communication problems, and abuse, and by less affect expression and support, than those of nondepressed controls (Birmaher et al. 1996).

Family factors associated with depression in adolescents are related to parental psychopathology and family interactions. Parental depression is one of the principal risk factors for depression in adolescents (Warner et al. 1992). Moreover, several studies have pointed out that maternal depression is the main risk factor for adolescent depression (Marmorstein and Iacono 2004; McCauley and Myers 1992). This finding is not surprising, these researchers noted, considering that mothers generally have a greater role in child-rearing than fathers; thus, any form of maternal impairment may be of greater impact on the child. On the other hand, this maternal role as primary caretaker could also lead to onset of depression in the mother as result of seeing her child struggle with depression.

It is difficult to identify how parental depressive symptoms affect children, but there is a consensus about the presence of several moderators or mediators on this influence. These moderators or mediators include 1) genetic predisposition (Marton and Maharaj 1993); 2) parent-child interaction or attachment (Dmitrieva et al. 2004); 3) learned helplessness due to inconsistent reinforcement from the depressive parent (Seligman 1984); 4) family interactions (Marton and Maharaj 1993) and poor family functioning (Shiner and Marmorstein 1998); 5) physical abuse (Kaslow et al. 1990); and 6) marital conflicts (McCauley and Myers 1992). A depressed parent tends to have serious communication problems and has few abilities to solve conflicts (McCauley and Myers 1992).

Family expressed emotion (EE)—defined as the extent to which relatives express criticism, hostility, and emotional over-involvement—plays a critical role in youth depression. Although the relationship between these variables has not been widely studied, high parental EE in particular has been related to increased depressive symptoms in adolescents. McCleary and Sanford (2002) found that rates of depression in their sample of adolescents were significantly higher in the high-EE than in the low-EE group. Other studies have reported that families of depressed children have higher rates of 1) parental rejection, 2) lack of emotional expressiveness, 3) lack of family cohesion, 4) lack of emotional support, and 5) lack of marital harmony and social isolation (Shiner and Marmorstein 1998). Some studies have found that fathers of depressed children were not emotionally involved with them, while mothers alternate between rejection and excessive emotional involvement (Warner et al. 1992). However, other studies reported that mothers of depressed children were less emotionally involved and talkative with them than mothers of nondepressed children (McCauley and Myers 1992). Furthermore, high emotional expressiveness in families has been related to difficulties in recovery and high relapse rates (Sanford et al. 1995).

There are few studies focusing on family interactions and depression in Latino adolescents. In Puerto Rico, we have conducted several studies that support the strong relationship between parental and family variables and adolescent depression. The results from a clinical trial with 71 depressed adolescents revealed that 40% of them said their most frequent problem was one relating to their family (Padilla et al. 2002), and 70% considered their most frequent interpersonal problem was with one or both parents (Rosselló and Rivera-Orraca 1999).

In another study, Martínez and Rosselló (1995) reported a correlation of .40 ($P > .01$) between depression and family dysfunction. The findings of this study also showed that communication, emotional involvement, and accomplishment of tasks within the family were the areas with higher predictive value in the depressive symptoms of Puerto Rican children and adolescents. In a study of coping strategies and depression, Velázquez et al. (1999) found that strategies that strengthen family relationships and fit into the family lifestyle were the best predictors of change in youth depressive symptoms. These strategies include exhibiting behaviors focused on an open communication among family members, sharing activities, and following rules to keep family harmony. Results from this study suggest that the increased use of these coping strategies reduces depressive symptoms in Puerto Rican adolescents, reflecting a direct relationship between youth depressive symptoms and family dysfunction. It is evident that family factors have a predictive value in adolescent depression, suggesting that while youth are in a process of becoming independent from their families, the perception of emotional involvement and acceptance from family members is important to them.

Sáez and Rosselló (1997) evaluated the relationships among perception of family functioning, marital conflicts, and depression in adolescents. They found a positive, moderate, and statistically significant relationship between family dysfunction and depression in a community sample. In addition, they found a positive correlation between the perception of marital conflicts and depressive symptoms, although this correlation was low. Recently, Sáez and Rosselló (2001) found a stronger correlation between both variables in a study with a larger community sample. Additionally, in this study statistically significant correlations were reported among depression, family criticism, and parental acceptance.

The quality of family relationships was also a key factor affecting mood change in depressive adolescents (Rosselló and Rivera-Orraca 1999). The most frequent interpersonal dispute reported by the adolescents in this study, which included 71 adolescents in a clinical trial, was with both parents, followed by a dispute only with the mother and, then, with siblings. Among the reasons they gave for the disputes with their parents were high requirements about academic achievement, home chores, friends, and clothes. Other situations that generated conflict with parents were issues related to going out (e.g., curfews) and the perception of being overprotected and treated differently than a brother or sister.

More recently, Sáez (2003), in a study with 312 youth, evaluated family environment through the adolescent's perception of family emotional overinvolvement, family negative criticism, parental acceptance, and parental marital discord. All these variables had statistically significant correlations with youth depressive symptoms. The variables of family negative criticism, parental acceptance, and marital conflicts explained 36% of the variance in those symptoms.

These findings with Puerto Rican adolescents provide further evidence of the relationship between family variables and adolescent depression. In general, the results of these studies are consistent with those reported with samples of different ethnic groups (Sáez and Bernal 2003), suggesting that the influence of family relational processes on the onset and course of depression in adolescents is not specific to a particular ethnic group. However, given that family norms and values vary from culture to culture, it is possible that the way in which some aspects of family dynamics influence the adolescent could differ across cultural or ethnic groups. For example, Sáez (2003) found that family emotional overinvolvement had an inverse relationship to depressive symptoms in a community sample of adolescents. This result is incongruent with the EE literature, which consistently supports the positive relationship between EE and depression. It may be that because of *familismo,* emotional overinvolvement is not considered as intrusive in some Latino families. In contrast, family emotional overinvolvement could serve as protective factor against the development of depressive symptomatology. This explanation is supported by the findings of a study by Velázquez et al. (1999), in which the investigators report that strengthening family relationships and making an effort to fit into the family lifestyle are the coping strategies that predict a change in Puerto Rican adolescents' depressive symptoms.

In summary, although many studies support the association between family processes and the onset, course, and prognosis of depression in adolescents, few studies have addressed the directionality of the association. It is not clear whether dysfunctional family processes contribute to the development of symptoms of depression in adolescents or the presence of depressive symptoms in the adolescent lead to family dysfunction. It seems that these variables are mutually affected and that no specific temporal order can be established between them. However, in order to be conclusive, more longitudinal studies evaluating this relationship are needed. At present, most studies on family processes and depression in adolescents have a cross-sectional design, which does not allow the evaluation of temporality.

This issue, along with the way in which a particular family variable influences the emotional and behavioral functioning of an adolescent, should be further investigated, with cultural aspects taken into consideration.

Relational Processes and Adolescent Depression Psychosocial Intervention Outcome Studies

Nine of at least 20 psychosocial intervention outcome studies for adolescent depression published to date included a parent involvement condition in their protocols. Three of them included family sessions in their treatment approach (Brent et al. 1997; Diamond et al. 2002; Harrington et al. 1998), and the rest included a separate parent psychoeducational component for which they reviewed the skills the youth were learning in cognitive-behavioral therapy (CBT) sessions of the Coping With Depression (CWD-A) course (Clarke et al. 1999, 2001, 2002; Lewinsohn et al. 1990, 1996; Rhode et al. 2004). Although in most of these 20 psychosocial intervention studies (with the exception of those by Vostanis et al. [1996] and Clarke et al. [2002]) active treatments resulted in significant adolescent improvement in depressive symptoms compared with control groups, the use of a family systems orientation or the addition of a parent psychoeducational group component to a specific CBT protocol had no additional significant effect on symptom reduction when compared with other active interventions.

The only exception, reported by Lewinsohn et al. (1990), indicates that the adolescent plus parent group condition revealed fewer problems as assessed with the Child Behavior Checklist. However, in that study, as reported by Clarke et al. (1992), one of the characteristics of depressed youth treatment responders, identified using depression scores on the Beck Depression Inventory (BDI) from pre- to posttreatment, was parent involvement in treatment. Interestingly, although Clarke et al. (2001) found that the CBT plus parent component condition showed a significant preventive effect at 12-month follow-up (and, to a lesser degree, at 24-month follow-up) when compared with a usual-care condition, no significant group differences were reported in a second study with the same design (Clarke et al. 2002).

Given the variety of relational issues and processes associated with the onset, course, and complications of depressive disorders, it is surprising that most of the psychosocial treatment and prevention studies for adolescent depression did not report results on relational measures or did not include them as part of their assessment protocols. In fact, even in the nine studies whose design included a family system or a CBT plus parent group treatment condition, the inclusion of this type of outcome measure was scarce or nonexistent. With the exception of the study conducted by Wood et al. (1996), in which individual CBT was the active intervention, among the psychosocial intervention studies, only those with an interpersonal psychotherapy (IPT) condition included measures of social adaptation (Mufson et al. 1999, 2004; Rosselló and Bernal 1999), social problem-solving skills (Mufson et al. 1999), and family criticism and emotional overinvolvement (Rosselló and Bernal 1999). In those studies, the active intervention (i.e., IPT) was reported to produce a significant increase in social adaptation over a wait-list control condition (Rosselló and Bernal 1999), as well as a greater improvement in overall social functioning, functioning with friends, and specific social problem-solving skills over a clinical monitoring wait-list condition (Mufson et al. 1999). No significant improvement was observed in youth self-report of family variables (Rosselló and Bernal 1999). Also, no improvement in social adaptation was reported in the CBT study of Wood et al. (1996).

A particular characteristic of the Brent et al. (1997) study was that a family psychoeducational intervention was provided as part of all the treatment conditions: CBT, systemic behavior family therapy (SBFT), and nondirective support treatment (NST). This family psychoeducational component included information about the affective illness and how the family could help the depressed youth. Although they could not clearly show the effects of this intervention, the investigators felt that this parental involvement helped parents understand the seriousness of their adolescent's condition and contributed to a reduced attrition rate (only 10% dropped out). Interestingly, only one psychosocial intervention study for youth depression reported a lower attrition rate (Wood et al. 1996, with a rate of 9%).

Overall, a limitation of these outcome studies is that they rarely evaluate other domains of treatment beyond the adolescent's depressive symptoms. This is a particularly sensitive issue in the case of Latino youth, whose culture emphasizes the importance of the family and relational factors. Because of the cultural characteristics and values of our population (e.g., *personalismo, familismo,* and spirituality), family and other relational variables can be of particular importance to the treatment of depression in youth. Therapy is more likely to be effective when it is congruent with the culture and context of the population to whom it is administered (Bernal and Scharrón del Río 2001). As we discussed earlier, in Puerto Rican youth samples, the strong relationship between parental and family variables to adolescent depression has been documented (Martínez and Rosselló 1995; Sáez 2003; Sáez and Rosselló 1997, 2001). Data from a recent clinical trial (J. Rosselló,G. Bernal, C. Rivera, "Randomized Trial of CBT and IPT in Individual and Group Format for Depression in Puerto Rican Adolescents, manuscript submitted for publication, 2005) reveal a significant correlation between the primary caretaker/parent BDI score and the adolescent Children's Depression Inventory (CDI) score at pretesting. At posttesting, the parents' depression measure also correlated with the treated youth BDI score. An interesting and unexpected outcome was a significant reduction in parents' depression symptoms (as assessed with the BDI) and other symptoms of psychiatric distress (as assesssed with the Symptom Checklist–36), after control for pretest scores, as a function of treating the adolescents.

In the context of the well-known association between relationship issues/relational processes and youth depression, the findings and the limitations of the psychosocial treatment studies should encourage the evaluation of other domains of treatment beyond the adolescent's symptoms.

Identification of Gaps in the Research

IMPLICATIONS FOR EPIDEMIOLOGICAL AND ETIOLOGICAL RESEARCH

Given that Latinos now constitute the largest minority group in the United States, there is a need for epidemiological research that examines the prevalence of depression in minority youth. In particular, there is a need for research that takes into consideration the relational and social contexts that give meaning to the particular disorder. Too often, epidemiological research on depression solely considers mood, symptoms, and syndrome as the primary criteria for diagnosis without attention to the relational and social processes, as well as the cultural beliefs and values, that shape the experience of depression.

In an increasingly multicultural society, the nature of adolescent depression and the relational process associated to this construct need further attention. One fruitful avenue of etiological and epidemiological research may be in the study of the validity of mental health constructs such as depression in cross-ethnic, multi-ethnic, and single-ethnic groups. Indeed, careful study of the metric, structural, and conceptual equivalence of such constructs may help move the field forward. For example, the evaluation of depression is usually based on self-report scales or interview protocols that are based on symptom criteria, which are in turn based on particular constructs of depression developed from contemporary psychology and psychiatry. The assumption is of a common underlying construct of depression. A number of investigators have challenged this view, suggesting that there is no single universal conceptualization of depression (e.g., Kleinman and Good 1986; Marsella et al. 2002) and that the experiences, meanings, and expression of depression will vary based on the social—and we would add, relational and cultural—context.

Recently, a national study of depression among Latino and Anglo adolescents was published (Crockett et al. 2005). Confirmatory factor analysis of the Center for Epidemiologic Studies—Depression scale provided evidence of a four-factor model of depression for Anglo Americans and Mexican Americans but not for Cuban Americans and Puerto Ricans. The findings suggest that Cuban Americans and Puerto Ricans do not share a common frame of reference for the construct of depression as do Anglo Americans and Mexican Americans. Differences as to how depression is conceptualized are congruent with the notion that such constructs are shaped by cultural and social contexts. Thus, a serious gap in both the etiological and the epidemiological study of depression is in the evaluation of how notions of depression or different expression of symptoms vary for different cultural groups with a different set of values from the majority culture.

IMPLICATIONS FOR CLINICAL ASSESSMENT STRATEGIES, SPECIFIC MEASURES, AND DIAGNOSTIC CRITERIA

If the factor structure of depression for a particular ethnic or cultural group is different, then its conception will differ, as will the experience, symptom counts, and cut-off points to evaluate it. Thus, careful studies of metric, structural, and conceptual equivalence need to be conducted on all measures to be used for different groups.

As noted earlier, in spite of the importance of relational issues and processes in the etiology, course, complications, and prognosis of depression in adolescents, relational variables are not frequently included as part of the assessment protocols in clinical trials for depressed youth. Although it is important to include adolescent self-reports, parent reports, and even teacher reports of relational variables, more assessment strategies that include actual observations of family interactions, peer interactions, and parent-adolescent transactions should be included. However, it is important to note that these observational measures should only be coded using culturally adapted coding systems that respond to the specific values and relational issues of the culture in which the study is being conducted.

Among the domains that should be included in a clinical assessment protocol for depressed youth are parents' symptoms/psychopathology, peer relationships, adolescent-parent interactions, and family functioning variables. Exploration of these domains should broaden our understanding of depression and provide insight as to how to treat it. We know that psychosocial interventions can reduce depressive symptoms, but we have less information about whether these treatments can effect change in other domains of functioning, or whether improvement in these domains can help patients maintain gains or prevent relapse. This line of inquiry is particularly important for the study of youth depression from a perspective that incorporates the participation of family members, with the assumption that change occurs in broader functional domains (family, school, peers) that are essential for treatment success.

IMPLICATIONS FOR INNOVATIVE TREATMENT

Findings from the treatment and prevention outcome studies suggest that the inclusion of parents as part of the treatment of depressed adolescents warrants further study. Even though the nine studies including parent involvement conditions conducted to date did not report a significant additional decrease in youth depressive symptoms, there are many reasons to include parents in the treatment of depressed youth. As Kovacs and Sherrill (2001) noted, enlisting the cooperation of parents in treatment can go a long way toward ensuring adherence and retention. Parents can have an enhanced psychological and educational role in the management of their child's depression and serve as resources to help in minimizing the impact of depression on the parent-child relationship. Furthermore, the literature on the relationship between parental and child psychopathology (Goodyer 2001) suggests that the mental health of the parent should at least be taken into account, and perhaps treated. In addition, parents can sometimes misinterpret their adolescent's depressive symptoms and conduct as misbehavior and manipulation. If they have a better understanding of their child's condition, they can be more accepting of their adolescent and collaborate actively in his or her treatment. Finally, the inclusion of parents in their child's treatment should optimize the efficacy of already effective treatments. Involving parents in the treatment of youth can help address treatment resistance, accelerate the treatment effects for the adolescent, and maintain therapeutic changes.

A number of investigators recommend this avenue of research (Kazdin and Weisz 1998; Sanford et al. 1995). After a review of the empirical and clinical focus of child and adolescent psychotherapy research, Kazdin et al. (1990) established several priorities for treatment research. Noting the scant attention to parental influences that may moderate outcome, these authors recommended that research be conducted to ascertain whether parent involvement is critical in clinical work. Also, Kovacs and Basteaens (1995) recommend that empirical treatment studies of depressed youth provide rationales for parental participation and guidelines for an optimal and healthy involvement in their children's treatment. This possible contribution to the field could be of great value for clinical practitioners.

Kendall (1991) also argues for parental involvement in the treatment of depressed children. This facilitates changes in interaction patterns, communication, and family rules. It may help parents to identify the depressogenic thoughts and help their son or daughter to restructure them. Parents can also learn the desirability of encouraging pleasant activities and those actions that will help their children attain self-improvement goals.

In summary, research findings have been consistent in reporting that parent-child conflict and dysfunctional family environment are related to depressive symptoms in children and adolescents. The addition of psychoeducational interventions for parents that address issues of negative cognitive styles, parent-child conflicts, and communication could enrich and maximize the treatment effects for depressed youth. Furthermore, recent advances in statistical techniques should allow researchers to examine the rate of change over time in order to study the impact of parental involvement.

Finally, another implication regarding the importance of relational variables in youth depression is an increased call for the integration of cognitive and interpersonal psychotherapy, particularly with regard to Latinos (S. A. Aguilar-Guaxiola, R. F. Muñoz, J. Guzman, unpublished manuscript, 2001; Pérez 1999) because of the cultural value placed on interpersonal/social interactions. Some forms of CBT already include training in social, communication, and conflict resolution skills. Given that IPT is the only treatment for depressed adolescents that has demonstrated significant improvements in relational areas strongly associated with depressive symptoms, it is logical to think that the integration of its principles and those of CBT would result in the design of potentially more powerful treatments that are able to have an impact on broader areas of functioning.

Conclusion

We believe that psychosocial intervention outcome research could open a new and potentially fruitful pathway for an optimal study of youth depression if parental-involvement conditions, integration of CBT and IPT principles in treatment protocols, consideration of cultural or ethnic differences, and broadening of assessment domains to include relational issues and processes are assumed as the main guidelines for conducting future intervention studies. We hope that the discussion in this chapter may stimulate investigators to identify additional areas of work and to develop additional ideas that could potentially help close the gaps and surpass the shortcomings in the research literature about youth depression that we have identified.

References

Bernal G, Scharrón del Río MR: Are empirically supported treatments valid for ethnic minorities? Toward an alternative approach for treatment research. Cultur Divers Ethnic Minor Psychol 7:328–342, 2001

Birmaher B, Ryan ND, Williamson DE, et al: Childhood and adolescent depression: a review of the past 10 years, Part I. J Am Acad Child Adolesc Psychiatry 35:1427–1439, 1996

Blazer DG, Kessler RC, McGonagle KA, et al: The prevalence and distribution of major depression in a national community sample. The National Comorbity Survey. Am J Psychiatry 151:979–986, 1994

Brent DA, Holder D, Kolko D, et al: Clinical psychotherapy trial for adolescent depression comparing cognitive, family, and supportive treatments. Arch Gen Psychiatry 54:877–885, 1997

Canino G, Shrout P, Rubio-Stipec M, et al: The DSM-IV rates of child and adolescent disorders in Puerto Rico. Arch Gen Psychiatry 61:85–93, 2004

Clarke GN, Hops H, Lewinsohn PM, et al: Cognitive-behavioral group treatment of adolescent depression: prediction of outcome. Behav Ther 23:341–354, 1992

Clarke GN, Rohde P, Lewinsohn PM, et al: Cognitive-behavioral treatment of adolescent depression: efficacy of acute group treatment and booster sessions. J Am Acad Child Adolesc Psychiatry 38:272–279, 1999

Clarke GN, Hornbrook M, Lynch F, et al: A randomized trial of a group cognitive intervention for preventing depression in adolescent offspring of depressed parents. Arch Gen Psychiatry 58:1127–1134, 2001

Clarke GN, Hornbrook M, Lynch F, et al: Group cognitive-behavioral treatment for depressed adolescent offspring of depressed parents in a health maintenance organization. J Am Acad Child Adolesc Psychiatry 41:305–313, 2002

Crockett LJ, Randall BA, Shen Y, et al: Measurement equivalence of the Center for Epidemiologic Studies Depression Scale for Latino and Anglo adolescents: a national study. J Consult Clin Psychol 73:47–58, 2005

Diamond GS, Reis BF, Diamond GM, et al: Attachment-based family therapy for depressed adolescents: a treatment development study. J Am Acad Child Adolesc Psychiatry 41:1190–1196, 2002

Dmitrieva J, Chen C, Greenberger E, et al: Family relationships and adolescent psychosocial outcomes: converging findings from Eastern and Western cultures. J Res Adolesc 14:425–447, 2004

Goodyer IM: The Depressed Child and Adolescent, 2nd Edition. Cambridge, UK, Cambridge University Press, 2001

Hammen C, Rudolph KD: Childhood mood disorders, in Child Psychopathology, 2nd Edition. Edited by Mash EJ, Barkley RA. New York, Guilford, 2003, pp 233–278

Harrington R, Whittaker J, Shoebridge P: Psychological treatment of depression in children and adolescents. Br J Psychiatry 173:291–298, 1998

Kaslow NJ, Rehm, LP, Pollack SL, et al: Depression and perception of family functioning in children and their parents. Am J Fam Ther 18:227–235, 1990

Kazdin AE, Weisz J R: Identifying and developing empirically supported child and adolescent treatments. J Consult Clin Psychol 66:19–36, 1998

Kazdin AE, Bass D, Ayers WA, et al: Empirical and clinical focus of child and adolescent psychotherapy research. J Consult Clin Psychol 58:729–740, 1990

Kendall PC: Guiding theory for therapy with children and adolescents, in Child and Adolescent Therapy: Cognitive-Behavioral Procedures. Edited by Kendall PC. New York, Guilford, 1991, pp 3–22

Kessler RC, Walters EE: Epidemiology of DSM-III-R major depression and minor depression among adolescents and young adults in the National Comorbidity Survey. Depress Anxiety 7:3–14, 1998

Kleinman A, Good B: Culture and Depression: Studies in Anthropology and Cross-Cultural Psychiatry of Affect and Disorder. Berkeley, University of California Press, 1986

Kovacs M, Basteaens LJ: The psychotherapeutic management of major depressive and dysthymic disorders in childhood and adolescence: issues and prospects, in The Depressed Child and Adolescent: Developmental and Clinical Perspectives. Edited by Goodyer IM. Cambridge, UK, Cambridge University Press, 1995, pp 281–310

Kovacs M, Sherrill JT: The psychotherapy management of major depressive and dysthymic disorders in childhood and adolescence: issues and prospects, in in The Depressed Child and Adolescent: Developmental and Clinical Perspectives, 2nd Edition. Edited by Goodyer IM. Cambridge, UK, Cambridge University Press, 2001, pp 325–352

Lewinsohn PM, Clarke GN, Hops H, et al: Cognitive-behavioral treatment for depressed adolescents. Behav Ther 21:385–401, 1990

Lewinsohn PM, Clarke GN, Rhode P, et al: A course in coping: a cognitive-behavioral approach to the treatment of depression, in Psychosocial Treatments for Child and Adolescent Disorders: Empirically Based Strategies for Clinical Practice. Edited by Hibbs ED, Jensen PS. Washington, DC, American Psychological Association, 1996, pp 129–135

Marmorstein NR, Iacono WG: Major depression and conduct disorder in youth: associations with parental psychopathology and parent-child conflict. J Child Psychol Psychiatry 45:377–386, 2004

Marsella AJ: Cultural aspects of depressive experience and disorders, in Online Readings in Psychology and Culture (Unit 9, Chapter 4). Edited by Lonner WJ, Dinnel DL, Hayes SA, Sattler DN. Bellingham, WA, Center for Cross-Cultural Research, Western Washington University, 2003. Available at: http:www.ac.wwu.edu/~culture/marsella.htm). Accessed January 22, 2005.

Marsella AJ, Kaplan A, Suarez E: Cultural considerations for understanding, assessing, and treating depressive experience and disorder, in Comparative Treatments of Depression. Edited by Reinecke M, Davison M. New York, Springer, 2002, pp 47–78

Martínez A, Rosselló J: Depresión y funcionamiento familiar en niños/as y adolescentes puertorriqueños/as. Revista Puertorriqueña de Psicología 10:215–245, 1995

Marton P, Maharaj S: Family factors in adolescent unipolar depression. Can J Psychiatry 38:373–382, 1993

McCauley E, Myers K: Family interactions in mood-disordered youth. Child Adolesc Psychiatr Clin N Am 1:111–127, 1992

McCleary L, Sanford M: Parental expressed emotion in depressed adolescents: prediction of clinical course and relationship to comorbid disorders and social functioning. J Child Psychol Psychiatry 47:587–595, 2002

Mufson L, Weissman MM, Moreau D, et al: Efficacy of interpersonal psychotherapy for depressed adolescents. Arch Gen Psychiatry 57:573–579, 1999

Mufson L, Dorta KP, Wickramaratne P, et al: A randomized effectiveness trial of interpersonal psychotherapy for depressed adolescents. Arch Gen Psychiatry 61:577–584, 2004

Office of the Surgeon General: Culture, Race, and Ethnicity. A supplement to Mental Health. Report of the Surgeon General. Washington, DC, U.S. Public Health Service, August 2001

Padilla L, Dávila E, Rosselló J: Problemas presentados por un grupo de adolescentes puertorriqueños/as con depresión y por sus padres. Pedagogía 36:80–91, 2002

Pérez JE: Integration of cognitive-behavioral and interpersonal therapies for Latinos: an argument for technical eclecticism. Journal of Contemporary Psychotherapy 29:169–183, 1999

Potter LB, Rogler LH, Moscicki EK: Depression among Puerto Ricans in New York City: the Hispanic Health and Nutrition Examination Survey. Soc Psychiatry Psychiatr Epidemiol 30:185–193, 1995

Ramirez RR, Patricia de la Cruz G: The Hispanic Population in the United States: March 2002. Current Population Reports, P20-545. Washington, DC, U.S. Census Bureau, 2002. Available at: http://www.census.gov/prod/2003pubs/p20-545.pdf. Accessed June 24, 2003.

Rhode P, Clarke G, Mace DE, et al: An efficacy/effectiveness study of cognitive-behavioral treatment for adolescents with comorbid major depression and conduct disorder. J Am Acad Child Adolesc Psychiatry 43:660–668, 2004

Roberts RE, Roberts CR, Chen YR: Ethnocultural differences in prevalence of adolescent depression. Am J Community Psychol 25:95–110, 1997

Rosselló J, Bernal G: The efficacy of cognitive-behavioral and interpersonal treatments for depression in Puerto Rican adolescents. J Consult Clin Psychol 67:734–745, 1999

Rosselló J, Rivera-Orraca Z: Problemas interpersonales presentados por adolescentes puertorriqueños/as con depresión. Revista Puertorriqueña de Psicología 12:55–76, 1999

Sáez E: Influencia del Ambiente Familiar en los Síntomas de Depresión y del Desorden de Conducta en Adolescentes Puertorriqueños/as. Unpublished doctoral dissertation, University of Puerto Rico, Río Piedras, 2003

Sáez E, Bernal G: Depression and ethnic minorities: Latinos and Latinas, African-Americans, Asian-Americans, and Native-Americans, in Handbook of Racial Ethnic Minority Psychology. Edited by Bernal G, Trimble JE, Burlew AK, Leong FTL. Thousand Oaks, CA, Sage, 2003, pp 401–428

Sáez E, Rosselló J: Percepción sobre los conflictos maritales de los padres, ajuste familiar y sintomatología depresiva en adolescentes puertorriqueños/as. Revista Interamericana de Psicología 31:279–291, 1997

Sáez E, Rosselló J: Relación entre el ambiente familiar con los síntomas depresivos y los problemas de conducta en adolescentes puertorriqueños/as. Revista Interamericana de Psicología 35:113–125, 2001

Sanford M, Szatmari P, Spinner M, et al: Predicting the one-year course of adolescent major depression. J Am Acad Child Adolesc Psychiatry 34:1618–1628, 1995

Seligman M: Attributional style and depressive symptoms among children. J Abnorm Psychol 93:235–238, 1984

Shiner RL, Marmorstein NR: Family environments of adolescents with lifetime depression: association with maternal depression history. J Am Acad Child Adolesc Psychiatry 37:1152–1160, 1998

Velázquez M, Sáez E, Rosselló J: Coping strategies and depression in Puerto Rican adolescents: an exploratory study. Cultur Divers Ethnic Minor Psychol 6:65–75, 1999

Vostanis P, Feehan C, Grattan E, et al: A randomized controlled outpatient trial of cognitive-behavioral treatment for children and adolescents with depression: 9-month follow-up. J Affect Disord 40:105–116, 1996

Warner V, Weissman M, Fendrich M, et al: The course of major depression in the offspring of depressed parents. Arch Gen Psychiatry 49:795–801, 1992

Wood A, Harrington R, Moore A: Controlled trial of a brief cognitive-behavioral intervention in adolescent patients with depressive disorders. J Child Psychol Psychiatry 37:737–746, 1996

CHAPTER 14

ROLE OF COUPLES RELATIONSHIPS IN UNDERSTANDING AND TREATING MENTAL DISORDERS

Mark A. Whisman, Ph.D.

For many people, the relationship they have with their spouse or partner will be the most important interpersonal relationship they develop in their lifetime. Therefore, the quality of these relationships is likely to be an important factor in mental health and well-being. Indeed, having a satisfying marriage or relationship has been identified as one of the most important goals in life (Roberts and Robins 2000), and a recent study involving a population-based sample of people between ages 24 and 74 found that marital satisfaction was the strongest predictor of life satisfaction, surpassing satisfaction in other domains of life, including health, work, children, and sexuality (Fleeson 2004).

Because such importance is given to marital or other close relationships, it seems reasonable to assume that couples relationships will play an important role in the onset, maintenance, and treatment of mental health problems. This chapter, which includes research on couples relationships and mental disorders, is divided into four sections. In the first section, I review basic research on couples relationships and mental disorders. I then cover, in the second section, the association between couples relationships and treatments for mental disorders and address, in the third section, the efficacy of couples interventions in the treatment of mental disorders. In the fourth section, I highlight directions for future research on psychological and biological aspects of couples relationships and mental health.

Note that most of the research on couples relationships and mental health has been conducted with married individuals. Research on couples relationships and mental health involving nonmarital close relationships, such as cohabiting and same-sex couples, is needed. To avoid confusion, however, the term *marital* is used in this chapter to refer to results from studies based exclusively on married individuals, whereas the more generic term *couple* is used to refer to mixed samples of couples or the underlying theoretical concepts that may apply to many types of close, romantic relationships. Also, a comprehensive review of research on couples relationships and mental disorders is beyond the scope of this chapter. Therefore, this chapter is a selective, rather than an exhaustive, review of the literature on couples relationships and mental health.

Couples Functioning and Mental Disorders

Following Brown and Harris's (1978) seminal finding that lack of a confiding partner is a risk factor for major depression, a growing body of empirical research has documented that couples relationships are associated with a wide range of mental disorders. The most common relationship variable that has been studied is relationship quality, operationalized in terms of a self-report measure of one's global evaluation of the relationship (often labeled as *satisfaction, distress,* or *discord*). The typical research design involves comparing relationship quality for people with a particular psychiatric disorder with relationship quality for people without the disorder (or with relationship quality for people with a different disorder).

As has been reviewed elsewhere (Whisman and Uebelacker 2003), greater marital discord has been found among treatment-seeking samples of individuals with mood, anxiety, and substance use disorders. Although informative, studies on relational processes in treatment-seeking samples are limited in their generalizability, insofar as epidemiological studies suggest that only approximately 20% of people with a recent or current psychiatric disorder obtain professional help (e.g., Kessler et al. 1994). Thus, it is important to evaluate this association not only in treatment-seeking samples but also in population-based community samples.

A sizable body of literature has linked couples discord with psychiatric disorders in large and representative community samples. In a large population-based community sample from Ontario, Canada, 24.5% of people with an active (i.e., 12-month) psychiatric disorder reported troubled relationships with their spouses compared with 8.9% of persons without a psychiatric disorder (Goering et al. 1996). A reanalysis of the same data found that in comparison to troubled relationships with relatives or friends, not getting along with one's spouse was more strongly associated with psychiatric disorders (Whisman et al. 2000). Furthermore, results from a population-based sample of married individuals from New Haven, CT, found that persons without a psychiatric disorder reported significantly more active and satisfying marital interactions than did persons with any disorder (Fredman et al. 1988), and not getting along with one's spouse was associated with increased risk for specific psychiatric disorders—namely, depression (Weissman 1987) and panic disorder (Markowitz et al. 1989). Similarly, results from a multistage stratified sample of couples from Detroit, MI, found that marital discord was associated with increased risk for depression (McLeod and Eckberg 1993) and anxiety disorders, including panic disorder, phobias, and generalized anxiety disorder (McLeod 1994). In a stratified random community sample of individuals, marital problems were associated with sexual dysfunctions in women but not in men (Dunn et al. 1999). In one of the largest population-based studies conducted to date, involving more than 2,500 married individuals drawn from the United States, a categorical measure of marital discord was associated with a 3.1-fold increased risk for mood disorders, a 2.5-fold increased risk for anxiety disorders, and a 2.0-fold increased risk for substance use disorders (Whisman 1999; Whisman and Uebelacker 2003). Marital discord also was associated with 10 of 11 specific disorders, with odds ratios ranging from 1.8 for alcohol use disorders to 5.7 for dysthymia.

Because of the cross-sectional nature of these studies, we cannot determine whether marital discord is a cause, correlate, or consequence of psychiatric disorders. Although more limited in number, prospective studies indicate that marital discord predates, and is therefore potentially causally related to, the onset of psychiatric disorders. In a population-based sample of more than 900 married adults who did not meet criteria for 12-month major depressive episode (MDE) at baseline, a categorical measure of marital discord was associated with a 2.7-fold increased risk for MDE during the following 12 months (Whisman and Bruce 1999). In a more recent analysis of the same sample, this time involving individuals who did not have an active alcohol use disorder at baseline, baseline marital discord was associated with a 3.7-fold increased risk for developing an alcohol use disorder during the following 12 months (Whisman et al., in press). Furthermore, the association between baseline marital discord and MDE and alcohol use disorders remained significant when the investigators controlled for demographic variables and history of the disorder.

Investigators also have evaluated whether couples discord is associated with more global measures of distress and impairment. This perspective is in keeping with the definition of disorders included in DSM-IV-TR (American Psychiatric Association 2000), which, for most disorders, requires the presence of clinically significant distress or impairment in social, occupational, or other important areas of functioning. Specifying the clinical importance of relationship discord (and other relational disorders) has been identified as a first step in a program of research that is needed to inform how relational problems are treated in the upcoming fifth edition of DSM (First et al. 2002).

Existing research suggests that marital discord is associated with distress and impairment. For example, a study of African American women found that marital discord was a risk factor for suicide attempts (Kaslow et al. 2000), and a large body of literature indicates that marital discord affects parenting and parent-child relationships (for a review, see Cummings and Davies 2002). As with the research on mental health, investigators recently have begun to evaluate the association between couples discord and distress and impairment in nationally representative samples. For example, in a population-based sample of more than 2,500 married and cohabiting individuals, couples discord was associated with greater psychological distress, greater likelihood of suicidal ideation, poorer perceived physical health, greater social impairment in relationships with relatives and friends, and greater work impairment (Whisman and Uebelacker, in press). Moreover, with the exception of suicidal ideation, these associations remained significant when the investigators controlled for current (i.e., 12-month) mood, anxiety, and substance use disorders, suggesting that the associations were not secondary to their shared association with psychiatric disorders. Indeed, in the multivariate analyses controlling for psychiatric disorders, substance use disorders actually had fewer significant associations with distress and impairment than did relationship discord. Other population-based studies have similarly found that marital quality is associated with distress (e.g., Cotton et al. 2003), work loss (e.g., Forthofer et al. 1996), and job satisfaction (e.g., Rogers and May 2003).

Most existing studies on couples functioning and distress and impairment have been cross-sectional. Longitudinal research is needed to establish that couples discord predates, and is therefore potentially causally related to, distress and impairment. Existing prospective studies of the role of marital discord in predicting subsequent distress and impairment generally have focused on distress, as measured by symptoms of depression. Results from these studies generally have shown that marital discord predicts subsequent distress (e.g., Beach and O'Leary 1993; Beach et al. 2003) and that this association may be stronger for women (e.g., Dehle and Weiss 1998; Fincham et al. 1997). More recent studies that used hierarchical linear modeling suggested that marital discord and distress show a bidirectional within-subjects effect, in which discord and distress influence each other over time (Davila et al. 2003; Karney 2001).

It could be argued that insofar as relationship quality is based on self-report, associations between couples discord and mental health, distress, and impairment could be a result of shared method variance or a person's mental status at the time of assessment. That is, general demoralization associated with many mental health problems could result in a person viewing all things, including his or her relationship, in a negative fashion. Similarly, even in prospective studies, participants' negative views of their relationship might reflect a negative cognitive perspective that could be contributing to poorer mental health. However, several lines of evidence argue against such interpretations of existing studies. First, a high degree of covariation is seen between partners' ratings of their relationship quality (Beach et al. 2003), thus suggesting that relationship ratings provided by participants are more than just negatively biased reflections of their relationship. Second, partners' satisfaction has been shown to predict a person's own mental health in both cross-sectional (McLeod and Eckberg 1993) and prospective studies (Beach et al. 2003), again suggesting that it is not just a negative bias that is driving the association. Finally, observational ratings of couples' communication also have been shown to covary with participants' mental health (e.g., Johnson and Jacob 1997), thereby indicating that other people perceive the relationships of people with mental health problems differently from how they perceive the relationships of people without such mental health problems.

Couples Functioning and the Treatment of Mental Disorders

In addition to evaluating the cross-sectional and prospective association between couples functioning and mental disorders, researchers have examined the association between couples functioning and treatment outcome. The rationale behind these studies is that to the degree that couples functioning is associated with the maintenance or course of a disorder, persons in poorer relationships who are receiving treatments that do not specifically modify couples functioning will have poorer outcomes relative to persons in better relationships. To the extent that couples functioning provides information about prognosis and treatment outcome, it can be said to have *clinical utility*, which has been identified as a major criterion for future revisions of diagnoses in DSM (First et al. 2004).

Couples functioning is associated with outcome for pharmacological and individual therapies for depression. For example, in a sample of depressed married women, marital disputes at treatment onset predicted poorer outcome to maintenance psychotherapy and/or antidepressant drugs at posttreatment (Rounsaville et al. 1979) and follow-up (Rounsaville et al. 1980). Similarly, endorsing relationship difficulties as causal factors in depression was associated with decreased homework adherence, decreased perceptions of the helpfulness of treatment, and poorer outcomes in individual cognitive therapy for depression (Addis and Jacobson 1996). Poor marital adjustment also has been shown to be associated with outcome following treatment for depression. For example, marital discord assessed shortly after hospitalization predicted greater likelihood of 9-month relapse rate in a sample of formerly hospitalized depressed inpatients (Hooley and Teasdale 1989), and baseline marital discord was associated with negative outcome in an 18-month longitudinal study of individuals with nonmelancholic depression (Hickie and Parker 1992).

Other studies have found a more complex association between marital discord and treatment outcome. For example, in a study of depressed outpatients receiving psychotherapy or medication, greater marital discord at the beginning of treatment was modestly associated with negative outcome immediately following treatment, whereas greater marital discord at the end of treatment was strongly associated with negative outcome during follow-up (Whisman 2001). Similarly, 6-month recovery from depression in an inpatient sample of depressed women was predicted by spouses' (but not patients') ratings of the marriage at baseline and patients' (but not spouses') ratings of the marriage at follow-up (Goering et al. 1992). Finally, marital quality also has been shown to predict speed of recovery from a depressive episode in a community sample (McLeod et al. 1992).

Marital functioning also has been shown to be predictive of outcome following treatment for alcohol use disorders. For example, marital conflict has been identified in retrospective studies as a cause for relapse (Maisto et al. 1988), and marital functioning has been shown in prospective studies to predict the likelihood of relapse and time to relapse among alcoholic patients in treatment (Maisto et al. 1998; O'Farrell et al. 1992, 1998).

Finally, marital functioning has been associated with outcome following treatments for anxiety disorders. For example, in a study of predictors of outcome following psychotherapy for married or cohabiting individuals with generalized anxiety disorder, increasing levels of relationship tension and friction were strongly associated with a reduced likelihood of improvement (Durham et al. 1997). Most of the research on marital functioning and treatment outcome for anxiety disorders has been conducted for panic disorder with agoraphobia. A recent review concluded that questionnaires specific to agoraphobic issues in couples' relationships or behavioral coding of couples' interactions appeared to be stronger predictors of outcome than were general measures of relationship quality, perhaps because of the denial or avoidance of problems or conflicts that is characteristic of panic disorder with agoraphobia (Marcaurelle et al. 2003).

Another area of research that has been evaluated with respect to individual-based treatments is the effect of these treatments on couples functioning. If couples discord is a by-product of a disorder, then improvements in the disorder should result in improvements in relationship functioning. However, results from existing studies suggested that individual-based treatments did not result in improvements in relationship functioning. For example, couples discord did not significantly decrease following individual-based treatments of depression (e.g., Beach and O'Leary 199; Jacobson et al. 1991) and substance use disorders (e.g., Fals-Stewart et al. 1996).

Couples Therapy for Mental Disorders

Historically, couples therapy has been evaluated primarily as a treatment for couples discord, and existing research suggests that couples therapy is effective in improving relationship quality. For example, Shadish and Baldwin (2003) reviewed six previous meta-analyses of studies comparing couples therapy with no-treatment control groups. According to these study results, they reported an overall mean effect size of 0.84 for couples therapy, which suggests that the average person receiving couples therapy was better off at the end of therapy than were 80% of the individuals in the no-treatment control group. They noted that the effect size for couples therapy was reasonably comparable to that for social, educational, and medical treatments for various conditions.

More recently, couples therapy also has been evaluated as a treatment for mental health problems (for more detailed reviews of these studies, see Baucom et al. 1998; Snyder et al. 2006). First, couples therapy has been studied as a treatment for major depression. In a recent review of nine studies that evaluated the efficacy of couples therapy for depression, Gupta et al. (2003) concluded that behavioral couples therapy (BCT), evaluated in three clinical trials, appeared to be efficacious in treating depression that co-occurs with couples distress. Furthermore, BCT results in significant improvements in marital discord. Other modalities of couples therapy have been evaluated in too few studies to draw firm conclusions about their efficacy, although initial results support their efficacy in treating depression.

Second, couples therapy has been evaluated as a treatment for substance use disorders. A recent review of the existing research indicated that BCT was effective in the treatment of alcoholism and drug abuse; BCT for alcoholism and drug abuse "produces more abstinence and fewer substance-related problems, happier relationships, fewer couple separations and lower risk of divorce than does individual-based treatments" (O'Farrell and Fals-Stewart 2000, p. 51). Furthermore, compared with traditional individual-based treatments, BCT resulted in "significantly (a) higher reductions in partner violence, (b) greater improvements in psychosocial functioning of children who live with parents who receive the intervention, and (c) better cost-benefit and cost effectiveness" (Fals-Stewart et al. 2005, p. 229).

Third, couples interventions have been evaluated in the treatment of panic disorder with agoraphobia. In a recent review of the efficacy of including a spouse or partner as co-therapist during in vivo exposure, Marcaurelle et al. (2003) concluded that partner-assisted exposure might be most appropriate for couples with good communication skills and relatively high relationship quality, whereas the literature on communication and problem-solving treatments suggested that this treatment may be most beneficial for couples with poor communication and problem-solving skills. Other reviewers have similarly concluded that if couples therapy will be included as an adjunct to exposure therapy, then specifically targeting couples relationships would likely be more effective than general interpersonal skills training (Daiuto et al. 1998).

Finally, evidence is emerging that couples therapy may be beneficial in the treatment of other psychiatric disorders. Specifically, two studies have evaluated partner-assisted exposure for obsessive-compulsive disorder, but the results of the two studies were contradictory, and several studies have suggested that general couples therapy interventions are "possibly efficacious" in the treatment of orgasmic disorder and hypoactive sexual disorder in women (for a review of these studies, see Baucom et al. 1998).

Directions for Future Research

Empirical studies conducted to date provide a solid foundation for the importance of couples relationships in the onset, course, and treatment of mental disorders. At the same time, in several areas, future research could help increase understanding of the role of couples relationships. In this section, I discuss directions for future research, with an emphasis on research that could be informative with respect to the DSM revision process.

As discussed by First et al. (2004), changes in DSM-IV (American Psychiatric Association 1994) focused largely on improving diagnostic reliability and validity. The emphasis on validity of psychiatric diagnosis can be traced to Robins and Guze (1970), who proposed several criteria for establishing validity, including clinical description, laboratory studies, delimitation from other disorders, follow-up studies, and family studies. More recently, Kendell and Jablensky (2003) proposed that a diagnostic category be described as valid only if one of two conditions were met. The first condition for establishing validity would be to document that natural boundaries (i.e., "zones of rarity") existed between it and other disorders and between it and normality. Although there is preliminary support for a natural boundary between discord and "normal" variations in relationships with respect to marital quality (Beach et al. 2005), future research is clearly needed to evaluate natural boundaries between different kinds of relationship "disorders" (such as relationship discord with and without violence), between relationship discord and psychiatric disorders, and between discordant and nondiscordant relationship subtypes within psychiatric disorders. The second condition proposed by Kendell and Jablensky (2003) for establishing validity would be to document that clear, qualitative differences exist between one diagnostic category and other diagnostic categories with similar syndromes. As an example of this type of research, Spotts et al. (2004) evaluated whether there were shared or independent genetic bases for marital quality, social support, and depressive symptoms. Relevant to the current discussion, when a combination of wives' and husbands' reports of marital quality was used, nonshared environmental influences seemed to be important in explaining the covariation between depression and marital quality, which the authors interpreted as evidence that husbands have an important influence on wives' depression. As such, these findings are consistent with the perspective that there may be qualitative differences between marital quality and depression with respect to their genetic basis, which would provide support for the second criterion for diagnostic validity. Future research is needed to expand on these types of analyses in men, in comparisons with other psychiatric disorders, and in comparisons with defining features of couples discord in addition to genetics.

In addition to researching the diagnostic validity of relationship discord, future research is needed to evaluate the clinical utility of couples discord because empirical advances in terms of clinical utility have been identified as important for revisions for DSM-V (First et al. 2004). For example, Kendell and Jablensky (2003) proposed that a construct has diagnostic utility, in part, if it provides testable propositions about biological and social correlates. Thus, understanding the role of couples discord in influencing biological processes and underlying neural bases of psychiatric disorders would help to advance understanding of the diagnostic utility of couples discord. For example, researchers could evaluate the systems in the brain involved in relationship discord and other relational processes that give rise to mental disorders, distress, and impairment. This type of research has found that brain activity associated with social exclusion is similar to brain activity associated with physical pain (Eisenberger et al. 2003), and among persons grieving a romantic relationship breakup, remembering one's ex-partner is associated with altered brain activity in regions identified with sadness (Najib et al. 2004). Similar kinds of studies that use couples events or stimuli could be informative regarding the neural pathways by which couples functioning may contribute to mental health outcomes. Furthermore, clinical research of persons in treatment is needed to understand how changes in couples functioning result in changes in psychological and biological functioning within a person, which contribute to treatment outcome. For example, it has been shown that individual-based treatments (e.g., behavioral or interpersonal treatments) result in changes in brain functioning similar to those seen following pharmacological treatment (e.g., Baxter et al. 1992; Furmark et al. 2002; Martin et al. 2001). However, changes in brain functioning and other biological processes have yet to be evaluated for persons with psychiatric disorders who receive couples therapy, and future research in this area would be informative in detecting specific mechanisms by which changes in couples functioning result in changes in mental disorders.

Identifying the biological and social correlates of a condition, however, is only one aspect of diagnostic utility. First et al. (2004) suggested that "the merits of a proposed change to DSM can be evaluated by considering 1) its impact on the use of DSM, 2) whether it enhances clinical decision making, and 3) whether it improves clinical outcomes" (p. 948). With respect to the last two criteria, research reviewed in this chapter indicates that couples discord is predictive of poorer prognosis and outcome for some disorders: most notably, mood and substance use disorders. As noted by First et al. (2004), "Most changes that entail the addition of a new disorder or new subtype are intended to highlight a homogenous (and previously unidentified) group of patients that require special clinical attention" (p. 950). Existing research suggests that individuals with major depression and substance use disorders who are in discordant relationships are such a subtype because they have poorer outcomes to traditional treatments. In comparison, the role of couples discord in the prognosis for and outcome of other disorders is largely unknown, and therefore, continued research on the role of couples discord in the course and out-come of these and other types of psychiatric disorders would help solidify the clin-ical utility of couples discord with respect to clinical decision making.

Research is also needed in the development and evaluation of effective treat-ments for people with mental disorders who are in discordant relationships. It seems logical first to consider interventions that directly target couples discord as potentially helpful for such individuals, and indeed, empirical support exists for this perspective for mood and substance use disorders and, to a lesser degree, for some anxiety and sexual disorders. In comparison, couples functioning has been associated with several disorders for which no published studies have evaluated the effect of couples interventions. For example, given that relationship discord is as-sociated with both increased risk for generalized anxiety disorder (e.g., McLeod 1994; Whisman 1999) and poorer outcome for generalized anxiety disorder (Durham et al. 1997), couples therapy may be helpful for patients with general-ized anxiety disorder. In developing couples-based interventions for other disor-ders, it may be helpful to keep in mind Baucom et al.'s (1998) distinction between partner-assisted interventions (in which the partner is a surrogate therapist or coach), disorder-specific interventions (in which the focus is on relationship fea-tures that are believed to influence the disorder or its treatment), and general couples therapy interventions (in which the focus is on improving relationship functioning in general). Thus, a new form of couples therapy for each specific disorder need not be developed to incorporate a therapeutic focus on improving relationship functioning. For some conditions, general relationship skills training (e.g., commu-nication training) may be added to existing treatments, which may result in improved outcome without substantial increases in cost.

Clinical decision making could also be facilitated if it were shown that couple discord moderated the outcome of different types of treatment for a given disor-der. For example, if it were shown that persons with couples discord responded better to treatment A than to treatment B, then the presence of couples discord would be useful in determining treatment choice. Unfortunately, most existing re-search on the role of couples discord in outcome of psychiatric disorders has eval-uated its effect on outcome for only one treatment or outcome collapsed across treatments. Therefore, future research evaluating couples discord as a moderator of treatment outcome would be informative with respect to its clinical utility vis-à-vis clinical decision making.

Conclusion

I have provided an overview of research linking couples functioning with the on-set, course, and treatment of psychiatric disorders. Specifically, existing research suggests that 1) couples discord is associated with mental disorders, distress, and impairment; 2) couples discord is predictive of onset of mental disorders and increase in distress; 3) couples discord is predictive of poor outcome of individual-based treatments for mental disorders; 4) individual-based treatments for mental disorders do not improve couples discord; and 5) couples-based approaches are effective in treating mental disorders. I have made several suggestions for directions for future research, with a particular emphasis on research that could inform the discussion of how relationship disorders are treated in DSM-V (First et al. 2002, 2004). Regardless of how couples discord and other relational disorders are treated in the DSM revision process, continued research on couples relationships in general, and on couples discord in particular, is needed to understand more fully the onset, course, and prevention and treatment of mental disorders and clinically significant outcomes such as distress and impairment.

References

Addis ME, Jacobson NS: Reasons for depression and the process and outcome of cognitive-behavioral psychotherapies. J Consult Clin Psychol 64:1417–1424, 1996

American Psychiatric Association: Diagnostic and Statistical Manual of Mental Disorders, 4th Edition. Washington, DC, American Psychiatric Association, 1994

American Psychiatric Association: Diagnostic and Statistical Manual of Mental Disorders, 4th Edition, Text Revision. Washington, DC, American Psychiatric Association, 2000

Baucom DH, Shoham V, Mueser KT, et al: Empirically supported couple and family interventions for marital distress and adult mental health problems. J Consult Clin Psychol 66:53–88, 1998

Baxter LR, Schwartz JM, Bergman KS, et al: Caudate glucose metabolic rate changes with both drug and behavior therapy for obsessive-compulsive disorder. Arch Gen Psychiatry 49:681–689, 1992

Beach SRH, O'Leary KD: Treating depression in the context of marital discord: outcome and predictors of response of marital therapy versus cognitive therapy. Behav Ther 23:507–528, 1992

Beach SRH, O'Leary KD: Marital discord and dysphoria: for whom does the marital relationship predict depressive symptomatology? J Soc Pers Relat 10:405–420, 1993

Beach SRH, Katz J, Kim S, et al: Prospective effects of marital satisfaction on depressive symptoms in established marriages: a dyadic model. J Soc Pers Relat 20:355–371, 2003

Beach SRH, Fincham FD, Amir N, et al: The taxometrics of marriage: is marital discord categorical? J Fam Psychol 19:276–285, 2005

Brown GW, Harris T: Social Origins of Depression: A Study of Psychiatric Disorder in Women. London, England, Tavistock, 1978

Cotten SR, Burton RPD, Rushing B: The mediating effects of attachment to social structure and psychosocial resources on the relationship between marital quality and psychological distress. J Fam Issues 24:547–577, 2003

Cummings EM, Davies PT: Effects of marital conflict on children: recent advances and emerging themes in process-oriented research. J Child Psychol Psychiatry 43:31–63, 2002

Daiuto AD, Baucom DH, Epstein N: The application of behavioral couples therapy to the assessment and treatment of agoraphobia: implications of empirical research. Clin Psychol Rev 18:663–687, 1998

Davila J, Karney BR, Hall TW: Depressive symptoms and marital satisfaction: within-subject associations and the moderating effects of gender and neuroticism. J Fam Psychol 17:557–570, 2003

Dehle C, Weiss R: Sex differences in prospective associations between marital quality and depressed mood. J Marriage Fam 60:1002–1011, 1998

Dunn KM, Croft PR, Hackett GI: Association of sexual problems with social, psychological, and physical problems in men and women: a cross sectional population survey. J Epidemiol Community Health 53:144–148, 1999

Durham RC, Allan T, Hackett CA: On predicting improvement and relapse in generalized anxiety disorder following psychotherapy. Br J Clin Psychol 36:101–119, 1997

Eisenberger NI, Lieberman MD, Williams KD: Does rejection hurt? An fMRI study of social exclusion. Science 302:290–292, 2003

Fals-Stewart W, Birchler GR, O'Farrell TJ: Behavioral couples therapy for male substance-abusing patients: effects on relationship adjustment and drug-using behavior. J Consult Clin Psychol 64:959–972, 1996

Fals-Stewart W, O'Farrell TJ, Birchler GR, et al: Behavioral couples therapy for alcoholism and drug abuse: where we've been, where we are, and where we're going. Journal of Cognitive Psychotherapy 19:229–246, 2005

Fincham FD, Beach SRH, Harold GT, et al: Marital satisfaction and depression: different causal relationships for men and women? Psychol Sci 8:351–357, 1997

First MB, Bell CC, Cuthbert B, et al: Personality disorders and relational disorders: a research agenda for addressing crucial gaps in DSM, in A Research Agenda for DSM-IV. Edited by Kupfer DJ, First MB, Regier DA. Washington, DC, American Psychiatric Publishing, 2002, pp 123–199

First MB, Pincus HA, Levine JB, et al: Clinical utility as a criterion for revising psychiatric diagnoses. Am J Psychiatry 161:946–954, 2004

Fleeson W: The quality of American life at the end of the century, in How Healthy Are We: A National Study of Well-Being at Midlife. Edited by Brim OG, Ryff CD, Kessler RC. Chicago, IL, University of Chicago Press, 2004, pp 252–272

Forthofer MS, Markman HJ, Cox M, et al: Associations between marital distress and work loss in a national sample. J Marriage Fam 58:597–605, 1996

Fredman L, Weissman MM, Leaf PJ, et al: Social functioning in community residents with depression and other psychiatric disorders: results of the New Haven Epidemiologic Catchment Area study. J Affect Disord 15:103–112, 1988

Furmark T, Tillfors M, Marteinsdottir I, et al: Common changes in cerebral blood flow in patients with social phobia treated with citalopram or cognitive-behavioral therapy. Arch Gen Psychiatry 59:425–433, 2002

Goering PN, Lancee WJ, Freeman JJ: Marital support and recovery from depression. Br J Psychiatry 160:76–82, 1992

Goering P, Lin E, Campbell D, et al: Psychiatric disability in Ontario. Can J Psychiatry 41:564–571, 1996

Gupta M, Coyne JC, Beach SRH: Couples treatment for major depression: critique of the literature and suggestions for some different directions. Journal of Family Therapy 25:317–346, 2003

Hickie I, Parker G: The impact of an uncaring partner on improvement in non-melancholic depression. J Affect Disord 25:147–160, 1992

Hooley JM, Teasdale JD: Predictors of relapse in unipolar depressives: expressed emotion, marital distress, and perceived criticism. J Abnorm Psychol 98:229–235, 1989

Jacobson NS, Dobson K, Fruzzetti AE, et al: Marital therapy as a treatment for depression. J Consult Clin Psychol 59:547–557, 1991

Johnson SL, Jacob T: Marital interactions of depressed men and women. J Consult Clin Psychol 65:15–23, 1997

Karney BR: Depressive symptoms and marital satisfaction in the early years of marriage: narrowing the gap between theory and research, in Marital and Family Processes in Depression: A Scientific Foundation for Clinical Practice. Edited by Beach SRH. Washington, DC, American Psychological Association, 2001, pp 45–68

Kaslow NJ, Thompson MP, Brooks AE: Ratings of family functioning of suicidal and non-suicidal African American women. J Fam Psychol 14:585–599, 2000

Kendell R, Jablensky A: Distinguishing between the validity and utility of psychiatric diagnoses. Am J Psychiatry 160:4–12, 2003

Kessler RC, McGonagle KA, Zhao S, et al: Lifetime and 12-month prevalence of DSM-III-R psychiatric disorders in the United States: results from the National Comorbidity Survey. Arch Gen Psychiatry 51:8–19, 1994

Maisto SA, O'Farrell TJ, Connors GJ, et al: Alcoholics' attributions of factors affecting their relapse to drinking and reasons for terminating relapse episodes. Addict Behav 13:79–82, 1988

Maisto SA, McKay JR, O'Farrell TJ: Twelve-month abstinence from alcohol and long-term drinking and marital outcomes in men with severe alcohol problems. J Stud Alcohol 59:591–598, 1998

Marcaurelle R, Belanger C, Marchand A: Marital relationship and the treatment of panic disorder with agoraphobia: a critical review. Clin Psychol Rev 23:247–276, 2003

Markowitz JS, Weissman MM, Ouellette R, et al: Quality of life in panic disorder. Arch Gen Psychiatry 46:984–992, 1989

Martin SD, Martin E, Rai SS, et al: Brain blood flow changes in depressed patients treated with interpersonal psychotherapy or venlafaxine hydrochloride: preliminary findings. Arch Gen Psychiatry 58:641–648, 2001

McLeod JD: Anxiety disorders and marital quality. J Abnorm Psychol 103:767–776, 1994

McLeod JD, Eckberg DA: Concordance for depressive disorders and marital quality. J Marriage Fam 55:733–746, 1993

McLeod JD, Kessler RC, Landis KR: Speed of recovery from major depressive episodes in a community sample of married men and women. J Abnorm Psychol 101:277–286, 1992

Najib A, Lorberbaum JP, Kose S, et al: Regional brain activity in women grieving a romantic relationship breakup. Am J Psychiatry 161:2245–2256, 2004

O'Farrell TJ, Fals-Stewart W: Behavioral couples therapy for alcoholism and drug abuse. J Subst Abuse Treat 18:51–54, 2000

O'Farrell TJ, Cutter HSG, Choquette KA, et al: Behavioral marital therapy for male alcoholics: marital and drinking adjustment during the two years after treatment. Behav Ther 23:529–549, 1992

O'Farrell TJ, Hooley J, Fals-Stewart W, et al: Expressed emotion and relapse in alcoholic patients. J Consult Clin Psychol 66:744–752, 1998

Roberts BW, Robins RW: Broad dispositions, broad aspirations: the intersection of personality traits and major life goals. Pers Soc Psychol Bull 26:1284–1296, 2000

Robins E, Guze SB: Establishment of diagnostic validity in psychiatric illness: its application to schizophrenia. Am J Psychiatry 126:983–987, 1970

Rogers SJ, May DC: Spillover between marital quality and job satisfaction: long-term patterns and gender differences. J Marriage Fam 65:482–495, 2003

Rounsaville BJ, Weissman MM, Prusoff BA, et al: Marital disputes and treatment outcome in depressed women. Compr Psychiatry 20:483–490, 1979

Rounsaville BJ, Prusoff BA, Weissman MM: The course of marital disputes in depressed women: a 48-month follow-up study. Compr Psychiatry 21:111–118, 1980

Shadish WR, Baldwin SA: Meta-analysis of MFT interventions. J Marital Fam Ther 29:547–570, 2003

Snyder DK, Castellani AM, Whisman MA: Current status and future directions in couple therapy. Annu Rev Psychol 57:317–344, 2006

Spotts EL, Neiderhiser JM, Ganiban J, et al: Accounting for depressive symptoms in women: a twin study of associations with interpersonal relationships. J Affect Disord 82:101–111, 2004

Weissman MM: Advances in psychiatric epidemiology: rates and risks for major depression. Am J Public Health 77:445–451, 1987

Whisman MA: Marital dissatisfaction and psychiatric disorders: results from the National Comorbidity Survey. J Abnorm Psychol 108:701–706, 1999

Whisman MA: Marital adjustment and outcome following treatments for depression. J Consult Clin Psychol 69:125–129, 2001

Whisman MA, Bruce ML: Marital distress and incidence of major depressive episode in a community sample. J Abnorm Psychol 108:674–678, 1999

Whisman MA, Sheldon CT, Goering P: Psychiatric disorders and dissatisfaction with social relationships: does type of relationship matter? J Abnorm Psychol 109:803–808, 2000

Whisman MA, Uebelacker LA: Comorbidity of relationship distress and mental and physical health problems, in Treating Difficult Couples: Helping Clients With Coexisting Mental and Relationship Disorders. Edited by Snyder DK, Whisman MA. New York, Guilford, 2003, pp 3–26

Whisman MA, Uebelacker LA: Distress and impairment associated with relationship discord in a national sample of married or cohabiting adults. J Fam Psychol (in press)

Whisman MA, Uebelacker LA, Bruce ML: Longitudinal association between marital discord and alcohol use disorders. J Fam Psychol (in press)

PART IV

SUMMARY AND IMPLICATIONS FOR FUTURE RESEARCH

CHAPTER 15

RECOMMENDATIONS FOR RESEARCH ON RELATIONAL DISORDERS AND PROCESSES

A Roadmap for DSM-V

David J. Miklowitz, Ph.D.
Steven R. H. Beach, Ph.D.
David Reiss, M.D.
Marianne Z. Wamboldt, M.D.
Richard E. Heyman, Ph.D.
Nadine J. Kaslow, Ph.D.

The current version of the *Diagnostic and Statistical Manual of Mental Disorders*, DSM-IV (and its text revision, DSM-IV-TR [American Psychiatric Association 2000]), contains significant advances over prior versions with regard to the inclusion of relationship problems and disorders. As highlighted in previous chapters in this volume, the limitations of DSM-IV do not stem from a failure to recognize the connections between the relational context and psychiatric disorders. Indeed, DSM-IV already highlights relational context in the "V codes" of Axis I (e.g., Partner Relational Problem, Sibling Relational Problem, Parent-Child Relational Problem), by listing categories of psychosocial problems on Axis IV (e.g., problems with primary support group, problems related to social environment), and in the Global Assessment of Functioning (GAF) scale on Axis V and the Global Assessment of Relational Functioning (GARF) scale in Appendix B. However, these categories and scales do not incorporate advances that have occurred in the empirical science of relationships since DSM-IV was developed.

In view of the empirical data now available, the descriptions of relational context provided by the DSM-IV V-codes are overly vague and general. As such, they have become an impediment, rather than an aid, to appropriate clinical conceptualization. At a minimum, these descriptions need to be elaborated so they can illuminate significant connections between the social environment and particular disorders and provide guidance about the boundaries between disorder and normal variations in relationship functioning. In addition, the V-codes, problems on Axis IV, and the GAF and GARF scales have been underutilized by epidemiologists and are given brief consideration, at best, in basic courses on the DSM. This suggests the value of changes in DSM-V that will make the codes and scales clearer, more specific, more reliable, and more useful to both researchers and clinicians. Fortunately, there appears to be a willingness to address the relative exclusion of key relational processes in the development of DSM-V.

The foregoing chapters have established the relevance of relational processes in understanding the emergence of psychiatric disorders; their associated biobehavioral markers; their etiology, course, and treatment; and the amelioration of burden on caregivers. Each chapter suggests the importance of systematic description of relational problems *as a part of a comprehensive assessment of most clinical disorders.* The purpose of this final chapter is to make recommendations for research to expand our understanding of how relational processes contribute to mental health outcomes and to the clinical utility of relational diagnoses in the DSM system. The recommendations focus on key areas of investigation over the next 5 years until the anticipated publication of DSM-V in 2011. The end goal is to have a set of data-based recommendations to inform the crafting of DSM-V.

In framing our recommendations, we were guided by several questions:

1. What is the overall rationale for integrating relational processes, formulations, or disorders into DSM-V?
2. How should we validate proposed changes to DSM-V that involve relational processes?
3. What applied research would be helpful in providing guidance for the next DSM revisions, in terms of research on measurement and assessment, basic processes, etiology, prognosis, and treatment?

We hope to provide a template for organizing research in relational disorders during the development of DSM-V.

A Philosophical Framework for Relational Research

Kendler (2005), speaking for a broad range of clinical scientists in a recent essay on understanding the evolution of psychiatric disorders, emphasizes the integration of multiple disciplines, perspectives, and levels of analysis in understanding the complex etiology of disorders. This model is consistent with our position that relational processes are essential components of a nexus of influences on psychiatric disorders. Relational causal factors must be integrated with epidemiological, genetic, neurobiological, psychological, and cultural explanations for mental illness.

Kendler's essay begins with the recognition that human subjective experience is inextricably linked with brain functioning. The "mental" and "biological" worlds are not separable but instead reflect different ways of understanding the same system. All psychiatric disorders are necessarily biological, in the same way that all mental processes are biological. The mental and biological mutually influence each other: subjective experiences have an impact on a person's biology and behavior in the world, and biological processes influence a person's subjective experiences (Kendler 2005).

To expand on Kendler's conceptualization, a person's emotions, thoughts, and impulses will affect his or her brain and behavior, which in turn will affect his or her relationships with others. In turn, relationships affect the mind-brain system, which then influences a person's behaviors and affects his or her relationships. Thus, thinking about psychiatric disorders as biological is not an alternative or "more basic" explanation of psychiatric disorders. Rather, when evidence warrants it, biological and relational data must be integrated into a more comprehensive understanding of etiology and disease course. This perspective argues for a comparable integration in the process of systematic assessment of clinical problems. Further, research need not focus on only one component of the causal chain. Instead, empirical investigations should be focused on "lots of small explanations, from a variety of explanatory perspectives, each addressing part of the complex etiological processes leading to disorders…etiological pathways will be complex and interacting, more like networks than individual linear pathways" (Kendler 2005, p. 435).

Perhaps most relevant to the study of relational processes, Kendler emphasizes "integrative pluralism," which requires examining multiple perspectives on the etiology, prognosis, or treatment of psychiatric problems. Examples of this perspective include studies of how genetic vulnerabilities increase the likelihood of exposure to certain noxious environments and, recursively, how these environments modify genetic and biological expression. For example, genetic risk for major depression puts a person at risk for interpersonal, marital, and family problems, which are in themselves risk factors for depression (Kendler and Karkowski-Shuman 1997). Likewise, stress has its greatest impact on depressive symptoms in the presence of certain genetic vulnerabilities, such as functional polymorphisms in the promoter region of the serotonin transporter gene (Caspi et al. 2003).

Finally, Kendler emphasizes "patchy reductionism" (Schaffner 1998), in which research on smaller but overlapping causal models at different levels of analysis (e.g., genetic, epidemiological, neural, psychological, relational) are integrated and patched into a larger causal framework. Over time, interweaving these causal models should result in a greater etiological understanding of mind-brain dysfunctions. The behavior of people embedded in relationships is one explanatory level of analysis. Integrating this level of explanation with other levels will provide a more complete picture of the complex pathways to psychiatric disorders.

Validating Proposed Changes for DSM-V

Kendler's perspective provides important guidelines for continuing research on relational processes and the inclusion of relational formulations in DSM-V. But how does one go about validating changes to a diagnostic system, whether these changes include relational formulations, relational specifiers, relational diagnoses, axes, or V-codes (hereafter referred to under the general heading of "relational disorders")?

Methods for validating relational disorders can follow the same process of validation as individual diagnoses. A good starting point is the scheme first expressed by Robins and Guze (1970) and more recently amended by First et al. (2004), with the additional complexity that the clinician must diagnose units consisting of more than one person.

PRECISE CLINICAL DESCRIPTION

First, relational disorders must be described in clearly operationalized terms. This requires research on *assessment modules* to operationalize, for example, bidirectional patterns of interaction, disturbances in emotional climate, presence of attachment problems or abusive relationships, or dyadic relational discord. Later in this chapter we make specific recommendations for research on assessment modules (see "Developing Relational Assessment Protocols").

Studies need to determine whether or not clinicians who observe the same interpersonal processes make the same relational diagnoses. Likewise, if relational processes become a separate axis, research must ascertain whether clinicians apply the axis consistently and reliably. Studies of the test-retest reliability of relational disorders or formulations (in the absence of treatment) are equally necessary.

DELINEATION OF SYNDROMES FROM NEAR-NEIGHBOR DISORDERS

Studies of new relational disorders or formulations must attempt to establish what distinguishes them from one another and from individual disorders that have relational consequences. Thus, "disorder of parent-child conflict management" must be reliably distinguishable from "disorder of parent-child attachment," and "feeding problem of infancy" must be distinguishable from major depressive disorder in the mother. Of course, some of these disorders can be comorbid with one another, but we must first establish that they can be reliably distinguished.

"COMMON FATE" STUDIES

It will be critical to determine whether persons in the same relational disorder categories have a common fate, and if not, whether different diagnostic subtypes follow predictable trajectories. For example, some individuals with dyadic relationship discord will have the same outcome (e.g., divorce), whereas others will show improvements in relational satisfaction depending on the balance of intervening risk, protective, and treatment variables. Longitudinal, theory-driven research is needed to determine how relationship problems unfold over time and lead to predictable outcomes.

In a related vein, longitudinal studies should determine the role of relational problems in the maintenance of individual disorders. For example, an individual major depressive episode may develop into longer-term dysthymic disorder when relational discord is present. Children with conduct disorder may develop life-course persistent antisocial behavior if parent-offspring abuse is present. Thus, relational formulations may become useful for understanding the prognosis of individual pathologies. In parallel, longitudinal studies should examine the ways in which individual disorders modify the outcomes of relationship problems. For example, the severity of a person's schizophrenia-spectrum disorder may modify the trajectory of a relational disorder over time.

PATHOGENIC VALIDITY

Do relationship patterns play a well-specified part in the causal nexus leading to individual psychopathology? Domains of investigation relevant to pathogenic validity may include quantitative behavioral genetics, laboratory studies of biobehavioral markers, family history studies, and investigations of psychosocial factors. The evidence for pathogenic validity may include 1) predictive studies (relationship X predicts disorder Y); 2) prevention or treatment studies (changing relationship X changes disorder Y); or 3) predictive, treatment, or prevention studies (X is linked to another component of the causal nexus, leading to disorder Y; e.g., cortical regulation of amygdala function). Hopefully, these investigations will identify common sets of correlates that are not part of the actual criteria for the relational disorders themselves.

For example, let us assume caregivers' high expressed emotion (EE) attitudes and behaviors (criticism, hostility, and emotional overinvolvement) were proposed as a relational specifier in major depressive disorder, bipolar disorder, or schizophrenia-spectrum disorders. Research on EE should then include questions such as the following: Do individuals who are at risk for depression and who are paired with high-EE relatives have identifiable patterns of neural activation when criticized (Hooley et al. 2005)? Do people diagnosed with bipolar disorder share common genetic vulnerabilities with parents who hold high-EE attitudes (e.g., genes that predispose to emotional dysregulation)? To what extent do high-EE patterns of relationship functioning reflect shared versus nonshared environmental factors in identical versus fraternal twins with schizophrenia? Do interventions that have the effect of reducing levels of EE decrease the chances that a depression-prone partner will have a recurrence?

UTILIZATION VALIDITY

Finally, research needs to examine the clinical utility of relational disorders, dimensions, specifiers, or elaboration of embedded relational criteria. Following the recommendations of First and colleagues (2004), we need to empirically demonstrate that modifications to DSM-V lead to measurable improvement in the assessment or treatment of persons who need mental health care. Relational formulations must have *user acceptability*. Such a conceptualization must help the clinician to 1) conceptualize the problem being presented; 2) communicate relevant clinical information to the patient, the family, or other practitioners; 3) make appropriate decisions about assessments; 4) choose effective interventions; and 5) predict future clinical management needs. Thus, for example, we need to demonstrate that adding dyadic relational disorder to the DSM-V leads to better treatment choices—and, ultimately, better outcomes—for persons with recurrent major depressive illness than would be achieved by simply applying the diagnosis of major depressive episode. In parallel, if we know that a person with major depressive disorder scores high on the relational specifier "presence of social, familial, and neighborhood support," we may be able to predict that he or she will require less intensive pharmacological treatment (or psychosocial intervention) than will a patient who scores low on this specifier.

Demonstrating utilization validity will require field trials of proposed criteria for relational disorders. An example of such a trial would be to survey practicing clinicians by using case vignettes that are presented with and without relational specifier information. The dependent variables in such a trial might include the clinician's diagnostic formulation, the proposed treatment regimens, the clinician's confidence in his or her assessment of the patient's future clinical needs, and the clinician's ratings of the utility of the additional relational data. Similar studies have been recommended for validating new criteria for individual DSM-V disorders (First et al. 2004).

Key Issues Requiring Focused Research in Developing DSM-V

In the following sections, we offer specific recommendations for research on relational disorders and processes. It is hoped that these recommendations will stimulate research to empirically justify the inclusion of relational disorders in the DSM-V.

PLACING RELATIONAL RESEARCH IN A BROADER NEXUS OF INFLUENCES ON PSYCHOPATHOLOGY

Thus far, the DSM nosology has remained descriptive. Individual disorders are characterized by their overt clinical manifestations without reference to what is known about biological or social processes that influence the onset, duration, or recurrence of disorders. This descriptive stance has posed serious problems for the nosology. Perhaps most importantly, it may hinder research, since nosological criteria do not map easily onto research on social or biological processes.

Recent research has raised many questions about these categories and their boundaries. For example, the genetic factors that increase vulnerability for general anxiety disorder are virtually identical to those that lead to vulnerability for major depressive disorder, although they may have separate environmental determinants (Kendler 1996; Kendler et al. 1992; Roy et al. 1995). This leads to the question of whether these two are distinct disorders, especially since people diagnosed with both disorders can respond to antidepressants. Finally, a nosology based only on description and consensus cannot be verified by more precise methods of psychological, relational, or biological testing.

There is serious interest in reopening the nosology to encompass more than descriptive criteria and to use what is known about etiology to reformulate diagnostic concepts. A dramatic example is in recent proposals concerning personality disorders. There is growing consensus to pool biological, developmental, and psychological data in diagnosing personality problems with four or five well-researched dimensions of personality functioning, rather than the three general classes of personality categories now in force.

It is in this context that linking relational disorders and selected areas of biological research becomes crucial for the diagnostic enterprise. Studies that forge these links promise to inform a nosology in which boundaries of diagnoses are established by both descriptive criteria and a growing knowledge of the nexus of the causes of clinical syndromes. In this spirit, participants in the relational disorders conference have examined possible links between current relational and current biological research on early deprivation and trauma, long-term pair bonding, and severe psychological distress including depression. Drawing on the scientific backgrounds of a subgroup of participants, and material presented at the conference (see Lim and Young, Chapter 2, this volume), conferees sketched out a series of studies that could be designed and executed well before the next edition of DSM. These recommendations illustrate the strategies of feasible research that would advance our understanding of the causal nexus of psychiatric syndromes, as well as provide clues to how risk factors and clinical manifestations of disorder might be described in future manuals.

To illustrate how such research might be conducted, conferees sought to design an experiment. Those engaged in the process were a mix of seasoned clinical researchers and teachers, experts in human family relationships, and (perhaps most importantly) basic researchers in the neurobiology of social behavior. The experiment they designed—examining early deprivation and later social bonding in prairie voles—illustrated a critical cycle: how questions of great clinical importance might be addressed, in part, through thoughtful use of animal models. Further, it illustrated how animal models might suggest ways to integrate analysis of family relationships, neurobiology, and the development of psychopathology.

The experiment could proceed in several steps:

1. Seventy vole pups are "recruited" for the study. Forty pups are periodically separated from their adult caretakers very early in development (separated [S] pups). Thirty pups are reared in normal fashion (non-separated [NS] pups). Behavioral indicators are closely followed for evidence of social engagement, fearfulness, and behavioral analogs of depression. When the pups reach adulthood, four groups of pairs are experimentally arranged as follows: 10 S-S pairs; 10 S-NS pairs; 10 S without pair bonding; 10 NS-NS pairs. The protective and even therapeutic effects of successful pair bonding can then be examined experimentally, with inclusion of measures of anxiety, depression, and affiliative behaviors.

2. If pair bonding has a combined therapeutic and protective effect, the S animals in S-NS pairs should show behavioral functioning that approximates those in the NS-NS pairs and considerably better functioning than the S-alone animals. What is unknown is whether S-S pairs might, despite their history of deprivation, be able to bond and afford each partner some restoration of functioning. If they cannot, examination of the oxytocin, vasopressin, and corticotropin-releasing factor systems would provide clues as to their difficulties, perhaps providing a mechanism for pharmacological manipulation. Moreover, the neurobiology of successful protection of S pups in successful S-NS pairings is then open to systematic investigation.

3. Another yield can be contemplated from this experiment. It is likely that even without a double insult (separation and no protective bonding) some of the S alone or S-S pups would not show evidence of behavioral abnormalities. These are the "resilient" pups. Comparing resilient and nonresilient pups—both exposed to the same environmental risks—may provide leads to the role of vasopressin, oxytocin, and corticotropin releasing factor mechanisms that underlie resilience.

The proposed experiment illustrates the power of testing hypotheses derived from human intervention research, but by using an animal model, which allows greater control and range of manipulation. The investigation built on one of several promising animal models: pair bonding in prairie voles (see Lim and Young, Chapter 2, this volume). Although primate models are attractive for studying maternal-child relationships, few primate species evidence long-term adult pair bonding. Prairie voles mate for life, and a good deal of the neurobiology underlying this social bond has been elucidated. This model offers an opportunity for understanding how successful pair bonding might be impaired if one or both partners has suffered early deprivation. Even more importantly, it affords an opportunity to understand more fully why and how pair bonding may offset the effects of early deprivation. Such an understanding would provide substantial insight into the mechanisms by which successful marriage reduces partners' vulnerability to depression and other psychopathology (see Whisman, Chapter 14, this volume).

What are the advantages of a strategy that combines carefully crafted clinical questions about relational disorders with sophisticated animal models of the neurobiology of social relationships? First, animal models allow longitudinal observations across key developmental periods that are expensive, difficult, or impossible to obtain in humans. Second, true experiments, with random assignment of animals to varying social environments, are possible. Third, and as a consequence of the first two, it is possible to distinguish the influence of distinctly different environmental traumas. In the case of our proposed study, we can distinguish the effects of early parental deprivation from later marital difficulties. Fourth, neurobiological investigations can be carried out in animals that are impossible in humans, including brain dissections, gene knockouts, and viral vector genes transfers.

Research with deep and broad experience in the study of human relations and human development is crucial in the design and evaluation of these studies. The utility of animal models hinges on the relevance of the social behaviors and developmental lines they measure. Ultimately, the relevance of these measurements will emerge as part of cross-talk between animal and human researchers. For example, studies are already under way linking early childhood deprivation and trauma with adult depression that include studies of the corticosteroid regulatory systems. Moreover, human investigations of oxytocin in the cerebrospinal fluid and oxytocin administration by nasal spray should enhance this cross-talk.

Given the centrality of this cross-talk to understanding and assessing psychopathology, conferees strongly recommended changes in research priorities and policy at the National Institutes of Health and other funding agencies. A series of initiatives could favor this kind of investigation:

1. Conferences that bring together animal and human researchers for the express purpose of collaborating in the design of closely linked studies
2. Requests for proposals designed around these concepts
3. Funding mechanisms that would support animal and human studies within the same studies
4. Clinical trials of interventions with human relationships to add relevant neurobiological indicators to more conventional indicators of therapeutic process and outcome

DEVELOPING RELATIONAL ASSESSMENT PROTOCOLS

Identifying Key Constructs

There were several themes regarding assessment that were touchstones for conferees. First, in addition to developing measures of global family function (e.g., GARF scale; American Psychiatric Association 2000), there is a need to isolate key constructs and provide unifying measurement recommendations that can foster research coherence, enhance clinical usefulness, and spawn translational collaborations. Criticism/hostility appears to be a key component of a risk factor for less adaptive functioning in several relational literatures, such as that on EE (see Brown, Chapter 7, this volume; Hooley et al., Chapter 11, this volume), couples dysfunction (e.g., Heyman 2001), and child conduct disorder (e.g., Reid et al. 2002). Conversely, the construct of secure attachment, or reciprocal friendly warmth with a balance between autonomy and connection, is seen as a protective variable or an indicator of adaptive functioning (see Benjamin et al., Chapter 10, this volume). Finally, relational conflict was noted as both a potential risk factor and a potential protective factor, depending on whether or not the conflict is able to be adequately resolved (Cummings et al. 2003). The literature citing poor problem-solving skills in couples (e.g., Clements et al. 2004) and confusing communications in family systems (e.g., Tienari et al. 2004) as risk factors for poor outcome may indicate that these skills are essential in providing resolution to the inevitable conflicts that occur in close relationships. Thus, the constructs of *criticism, attachment,* and *conflict resolution* were deemed to be the most developed and validated for pushing forward into a more standardized assessment schema.

Research on Expressed Emotion

In keeping with the first theme, there was considerable agreement that research on EE, especially criticism and hostility, should be emphasized in the development of DSM-V. EE has emerged as perhaps the most well-validated relational construct, with 23 of 26 prospective studies showing an association between high-EE attitudes and relapses of psychosis in persons diagnosed with schizophrenia, and nine studies showing linkages between EE and relapses of mood disorder (see the meta-analysis by Butzlaff and Hooley [1998]). EE has profound implications for the understanding of the etiology, prognosis, and treatment of mental disorders, but many questions remain.

Until very recently, EE research was entirely psychosocial in approach, and this may have limited its appeal in the medical model–based DSM system. The research paradigm of Hooley and associates (2005), in which persons with a history of depression listen to audiotapes of maternal criticisms while undergoing a functional magnetic resonance imaging procedure, takes us one step closer to understanding the mediating biological mechanisms by which high parental criticism is linked to relapse. Other paradigms, such as examinations of the roles of neurotransmitter or neurohormonal systems (e.g., as measured by salivary cortisol levels) when at-risk persons are interacting with high-EE versus low-EE family members, may further clarify these mediating processes.

A second area is the extent to which knowledge of a family's EE status should influence treatment recommendations for persons with major psychiatric disorders. When a family of a person diagnosed with depression, bipolar disorder, or schizophrenia is high-EE, does it follow that the treatment must be family- or couple-oriented, or is it equally effective to apply cognitive-behavioral or interpersonal therapy with an emphasis on family relationships? Does individual or group treatment of the high-EE relative lead to a better outcome of the target patient's disorder, even if the patient is not directly involved?

Third, what are the best ways of assessing EE in clinical practice? Very few clinicians are able to administer and score the Camberwell Family Interview. Questionnaire methods, such as the Perceived Criticism scale (Hooley and Teasdale 1989), especially if accompanied by direct observations of family interactions, may be sufficient. Studies that examine the incremental validity of various questionnaire and observational assessments for predicting patients' symptom trajectories are essential for transporting the EE technology into community settings.

Finally, the role of EE in the etiology of psychiatric disorders has been neglected. EE may reflect a poor temperamental fit between a mother and an at-risk offspring. It may reflect a parent's difficulty with affective regulation when his or her child first shows signs of behavioral disturbance (Miklowitz 2004). In combination with other genetic, biological, and psychological processes, parental EE may predict the onset of certain types of psychiatric disorders in children. For example, in the presence of the cascade of events that leads to the first onset of schizophrenia, high-EE parental attitudes may serve as a stress trigger.

Several recent studies illustrate these points. McFarlane (see Chapter 5, this volume) examined the role of biological and socioenvironmental factors in the early and later prodromal phases of psychosis among at-risk persons. The design involved an open trial of community-based family-aided intervention and low-dose atypical antipsychotic medications. At 12-month follow-up, McFarlane and colleagues observed low rates of conversion to full-blown schizophrenia when at-risk persons received comprehensive family and pharmacological treatment. Interestingly, EE, when measured in the prodromal phase, consisted almost entirely of parental emotional overinvolvement rather than criticism. These results suggest that criticism may not appear at the onset of the disorder but may emerge later as the illness becomes more recurrent and chronic. These findings are consistent with those of Hooley and Richters (1995), who observed in a cross-sectional study that levels of parental criticism increased with the number of illness episodes in the offspring with schizophrenia. Prevention designs may determine that early intervention decreases the likelihood of affective negativity in caregiver-patient interactions, which may in turn lead to a less deteriorative course of illness for the patient.

A recent twin study by Caspi and coworkers (2004) examined mothers of 565 5-year-old monozygotic twin pairs. The investigation was able to discriminate in each family the twin to whom the mother expressed the highest levels of EE and the twin to whom she expressed the most warmth. The member of the twin pair who received greater negativity and less warmth developed more antisocial behavior problems. After taking genetic influences into account, Caspi et al. were able to conclude that maternal EE was causally related to the onset of antisocial behavior problems. Determining the role of EE in the onset of disorder—especially in studies that use longitudinal designs and that include quantitative estimates of the role of genetic factors—may help guide future preventative intervention efforts in research and clinical settings.

Research Using Multiple Methodologies and Reporters

A second theme in developing assessment protocols was that relational patterns should be measured in a specific relationship, across settings, and, if possible, across time, using multiple methods (brief questionnaire, clinical interview, family observation) and multiple reporters. The key relational constructs noted earlier currently have a panoply of methods of assessment and operationalization (e.g., the hostility/criticism construct; see Kerig and Baucom 2004; Kerig and Lindahl 2001), which makes it necessary to create and test the viability of an omnibus observational measure of the construct that could be used across intra- and intergenerational relationships. Such research could explore the core and most valid elements of the construct (e.g., testing Gottman and colleagues' [1998] hypothesis that *contempt and belligerence* may have more impact than *angry affect*). Similarly, consensus should be reached on developmentally appropriate and standard methods of assessing *attachment* in dyadic relationships.

Measures of relational assessments currently are being reviewed for recommendation in the second edition of the *Handbook of Psychiatric Measures* (Holm et al., in press), and this resource will serve as a way to start the dialogue of standardization. Conferees also recommended a second conference focused on obtaining consensus on measurement strategies for these key constructs as a way of moving the research agenda forward.

Valid Assessments of Key Constructs

A third theme of developing assessment protocols that unifies the first two is the need for valid assessments of key constructs that can be used for epidemiological and clinical purposes (i.e., are less time consuming and/or do not require extensive training or equipment), again across time with multiple methods and reporters. This may be accomplished by sharpening our knowledge of the core elements of the construct or by certifying brief measures as screeners (i.e., with acceptable sensitivity and good specificity), with those individuals screened as positive receiving more in-depth assessment (see Hooley et al., Chapter 11, this volume). There is a need for more normative data, both for the population and for key demographic and clinical groups (i.e., groups differentiated by age, gender, ethnicity, family composition, and clinical status). The clinical utility of family measures would be improved by providing clinical cut-off scores with associated operating characteristics (e.g., sensitivity and specificity), as well as measurements sensitive to change for use in assessing outcomes of interventions. Standardized measures that assess specific constructs would be most useful to integrate with neurobiological assessments to allow examination of key gene–environment interactions or the strength of certain relationship patterns in protecting against or exacerbating underlying neurobiological vulnerabilities.

Use of Retrospective Measurement

A fourth theme of developing assessment protocols, as discussed by Brown (see Chapter 7, this volume) is that further work should be conducted on the utility of cross-sectional and retrospective measures. Brown's hypothesis is that the individualized meaning or "metabolism" of trauma (as found in retrospective reports) is more predictive of key outcomes than are potentially more veracious historical data. This hypothesis may have important translational implications (i.e., Do retrospective reports, compared with historical data, relate more closely to dysfunctional processes identified by neuroimaging?). It is possible that verified historical trauma (e.g., from data collected in a prospective longitudinal study) may lead to different results than current retrospective report of past trauma. This is an area where existent data from longitudinal studies may be mined to establish the relationships between these measures and to determine their differential impact on measures of neuroendocrine functioning. Measurement techniques from attachment research (e.g., on coherence of current narrative process as opposed to content) may be useful to integrate in this literature (Main 2000), as would internalized representations of past relationships (see Chapter 10, Benjamin, this volume). In summary, this program of research could clarify whether differential processing of toxic environments and traumas create biological vulnerabilities, and in turn whether these biological vulnerabilities predict future psychopathology in at-risk persons who do not initially have psychiatric disorders.

Taxometric Validity

A final theme of developing assessment protocols involves increased efforts on investigating the *taxometric* validity of disordered relationships (see Beauchaine and Beach, Chapter 8, this volume). Heyman and Slep (Chapter 9, this volume) used partner abuse as an example of a putative relational disorder that many researchers believe is a distinct relational disorder. Similar work could be proposed and conducted for child maltreatment, couple disorder, and parent-child disorders. Findings from taxometric analyses could then be examined by researchers and clinicians alike for guidance on specific measures with associated cut-points. The research cycle would then likely iterate through the first four themes to improve measurement of the taxonic indicators.

Recommendations for Treatment and Prevention Research

Considerable progress has been made in specifying efficacious relational interventions that change key relational processes and, as a consequence, reduce the symptoms of psychiatric disorders, risk of disorder onset, or risk of relapse. This success suggests the importance of a strong continuing focus on the utility of specific, targeted relational interventions for serious mental disorders. Relational interventions may be delivered as monotherapy, with a goal on improving the outcomes of specific disorders (e.g., drug abuse, depression), or in conjunction with pharmacotherapy to improve long-term outcome and reduce family burden (as in schizophrenia). The preceding chapters in this book suggest a number of avenues for continued development of relational interventions, including programs designed to reduce EE, enhance parenting, alleviate relationship discord, or utilize marital relationships to enhance immediate and long-term outcomes.

For the treatment of severe mental illness and and substance abuse (including alcohol abuse), there is strong evidence that relational processes are pivotal for both short-term and long-term improvement. But additional work is necessary to reliably identify particular relational phenotypes that can guide clinical recommendations. There is a paucity of research detailing the extent to which well-specified relational variables predict treatment response and the maintenance of treatment gains. It is also unclear whether specific relational indicators identify relational interventions as optimal or essential for effective treatment.

Expressed emotion has provided very promising leads regarding the potential for the relational environment to modify long-term outcomes in severe mental illness. As indicated earlier, focused research on short-hand methods of assessing EE could increase the use of this construct to guide treatment recommendations. A second area, relationship discord, also has a well-established measurement tradition and, with a small amount of focused research, could be more widely used to guide intervention decision making. For example, it should be determined whether there is a discontinuity between marital/relationship discord and ordinary marital/relationship difficulties. Likewise, it should be determined whether some problems, such as physical violence, contribute to the onset or maintenance of mental illness beyond their association with marital/relationship discord.

A third area with a strong tradition of assessment research is assessment of parenting, and there is good potential for research on assessments of particular parenting relationships to lead to recommendations regarding intervention decision-making. For example, parent training can alleviate depression in mothers of conduct-disordered children (Sanders and McFarland 2000). The generalizability of this finding could be examined and thereby lead to new avenues of clinical intervention for many patients.

It is equally important that the routine assessment of relational *outcomes* be implemented across all treatments of mental illness in order to better establish the impact of psychosocial and pharmacological treatments on family burden. As was highlighted by Whisman (see Chapter 14, this volume), outcome research on severe mental illness often ignores the impact on family or other relational processes and so does not allow direct comparisons of interventions on relationship outcomes. Given the importance of disrupted relationships as a source of distress, morbidity, and mortality, this oversight should be corrected in future research so that we can better assess the true impact of illness and treatment on burden.

Complementing the highly targeted research efforts suggested above, studies also are needed to identify appropriate and effective methods for engaging partners and family members in relational treatments. This may be particularly important in cultures that place emphasis on family involvement (see Bernal et al., Chapter 13, this volume). The barriers to participation in an adequate course of treatment, even for highly motivated couples and family members, should be taken seriously. However, problems associated with implementing relational interventions may be compounded by the need to involve the spouse/partner or other family members in what may be seen by one or more persons as an individual problem. This involvement may prove particularly difficult if the spouse or family members already feel estranged. In addition, the requirement of relational interventions that all involved parties attend sessions in the face of competing demands such as work and child care entails important logistical problems. Focused research, targeted at expanding existing delivery models and providing a wider range of empirically supported options, is necessary to identify practical methods of delivering relational interventions across of range of disorders and circumstances. In addition, investigations aimed at marketing relational interventions will also be of considerable value.

Of particular importance for long-term progress in the integration of relational interventions with biological interventions is better understanding of the biological mechanisms linking relational interventions to positive outcomes over time. As is suggested by research on the basic biochemistry and neuroscience of relationships, studies that document the effects of relational interventions on biomarkers of stress, on brain activity pre-post intervention, and on gene expression may help elucidate these key mechanisms. It will also be important for research on intervention with the early family environment to examine biochemical mediators of effects and examine the extent to which such changes account for the effects of interventions on long-term outcomes. For example, examination of the extent to which early prevention programs with genetically at-risk children can change expression in the serotonergic system—and alter patterns of reactivity to stress or negative interpersonal events—would be of substantial theoretical relevance.

We also need to collect data on novel approaches to strengthening parenting and marital relationships as a way of preventing the onset of mental illness. Research should focus on the extent to which some family behaviors are adaptations to the patient's illness rather than factors that maintain the patient's illness. Likewise, empirical investigations are needed to better highlight nonpathological relational processes that can contribute to the etiology and maintenance of illness (e.g., nonforgiveness and blame maintenance processes). Research on the impact of preventative efforts to reduce divorce, family dysfunction, and marital/relationship dissolution could contribute greatly to the available repertoire of methods for preventing negative mental health outcomes.

Finally, neighborhood and other relevant social contexts should be better investigated as moderators of the effects of relational treatment effects. For example, do standard treatments for marital/relationship dysfunction vary as a function of socioeconomic status? A related area in need of study is better information identifying when relational treatments work, for whom, for what diagnoses, for what ages, or for what cultural groups. Similarly, there is a great need for research on family interventions that use culturally informed assessment methodologies that identify, for example, the relevant relational variables in each culture and when treatments should be culturally specific and when cross-cultural.

For all the areas discussed in this section, funding mechanisms should emphasize the use of existing data sources where possible. Many of these questions may be addressed through secondary analyses of outcome studies, epidemiological research, and longitudinal research projects already conducted. Strategies for identifying key data sets and encouraging their use by other researchers are an important way for funding agencies such as the National Institutes of Health to enhance research on relational processes in mental health.

Conclusion

Research prior to the publication of DSM-V should emphasize the role of relational processes and disorders in moderating or mediating the associations between individual disorders and outcomes. Relational processes can be viewed as one level of analysis in understanding the etiology, course, and treatment of individual disorders. Knowledge of these processes will enhance our understanding of genetic and neurobiological etiological pathways.

Changes to the DSM system that incorporate relational processes should undergo the same process of validation that is undertaken for individual disorders. Studies on assessment protocols should focus on the validation of key constructs taken from multiple perspectives and on the use of cross-sectional and retrospective as well as prospective methodologies.

Examples of key areas for relational research include examining the neurobiology of pair bonding and the effects of early trauma on successful attachment in animal models; ascertaining the interface between psychosocial and biological processes in prognostic studies using the EE construct; and conducting treatment and prevention research that integrates relational interventions with pharmacotherapy. Finally, empirical studies focused on relational interventions (including broader social networks) in preventing the onset of individual disorders, and the effects of such interventions on changes in biological risk markers (e.g., the serotonergic system), are critical to bringing relational formulations into a centralized position in our nosological system.

References

American Psychiatric Association: Diagnostic and Statistical Manual of Mental Disorders, 4th Edition, Text Revision. Washington, DC, American Psychiatric Association, 2000

Butzlaff RL, Hooley JM: Expressed emotion and psychiatric relapse: a meta-analysis. Arch Gen Psychiatry 55:547–552, 1998

Caspi A, Sugden K, Moffitt T, et al: Influence of life stress on depression: moderation by a polymorphism in the 5-HTT gene. Science 301:386–390, 2003

Caspi A, Moffitt TE, Morgan J, et al: Maternal expressed emotion predicts children's antisocial behavior problems: using monozygotic-twin differences to identify environmental effects on behavioral development. Dev Psychol 40:149–161, 2004

Clements M, Stanley SM, Markman HJ: Before they said "I do": discriminating among marital outcomes over 13 years. Journal of Marriage and the Family 66:613–626, 2004

Cummings EM, Goeke-Morey MC, Papp LM: Children's responses to everyday marital conflict tactics in the home. Child Dev 74:1918–1929, 2003

First MB, Pincus HA, Levine JB, et al: Clinical utility as a criterion for revising psychiatric diagnoses. Am J Psychiatry 161:946–954, 2004

Gottman JM, Coan J, Carrere S: Predicting marital happiness and stability from newlywed interactions. Journal of Marriage and the Family 60:5–22, 1998

Heyman RE: Observation of couple conflicts: clinical assessment applications, stubborn truths, and shaky foundations. Psychol Assess 13:5–35, 2001

Holm KE, Wamboldt F, Reiss D: Relational and family measures of risk and protective factors, in Handbook of Psychiatric Measures, 2nd Edition. Edited by Rush JA, First MB, Blacker D. Washington, DC, American Psychiatric Publishing (in press)

Hooley J, Richters JE: Expressed emotion: a developmental perspective, in Emotion, Cognition and Representation. Edited by Cicchetti D, Toth SL. Rochester, NY, University of Rochester Press, 1995, pp 133–166

Hooley JM, Teasdale JD: Predictors of relapse in unipolar depressives: expressed emotion, marital distress, and perceived criticism. J Abnorm Psychol 98:229–235, 1989

Hooley JM, Gruber SA, Scott LA, et al: Activation in dorsolateral prefrontal cortex in response to maternal criticism and praise in recovered depressed and healthy control participants. Biol Psychiatry 57:809–812, 2005

Kendler KS: Major depression and generalized anxiety disorder: same genes, (partly) different environments—revisited. Br J Psychiatry 168 (suppl 30):68–75, 1996

Kendler KS: Toward a philosophical structure for psychiatry. Am J Psychiatry 162:433–440, 2005

Kendler KS, Karkowski-Shuman L: Stressful life events and genetic liability to major depression: genetic control of exposure to the environment? Psychol Med 27:539–547, 1997

Kendler KS, Neale MC, Kessler RC et al: Major depression and generalized anxiety disorder: same genes, (partly) different environments? Arch Gen Psychiatry 49:716–722, 1992

Kerig PK, Baucom DH (eds): Couple Observation Coding Systems. Mahwah NJ, Lawrence Erlbaum, 2004

Kerig PK, Lindahl KM (eds): Family Observation Coding Systems. Mahwah, NJ, Lawrence Erlbaum, 2001

Main M: The organized categories of infant, child, and adult attachment: flexible vs inflexible attention under attachment-related stress. J Am Psychoanal Assoc 48:1055–1096, 2000

Miklowitz DJ: The role of family systems in severe and recurrent psychiatric disorders: a developmental psychopathology view. Dev Psychopathol 16:667–688, 2004

Reid JB, Patterson GR, Snyder J: Antisocial Behavior in Children and Adolescents: A Developmental Analysis and Model for Intervention. Washington, DC, American Psychological Association, 2002

Robins E, Guze SB: Establishment of diagnostic validity in psychiatric illness: its application to schizophrenia. Am J Psychiatry 126:983–987, 1970

Roy MA, Neale MC, Pedersen NL, et al: A twin study of generalized anxiety disorder and major depression. Psychol Med 25:1037–1049, 1995

Sanders MR, McFarland M: Treatment of depressed mothers with disruptive children: a controlled evaluation of cognitive behavioral family intervention. Behavior Therapy 31:89–112, 2000

Schaffner KF: Genes, behavior, and developmental emergentism: one process, indivisible? Philosophical Science 65:209–252, 1998

Tienari P, Wynne LC, Sorri A, et al: Genotype-environment interaction in schizophrenia-spectrum disorder: long-term follow-up study of Finnish adoptees. Br J Psychiatry 184:216–222, 2004

INDEX

*Page numbers printed in **boldface** type refer to tables or figures.*